SURGEONS
AT
GEORGETOWN

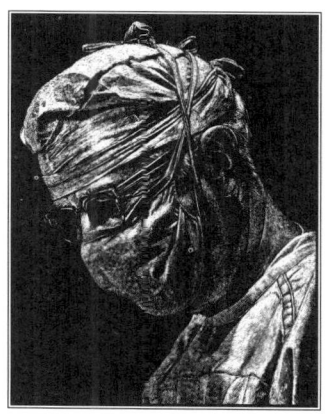

SURGEONS AT GEORGETOWN

Surgery and Medical Education
in the Nation's Capital 1849–1969

Patricia Barry

HILLSBORO PRESS
Franklin, Tennessee

Printed in the United States of America

05   04   03   02   01   1   2   3   4   5

Library of Congress Catalog Card Number: 2001088541

ISBN: 1-57736-236-5

Cover design by Gary Bozeman

Cover art by Thomas C. Lee

HILLSBORO PRESS
PROVIDENCE HOUSE PUBLISHERS
238 Seaboard Lane • Franklin, Tennessee 37067
800-321-5692
www.providencehouse.com

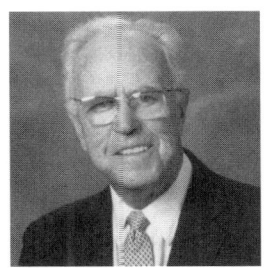

To the memory of
Robert J. Coffey, M.D., Ph.D.,
Chairman of Surgery,
Georgetown University Medical Center,
1947–1969.

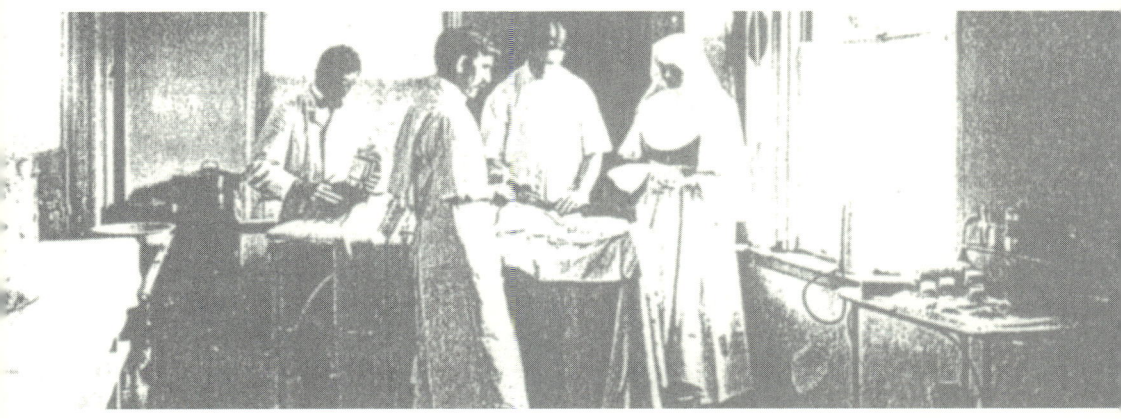

CONTENTS

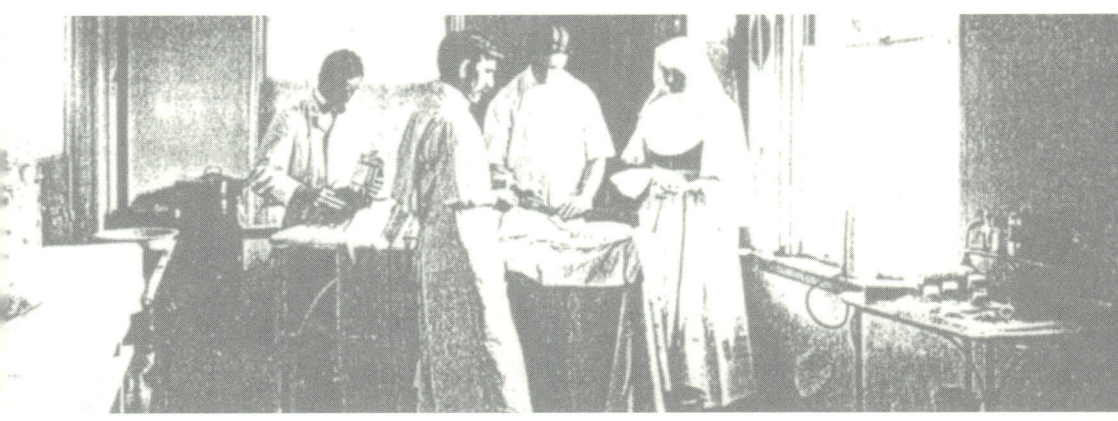

PREFACE & ACKNOWLEDGMENTS

ROBERT J. COFFEY'S association with Georgetown University School of Medicine spanned more than fifty years. It began in 1928 when he enrolled there as a medical student, attending lectures in the old building on H Street in downtown Washington, D.C. It ended with his retirement from surgical practice and teaching at age seventy-three in 1982. Even then, his interest did not cease. As a final gift to his alma mater, Dr. Coffey commissioned this history of surgery at Georgetown.

After his appointment in 1947 as the school's first full-time chairman of surgery in the then-new medical center on Reservoir Road, Robert Coffey laid the foundations of its modern surgery department. He was known— and is remembered—as an excellent surgeon and academic who received many honors; as an able administrator who hired first-rate faculty and made the department nationally recognized; and as an exacting instructor who put the fear of God into his residents but commanded their respect by demanding that they, too, strove for excellence in practicing surgery.

Dr. Coffey once said it was the "completeness and finality" of operative care that first attracted him to surgery. He was always decisive: an expert diagnostician who approached difficult procedures with confidence, gave patients of his best, and did not repine on occasions when he did not succeed. Such detachment, combined with a personal modesty not often recognized by residents who knew him mainly in the operating room, were evident in his approach to this book.

He could have written a memoir of his own years at Georgetown. Instead, looking to the wider picture, he commissioned a comprehensive history of surgery at Georgetown spanning 120 years, from the organization of the medical school in 1849 to the end of his own chairmanship in 1969. As the research gradually brought his distant predecessors to life, he became fascinated by their endeavors—perhaps seeing patterns of familiarity in their perennial struggles against constricting budgets, medical politics in the school and community, and the limitations on surgery of its time and place.

Sadly, Dr. Coffey did not live long enough to see the completed work. He died, aged eighty-six, at Georgetown University Hospital, early on the morning of January 26, 1995. Mourners at his funeral—family, friends, former colleagues, students, and patients—overflowed the Church of the Immaculate Conception in downtown Washington. Among them was his elder brother Jerome, who nearly seven decades earlier had studied medicine with him in the old H Street medical school building only a few blocks away.

Jerome Coffey, founder and director of the Hollywood Clinic, Florida, generously supported the continuing research and publication of this book. The result is a record of the contributions to Georgetown not only of Robert Coffey and his mid-twentieth century colleagues, but also of the many remarkable and dedicated surgeons who went before them.

Having no training in medicine and only one contact with surgery—at the sharp end of the knife—I am all the more indebted to the many people who helped with this book.

First and foremost, Robert J. Coffey himself. In hours of taped interviews he recalled his first-hand experiences of Georgetown and explained medical terms and procedures in simple English which even this listener, less prepared than the dimmest of his many past students, could understand. I realized what an excellent teacher he had been. Although his quick, get-the-job-done surgeon's nature must have deplored the slow progress of historical research, he never revealed impatience. He was a kindly mentor; I regret that he did not live to see this book, his long-held vision, in print.

Secondly, much gratitude is due to John Rose, dean of the medical school from 1963 to 1973. Having written and lectured on Georgetown's history himself, his interest in this book was generously abundant from the start. Out of his extensive experience as a student, professor, and dean, Dr. Rose provided much of the connective tissue that fleshed out mid-twentieth century documents. His critical help was also invaluable.

The Georgetown surgeons, former residents, and staff who contributed their memories and insights to the last chapter include John F. Potter, Alfred J. Luessenhop, John Dillon, Linda Langan Kildea, William Maxted, Peter Y. Evans, William Feiler, Robert B. Wallace, John Stapleton, La Salle D. Lefall Jr., Sister Eileen Niedfield, Kathryn D. Anderson, and, most of all, Thomas C. Lee. As Dr. Coffey's closest surgical associate and friend, Tom Lee filled many of the gaps left by Coffey's disinclination to talk much about himself.

Uncovering the history of Georgetown medical school from 1849 onwards meant piecing together evidence from thousands of documents and a variety of sources: Georgetown University Archives and Dahlgren Medical Library; National Library of Medicine; Library of Congress; National Archives; Smithsonian Institution; American College of Surgeons; American Medical Association; Historical Society of the District of Columbia; Martin Luther King Jr. Library, D.C.; Medical Society of the District of Columbia; Lloyd House Library, Alexandria; Jewish Historical Society of Greater Washington; Sons of the American Revolution. Librarians in all these institutions were always interested and eager to help—in particular Dr. Steven Greenberg, of the National Library of Medicine's history room, who could be counted on to track down the most obscure reference.

At Georgetown University, I relied on the expertise of its archivist, the late Jon Reynolds, and his assistants in the Special Collections Room of the Lauinger Library, especially Lynn Conway (now archivist); and the expertise of Afshin Nili, Betsy King, and the late Helen Badgoyan in the Dahlgren Medical Library. The work also benefitted enormously from the encouragement and criticism of Robert Emmett Curran, professor of history and author of the bicentennial history of Georgetown University.

    I am grateful to Patrice La Liberté, formerly of Georgetown University, for donating her superb professional editing skills; to my husband, John Barry, for his encouragement and ruthless red pen; and, in the production stages, to the staff of Providence House Publishers.

    Finally, my thanks go to the Coffey family: Dr. Coffey's brother Jerome, his wife Mary Catherine, his daughter Anne Proctor, and his son Robert Jr. Without their support, this book could not have been written.

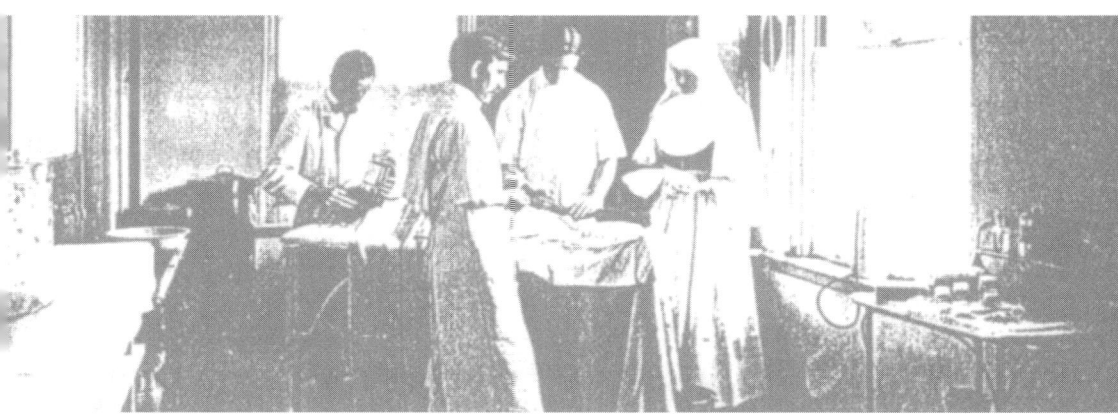

INTRODUCTION

TODAY, WE TAKE so much for granted. At the beginning of the twenty-first century, a whole range of illnesses that killed or disabled our ancestors are now preventable or easily cured, and many diseased organs can be repaired or replaced.

As with medicine and surgery, so with institutions. Today Georgetown University School of Medicine ranks as a leading medical school, each year attracting more than twelve thousand student applications from all over the world and graduating two hundred M.D.s on an annual budget of some $150 million. Yet most of its current faculty, students, and alumni have no idea how precarious was its progress through history, how often it only narrowly escaped bankruptcy and closure, and how long it battled against odds that defeated many other medical schools.

How Georgetown not only survived, but in some respects achieved international stature, is largely a chronicle of extraordinary individuals who willed it to happen. This history, therefore, focuses on the people—especially the surgeons among them—who drove Georgetown forward. Their stories give fascinating insights into the times and city in which they lived. They also mark significant milestones in the rise of medical education in the United States and in the progress of surgery worldwide.

Georgetown surgery has had its share of medical heroes: John Brown Hamilton, who founded the tiny laboratory which later expanded into the

National Institutes of Health; George Tully Vaughan, one of the first Americans to operate on the human heart, half a century before the advent of open-heart techniques; Charles A. Hufnagel, the first person to use plastics inside the body and inventor of the first artificial heart valves; Alfred J. Luessenhop, the originator of endovascular surgery.

But there were many others who, while achieving no special fame or "firsts," played full-blooded roles in the evolution of the medical school, Washington, and the nation itself—embroiling themselves in the carnage of the Civil War; fighting for civil rights during Reconstruction; founding local hospitals and national medical organizations; and, within the scope of this book, attending presidents from Lincoln to Nixon.

The subtext to these personal stories is the special difficulties faced by generations of medical educators in the nation's capital. The stateless District of Columbia, always oscillating uneasily between home rule and congressional control, has never enjoyed a sound economic base. That deficiency has often worked to the detriment of the city's three medical schools, to a degree unmatched elsewhere. For nearly one hundred years, without endowments or state subsidies, Georgetown's professors reached into their own pockets to keep the school going. Even today, the medical schools of Washington are circumscribed by its stateless geography, still vulnerable to the whims of Congress—which in some years has bestowed funds to help them and, in other years, has taken that assistance away.

Many other obstacles and dramas marked Georgetown's progress through peace and war, prosperity and depression, good fortune and ill luck. But always it was the individuals propelling that saga who stood out. They emerge from the past as remarkable people—sometimes courageous, sometimes flawed, always interesting—whose stories deserve to be told.

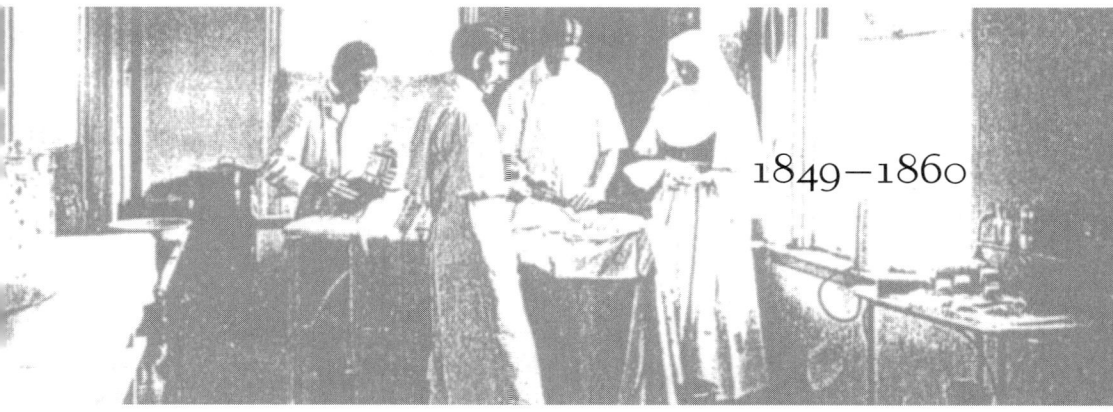

1849–1860

CHAPTER ONE

FOUR DOCTORS, FOUR ROOMS
The Founding of Georgetown Medical School

THE DAY WAS May 12, 1851. That Monday, the literate citizens of Washington browsed the pages of the *National Daily Intelligencer* to read the latest news from Europe. The Great Exhibition in London—the first World Fair and a celebration of the first fruits of the industrial revolution—was about to display all the new miracles of science and technology. The exhibition had, in fact, been opened by young Queen Victoria twelve days earlier. But with news taking two weeks to cross the ocean, the *Intelligencer* was still describing merely the preparations for that dazzling spectacle—and at such length that it is clear its readers hungered for every detail.[1]

Closer to home, a much more modest event—rating just a two-sentence advertisement in the same newspaper—was scheduled for that very afternoon at the Smithsonian Institution. As yet only half-built and surrounded by mud, the Smithsonian was a world away from the Great Exhibition on the spectrum of scientific elitism. But it had already seized the enthusiasm of people living in America's capital, and its every meeting attracted large audiences. In a city that was still tiny—"like an overgrown, tattered village which some late hurricane had scattered along the river's edge," one resident observed[2]—the embryonic Smithsonian was a symbol of culture and intellectual advancement, a promise of what Washington aspired one day to become.[3]

1

So on May 12, a large number of citizens made their way to the isolated building that rose like a castle above its surrounding pastureland. They crossed the Washington Canal—a waterway serving as the main sewage conduit for the city—by way of a narrow, iron bridge. They could see to their west the short stump of the Washington Monument, then only a fifth of its eventual height, and to their east the shallow wooden dome of the Capitol.4 Most wore the uniform of social standing, the women in silk bonnets and hoop skirts, the men in dark frock coats and high cravats, a few in the clerical black of the Jesuit order.

This "numerous and intelligent" crowd finally gathered in the new lecture theater of the Smithsonian, a room that occupied the entire east wing. They edged along the tiers of seats that curved in a bank above the lecturer's table, and sat down beneath brilliant chandeliers and a vaulted plaster ceiling that soared two stories above them.5 The Marine band struck up a few popular tunes and then, soon after 4:30 P.M., the ceremony began. The Reverend James Ryder, S.J., president of Georgetown College, rose to give his address on this special occasion: the opening of the college's first professional school, its medical department.

Ryder spoke without notes for almost an hour. According to the *Intelligencer,* he "pronounced a handsome and deserved eulogium on the medical profession, and expressed his conviction that the Faculty of the new institution would so conduct itself as to benefit their students and the community, while at the same time they would cherish a friendly spirit and maintain a noble rivalry with older institutions."6

Today, these words sound like worthy sentiments predictable to the occasion. But their pointedness was not lost on this audience, particularly not on the physicians who were the founding members of the new faculty in question: Noble Young, Charles Liebermann, Johnson Eliot, and Flodoardo Howard. Were these four doctors amused, embarrassed, or chagrined by Ryder's remarks? We do not know. But we can reasonably assume that they felt a certain ironic satisfaction. For had they really been able to "cherish a friendly spirit" to the "older institution" he was referring to, they would never have come together to found the medical department of Georgetown College, and this ceremony would not be taking place at all.

Until that moment, there had been only one medical school in the nation's capital, attached to Columbian College (the predecessor of George

Washington University), and only one general hospital, the Washington Infirmary. Seven years earlier Congress had granted the Columbian faculty the right to move its medical school into the new infirmary and use it as a teaching hospital.[7] That Act of 1844 had antagonized many physicians and surgeons in the city because it meant that only those nine who were members of the Columbian faculty had access to the hospital. Even worse, if any other doctor were obliged to send a private patient to the infirmary, he automatically lost both the management and fees of the patient's care.[8] In the eyes of the medical community, this was an injustice compounded by the fact that the infirmary was not a private facility; it was owned and largely funded by the federal government. From 1848 onwards, Congress appropriated between two thousand and six thousand dollars a year for its upkeep.[9]

Noble Young and Flodoardo Howard were two of those passionately opposed to Columbian's monopoly. Both were prominent Washington physicians. Howard had attended the first conference of the American Medical Association (AMA) in Philadelphia in May 1847, and with Young he had also attended the second in Baltimore in May 1848.[10] Both times they went as delegates of the Medical Society of the District of Columbia, a powerful organization founded in 1817, which granted doctors' licenses and served as a watchdog over professional standards locally. When the time came to appoint five delegates to the 1849 AMA conference, Young felt so strongly about the infirmary issue that he tried to persuade the society that none of the Columbian professors should be considered[11]—probably because Columbian, as a medical school, already had the right to send two delegates of its own.[12] The attempt failed, but the rancor remained.

Noble Young was not the kind of man to let so unsatisfactory a situation go unchallenged. Of Scottish-Irish descent, with a strong sense of humor and fondness for telling jokes, he was also decisive and blunt-spoken. According to his friend Samuel Busey, another Washington physician, he was "a cultivated and polished gentleman, a most congenial companion" who, nevertheless, "never professed love when he did not have it, nor concealed aversions when he had them."[13] During the spring and summer of 1849, Young discussed the problem of Columbian and the infirmary at length with Howard, Eliot, and Liebermann. All were good friends with rising careers. At forty-one, Young was the eldest and had the most medical experience, having received his medical degree in 1828, ten years ahead of Liebermann (now age thirty-seven), thirteen years ahead of Howard (thirty-five), and fourteen years ahead of Eliot (thirty-four). Liebermann had graduated in Germany, but the other three had all trained at Columbian—Eliot had even served as a junior faculty member there—so they were well acquainted with the faculty whose privileges they both envied and opposed.[14]

The solution, they finally agreed, was to form a medical school of their own. This was not quite so bold a move as it might appear today. In nineteenth century America, any doctor could start a school, and more than a few did. There were about forty medical schools in the United States by the late 1840s, many of them "proprietary" establishments owned and funded by one or more doctors who ran them as profit-making ventures.[15] Some were good enough by the standards of the time; others were wholly without merit. But the most prestigious were those which, like Harvard and Pennsylvania, were modeled on the European system and linked to established colleges and universities. So the four Washington doctors decided to try to form a medical department attached to a local college already chartered to award degrees. Georgetown, the only other such college besides Columbian in the District of Columbia, was the obvious choice. But Georgetown was a Jesuit institution, whereas the four themselves could not have represented a more ecumenical range of faiths: Young was a Catholic, Eliot an Episcopalian, Howard a Methodist, and Liebermann a Jew—indeed, he was the first Jewish physician in Washington. Clearly this breadth of belief was important to them, because their first impulse was to avoid Georgetown and apply instead to the University of Virginia.[16]

The person who changed their minds was John Carroll Brent, a Washington lawyer, an alumnus and benefactor of Georgetown College, and also a relative of Johnson Eliot. Brent persuaded them that they had nothing to fear from the Jesuits.[17] Therefore, on October 12, 1849, the four doctors sat down together in Young's office and composed a letter to President Ryder and his colleagues at Georgetown. It consisted of a single sentence: "Gentlemen: The undersigned are about to establish a Medical College in the District of Columbia, and respectfully ask that the right to confer the degree of M.D., granted to you by your charter, may be extended

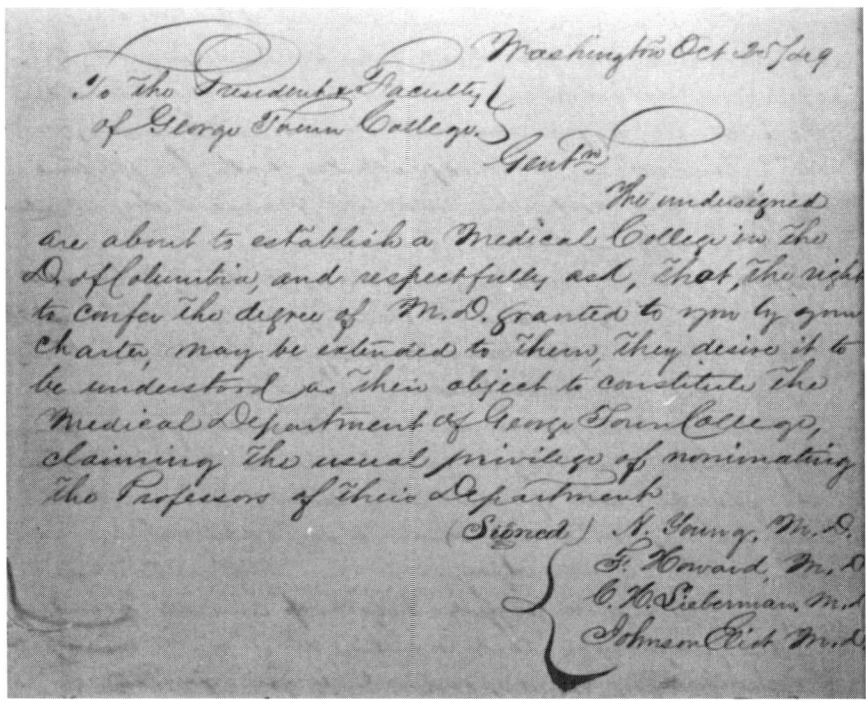

*The first formal action that led to the founding of
Georgetown University School of Medicine: the
four founders' briefly-worded request to Reverend
James Ryder, S.J., president of Georgetown College
as copied onto the first pages of the faculty minutes.
Courtesy of Georgetown University Archives.*

to them; they desire it to be understood as their object to constitute the
Medical Department of Georgetown College, claiming the usual privilege
of nominating the Professors of their Department."[18]

And so, conceived out of professional envy and frustration with local
medical politics, as well as a genuine desire to improve medical education
in Washington and a natural urge to further these four doctors' own
careers, an ambitious idea was set on paper. It took just sixty-six words to
lay the foundation of an institution which, over the decades that lay ahead,
would surmount extraordinary difficulties to become a medical school of

national stature—sending forth alumni who would eventually save lives and restore health by medical and surgical procedures undreamed of in 1849.

The timing was fortunate. Georgetown College, like the nation itself, was then just sixty years old and ripe for expansion. It had been founded in the historic year 1789, by the Reverend John Carroll, a man of outstanding ability and vision who was as wholeheartedly committed to the cause of American independence as he was to the Catholic Church. That same year, Carroll became the first Catholic bishop (later archbishop) of the entire United States, based in Baltimore; and he chose for his episcopal coat of arms an emblem of the Madonna framed by the thirteen stars of the first American states. Patriot, priest, and prelate, he was also committed to education. He had never forgotten that forty-two years earlier, when he was only twelve years old, his parents had been obliged to send him across the Atlantic to be educated by Jesuits in Europe, because Catholic schools were then suppressed in Maryland. Although he founded several other schools, colleges, and seminaries, Georgetown Academy, as it was first known, was always Carroll's favorite venture. It was the first Catholic college in the country, although from the start—perhaps because of Carroll's memories of intolerance—it accepted students of "every religious profession." He personally chose for its site a 1.5 acre hilltop overlooking the established tobacco port of "George Town" on the "Potowmack River," bought for seventy-five pounds sterling. It might have been less expensive if he had followed his wealthy family's urgings and used land they already owned a few miles away, but he fell in love with this hilltop—describing it as "one of the most lovely situations that imagination can frame." The family land that John Carroll, according to tradition, turned his back on was then a relative wilderness; five years later federal stonemasons began to erect the Capitol there.[19]

The Georgetown hilltop was to prove a wise choice in more ways than one. From their high windows, the teachers and students at the new college not only saw the embryonic capital city of Washington begin to take shape, but also watched in horror as it was burned by the British in August 1814. The following winter, Congress (uncomfortably ensconced in the only undamaged public building in town, the post office)[20] granted the college the right to confer degrees in "the arts, sciences, and liberal professions"—a charter which legally conferred university status on Georgetown and permitted the later addition of the medical department. The bill was signed by President James Madison on March 1, 1815.[21] Two months later Archbishop Carroll made the arduous journey from Baltimore to visit his beloved college for the last time; he died at home, aged eighty, the following December.

James Ryder became Georgetown's twentieth president in 1840. Born in Ireland and brought to the United States as a young boy by his widowed mother, Ryder was one of the most brilliant Jesuits of his generation. In 1820, after seven years at Georgetown College, he was selected to go to Rome for further training in the Society of Jesus; he was ordained there in 1824 and then sent to teach theology at the University of Spoleto. He returned to Georgetown as a professor of philosophy and theology in 1829. Though he frowned on intemperance—banning both alcohol and tobacco on campus during his presidency, to the indignation of faculty and students alike—Ryder was nevertheless a worldly man with a talent for getting on terms with the most influential men of his time and place. In Spoleto, he had been a friend of Archbishop Ferretti, later Pope Pius IX, and in Washington he became close to President John Tyler and many leading members of Congress and the city. Within the college, he was likewise an admired figure.[22]

When Ryder took charge in 1840, Georgetown, despite its charter, could still not claim to be a true university. It contributed little in the way of original scholarship; many of its professors were not of the highest quality; it had awarded degrees to an average of only four graduates a year over the previous decade; and it possessed no graduate or professional schools. Ryder, no doubt influenced by his five years at Spoleto, was determined to change this. As early as 1832, he had written of his conviction that Georgetown should be made "an integral part of a comprehensive university with chairs of Chemistry, Medicine and Law." An important step in furthering his ambition came when Ryder managed to recruit a number of Jesuit scholars expelled from Italy and Germany in the anti-Jesuit pogroms of 1847–48. Several were excellent teachers of mathematics, astronomy, physics, and chemistry—subjects exactly in tune with the burgeoning interest in science that characterized the 1840s. Another leap forward came in 1844 when Georgetown built its own astronomical observatory, funded by two Georgetown Jesuits who had donated their family inheritance.[23]

Those were two of the landmarks in Ryder's push to upgrade the college's academic status. The offer from that ambitious group of doctors in 1849 was a third. Whether it dropped on Ryder's desk out of the blue of that late October day, or whether he had already been alerted by Brent, it must have seemed a windfall. Certainly, he wasted no time in responding. Within nine days, and without seeking permission from Rome, Ryder met with the four physicians and consented to let them organize the medical department of Georgetown College.[24] It was an excellent deal for both sides: the college gained a professional school; and the medical school could begin by advertising itself as the adjunct of a respectable academic institution. No matter how much prestige accrued to each, however, the arrangement was still one of pure public relations. Ryder sought no academic control over the medical curriculum. He offered no rooms for the new department within the college, nor any small plot of land to erect a building on campus, nor funds of any kind to support it. Indeed, he made it clear from the outset that the medical school should "impose no condition or burden on the college."[25] It had to pay its own way. The physicians would not have expected anything else; for them, the goal was the Georgetown name, which they had been granted. Little more than the name, in fact, linked the college and the medical school for decades to come. Geographically, administratively, and financially, they would operate almost entirely independently of each other for nearly forty years and would not be truly united until 1930, eighty-one years later.

In the archives of Georgetown University today there is an old ledger bound in worn tan suede. Preserved and donated to the university in 1900 by Mary Llewellyn Eliot, the widow of Johnson Eliot, this ledger contains the minutes of faculty meetings over the school's first twenty-six years. The first pages are written in the sloping, and not always neat, script of Flodoardo Howard, who served as the faculty's first recording secretary. The entries are spare to the point of emaciation; as Mrs. Eliot noted dryly when she donated the book, "all matters of a personal nature were omitted."[26] But from them it is still possible to trace the story of how the four doctors set about creating a medical school from scratch.

They began on November 3, 1849, barely ten days after obtaining Ryder's consent, by nominating themselves the first professors of the new faculty: Noble Young, professor of the principles and practice of medicine; Flodoardo Howard, professor of obstetrics and diseases of women and children; Johnson Eliot, professor of anatomy; and Charles Liebermann, professor of surgery. (The only department in these days was the medical school itself; it would not become the School of Medicine, divided into a number of branch departments, until well into the twentieth century.) Ryder confirmed their appointments two days later.[27]

They must surely have had qualms about embarking on this venture. There was no guarantee of financial success. Moreover, all the burdens of teaching students and administering the school would have to be borne in the time left from their professional obligations as practicing physicians and other commitments to the local medical community. This was a time when competition between doctors was intense. The census returns for 1850 show that 104 physicians and 28 apothecaries were practicing in the District of Columbia (including the cities of Washington and Georgetown), which then had a population of 51,687—a remarkably high ratio of 1 doctor of medicine to 497 people.[28] This overabundance was repeated across the nation; everywhere, physicians' incomes had fallen sharply in recent years.[29] In Washington, as in every city, one or two physicians took the lion's share of the wealthiest patients. James Crowdhill Hall, for example, was then the city's most fashionable practitioner: he was said to have attended every president from Jackson to Lincoln, and every Supreme Court justice, every cabinet member, every prominent senator and representative in Congress, and most foreign embassies for many years.[30] Against such competition, the rewards went to those who seized their opportunities. The four who founded Georgetown medical school were such men.

Noble Young (1808–83), born in Baltimore and educated in Washington, not only had a large practice but also served as attending physician to various city institutions, including the penitentiary. (In later years, his standard joke in lectures was to refer to cases he had seen

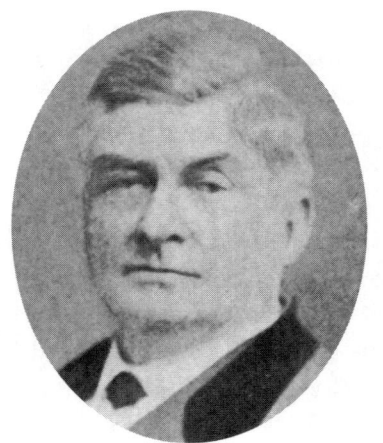

Noble Young, M.D., 1808–83. Courtesy of the Medical Society of the District of Columbia.

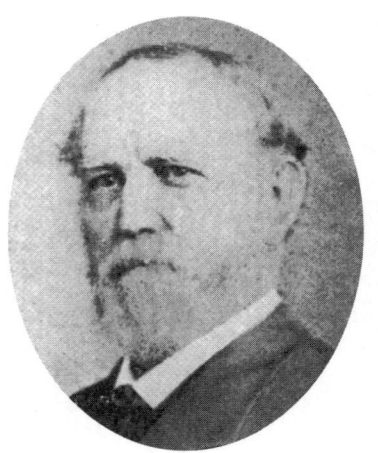

Flodoardo Howard, M.D., 1814–88. Courtesy of the Medical Society of the District of Columbia.

"when I was in jail" or "when I was in the workhouse."[31]) A prominent member of the Medical Society of D.C., he had already served as its vice president in 1839 and was at this time one of its board of examiners, which granted licenses to qualified doctors in the District of Columbia.[32] In 1849 he was successful enough to support a large household: his wife, Adelaide, their six young children, his father, and two household servants.[33]

Flodoardo Howard (1814–88), born in Virginia and educated in Maryland, had trained as a pharmacist for some years before studying medicine. Called a "plodding" man by Busey and, more affectionately, "Flodledardledo" by Young[34], he was building up his medical practice and supporting a young family, but was active in the society and had served as its librarian for five years.[35]

Johnson Eliot (1815–83), born in Washington, D.C., of a distinguished family who were early English colonists of Massachusetts and Maryland, was a modest and retiring man and a capable and kindly physician. He was serving as the society's treasurer and preparing for his marriage to Mary Llewellyn a few months later.[36]

But of the four founders, certainly the most interesting was Charles Heinrich Liebermann (1812–86), Georgetown's first professor of surgery. He was the odd man out—a foreigner, a Jew, a relative newcomer to

Washington—yet his influence on the others in the group, and upon the medical school, was decisive.

Liebermann was short in stature, bespectacled, and frail-looking even at thirty-seven, an appearance that belied the revolutionary fervor and hot-headed courage he had demonstrated as a young man.[37] He was born on September 15, 1812, in the Baltic city of Riga, the capital of Livonia (now Latvia), which was then, as at other periods in its history, under Russian domination. In 1830, Liebermann was eighteen years old and a student at the University of

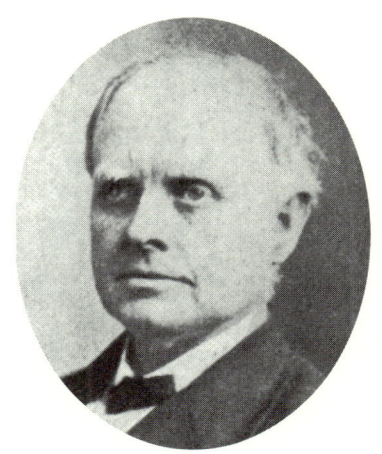

Johnson Eliot, M.D., 1815–83. Courtesy of Georgetown University Archives.

Dorpat, near St. Petersburg, when Polish nationalists attempted a major revolt against their Russian masters. Liebermann was among the students who rushed to join the cause. Armed with old muskets and farm scythes, they marched across the Polish border and were almost instantly arrested by the Russians, who dispatched them to a prison in Siberia. It was a harsh place where Polish aristocrats were chained and starved; but Liebermann's family commanded some influence, and he was soon released.

In the years that followed, he survived a succession of adventures and deprivations. There was an audience with Czar Nicholas I, who gave Liebermann a pardon that allowed him to return home to Riga—although the small print, he afterwards discovered, obliged him to remain under the surveillance of the secret police and give up all property and privileges. Later came another short spell in a Russian jail. But he also labored to complete his education, receiving a bachelor's degree in Dorpat in 1836 and a medical degree in 1838 at the University of Berlin. The German licensing system required a further two years' clinical experience before he could qualify to practice medicine. Liebermann was fortunate enough to spend those two years studying under the Austrian surgeon Johann Dieffenbach, one of the fathers of both ophthalmic and plastic surgery. Liebermann was there in the operating room when Dieffenbach performed

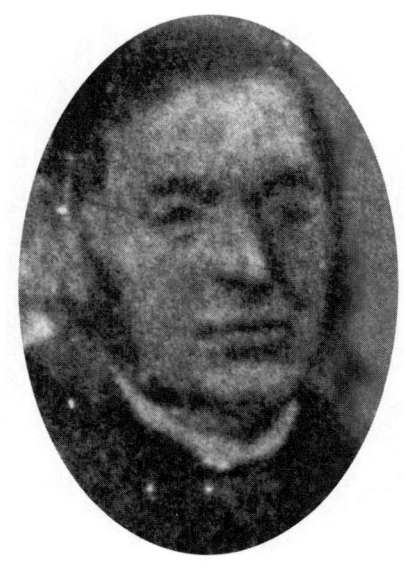

Charles Liebermann, M.D., 1813–86. Detail of painting by Alonzo Chappell. Courtesy of Brown University.

the world's first operation to correct strabismus (eye squint), and he learned techniques that would prove invaluable throughout his later career. In June 1840, Liebermann received his qualifying diplomas and immediately set off on a trip to Holland and England. But in Hamburg he saw an American clipper about to set sail for Boston and decided to see something of the United States before returning home.

The twenty-eight-year-old Liebermann landed in Boston in the early fall of 1840, in the midst of William Henry Harrison's "log cabin and hard cider" presidential campaign. Relishing the excitement of an American election, Liebermann visited New York and then decided on a brief visit to Washington. He stayed for the rest of his life.

Liebermann neither spoke nor understood more than a few words of English. But in this land of immigrants there were many who spoke the languages of central and Eastern Europe. One Russian, hearing of Liebermann's experiences with Dieffenbach and the new operation for strabismus, brought to him a local butcher, a large man whose eyes, Liebermann later told a colleague, "were looking in every direction but the right one."[38] Liebermann operated on the man and corrected the deformity. It was a first in America, according to Dieffenbach himself: "Dr. Liebermann . . . was, after myself, the third physician in Europe and the first one in the United States who, as early as October last (1840), performed the operation for strabismus with complete success."[39] Word of Liebermann's skill spread so rapidly in this small community—in 1840 fewer than twenty-four thousand people lived in the city of Washington itself[40]—that another case arrived at his lodgings almost immediately.

Within two or three months, Liebermann was performing several of the operations he had learned from Dieffenbach—for club foot and cataracts, as well as strabismus. Finding himself with a promising surgical practice, despite his foreign manners and lack of English, Liebermann kept delaying his return home.

Soon, however, his future was settled in the most traditional way. In early 1841 he met and married sixteen-year-old Louisa Catherine Betzold of Alexandria; their first child, Mary, was born the following November. By then Liebermann—changing his given name from Carl to Charles—had set up an office in the basement of their home on the corner of Eleventh and F Streets NW. Advertising in the *Intelligencer*, he described himself as "ready at all times to advise or practice either medicine, surgery or midwifery, for the poor gratis, not excepting capital [life-threatening] operations."

To practice in the District of Columbia, Liebermann needed a license, but how he acquired it typified the lax regulations of those days. In 1839 the Medical Society had set up a licensing process, which required an applicant to come before the society's five examiners, "produce a diploma from some respectable medical college or society . . . furnish satisfactory evidence that he has studied physic and surgery three years, including one full course of medical lectures as usually taught at the medical schools, or four years without such a course of lectures," and pay a license fee of five dollars.[41] What actually happened to Liebermann he described some twelve years later when obliged to rebut a jealous accusation that he was not properly qualified to practice medicine:

> The Pole who then resided with me as a translator and who, I soon found, did not understand more English than myself, had the order to show my papers to anyone who might call. The visiting cards of Drs. Sewall, Causin, May and Hall [leading members of the society] I found at my office; Drs. Lindsly and Worthington [two of the society's current examiners] I went to see myself; to each of the latter I handed a $5 piece as requested, and to my knowledge none of them asked for my papers, nor has any of them examined me. Some two years after that, Dr. [Flodoardo] Howard brought me the license . . . which had remained all that time with Dr. Worthington, I having no idea of having been honored with such an instrument.

Charles Liebermann was the dominating figure in the planning of Georgetown medical school. Of that there can be no doubt. Noble Young was more powerful within the local medical community and more proficient in its politics. But Liebermann had qualifications far superior to his three colleagues, and, in particular, the experience of having studied at the University of Berlin, then one of the best medical schools in the world. He took a dim view of medical education in Washington—to the extent that, as Johnson Eliot's son later noted, "he continually spoke of [its] defects to his medical friends and urged upon them the formation of a new college."[42]

Most American medical schools of the time graduated their students after no more than eight months of study. Young men whose families could afford it were sent to Europe where the universities offered longer and more rigorous academic courses and excellent clinical training in nearby teaching hospitals, or to the few American schools that were modeled on the European pattern. Those who could afford no school—still the majority in the 1840s— apprenticed themselves to local physicians and picked up practical know-how on the job. This almost certainly gave a sounder foundation for the practice of medicine than the lesser American schools which, originally set up to supplement the system of apprenticeship, were now beginning to replace it.

The reformer Abraham Flexner, scourge of American medical education sixty years later, lamented that the student of this era "no longer read his master's books, submitted to his quizzing, or rode with him the countryside in his enjoyment of valuable bedside opportunities. All the training that a young doctor got before beginning his practice had now to be procured within the medical school. The school was no longer the supplement; it was every-thing." But the "everything" consisted of didactic lectures, meager facilities—not so much as a skeleton or a book in some schools—and often no clinical training whatsoever. "Competent and humane physicians," Flexner observed, "the country came to have—at whose and at what cost, one shud-ders to reflect; for the early patients of the rapidly made doctors must have played an unduly large part in their practical training."[43] The American Medical Association was organized in 1846 in an attempt to improve national standards of education and practice—as well as to combat the pervasive problem of outright quackery—but by 1849 it had barely got into its stride.

Liebermann was not one to conceal his opinions. "He was blunt in manner and speech," said one contemporary.[44] "He did not tire of speaking concerning the German methods of teaching medicine," said another.[45] So although no detailed record has come down to us, we can certainly assume that in those early faculty meetings, Liebermann would have been emphatic about the importance of providing, as the European schools did, clinical instruction to students. But for that they needed beds with patients in them—which, with Columbian monopolizing the city's only hospital, meant establishing some new facility of their own. The first step in this direction was taken by the four doctors at their second faculty meeting on November 13, 1849, when they asked Flodoardo Howard "to obtain a suitable house for a public dispensary and for anatomical purposes."[46] Within two weeks, Howard found a house only two blocks away from his own office, which the owner, John Seaver, was prepared to lease to them for $150 a year.[47] It was too small for more than a few beds, but it was a start.

Halfway through the nineteenth century, Washington was still a small country town. Its unpaved, unlit streets (with no house numbers or street signs before 1853) swarmed with the hogs and geese which served as official garbage collectors; its road surfaces turned into a congealed morass of mud after rain or snow, or into blinding dust in dry weather. Its citizens were accustomed to visiting Europeans comparing it derisively with other capital cities. The broad avenues of L'Enfant's grand plan were already laid out— "broad avenues that begin in nothing and lead nowhere" wrote Charles Dickens of what he called the "City of Magnificent Intentions"—but its great buildings and monuments, though designed in the most imposing classical style, were still largely unfinished. The property boom long anticipated by many early speculators was only just beginning. Houses were still scattered amid vacant lots and even fields of cattle.[48]

The modest building which the new Georgetown medical faculty rented from Mr. Seaver stood on the southeast corner of F and Twelfth Streets NW. Today that site is occupied by a multi-story office block in the heart of the city's downtown business district. But in 1849 most of F Street was still residential, and the small corner house stood on a double lot with plenty of open ground, so the premises could easily be extended.[49]

All they needed was money. By the end of December, with the lease signed and repairs to the building under way, the bills began to arrive. Each member of the faculty was asked to contribute $12. By this time, another professor had been appointed—Joshua A. Ritchie, a thirty-five-year-old graduate of Jefferson Medical College—so the first levy amounted to $60. A month later, the five jointly contributed a further $60, but still it wasn't enough.[50] In a pattern familiar to every future generation of Georgetown medical school administrators, the cost of putting the building in order escalated, and in mid-March of 1850 Noble Young reported that another $600 was needed. He spelled out the expenses: $150 for rent, $250 for fitting up the dispensary and lecture room, $100 for chemical apparatus ("the best that will answer for medical purposes"), and $100 for "fuel, stoves, lights and other necessary contingencies."[51]

At a time when doctors in Washington ordinarily charged one dollar or less per patient visit and five dollars for comprehensive maternity and obstetric care[52]—fees not always received—the scale of this expenditure stunned the group. They were so alarmed that Young felt it only fair to offer anyone the chance to drop out of the venture, which was still, he acknowledged, "more or less of an experiment" with no guarantee of success. "Any gentleman who cannot, or does not, desire to enter into such expenses will have at this, the only proper time, an opportunity to withdraw," he told them. To their credit, all chose to continue. But they also decided that vacant chairs should be filled "as soon as practicable"; more professors had to be brought on board to share the financial burden.[53]

Over the next six months, their plans changed radically. The faculty decided to use the old house on the corner simply as a six-bed dispensary and to erect a new building for the medical school itself on the adjoining vacant lot on F Street. The cost was estimated at fifteen hundred dollars but, despite the faculty's orders that the work "be governed by the strictest economy consistent with a plain and substantial structure," the final bill for constructing and furnishing it came to nearly twenty-eight hundred dollars.[54]

Nevertheless, the faculty went ahead with this costly project in the hope of aid from the U.S. Congress, which directly governed the District of Columbia and was the only source of public funds for the city. But when Liebermann went to the Capitol in September 1850 and requested a two thousand dollar appropriation, he was turned down.[55] So the professors, now numbering seven, paid for the new building themselves, each contributing four hundred dollars over a twelve-month period.[56]

Another disappointment to the faculty was Georgetown College's apparent lack of interest in their endeavors. President Ryder's involvement

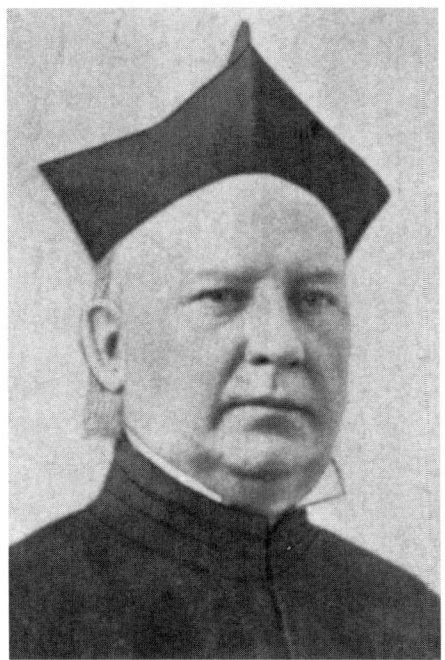

Reverend James Ryder, S.J., president of Georgetown College, 1848–51. Courtesy of Georgetown University Archives.

had so far been limited to writing letters to confirm the appointment of each new faculty member. But his early promise to provide someone from the college to teach chemistry in the medical department never materialized.[57] And although he had supported their efforts to win federal funding, writing to Congress to express his "lively interest in the success of their enterprise,"[58] they were convinced that another Georgetown Jesuit had sabotaged the attempt by privately testifying to the congressional committee that the college had no connection with the proposed medical school at all. Joshua Ritchie, a Georgetown alumnus who often served as liaison between the medical faculty and the college, was furious that the Jesuit in question had gone unrebuked for this hostile act.[59] It was not a propitious beginning. Yet there is every reason to suppose that Ryder himself—far more than most of his Jesuit colleagues—was committed to the concept of a medical department. In any event, he never lost an opportunity to promote Georgetown College.[60] Since the medical school was connected to the college and bore its name, Ryder wanted it to begin in a way that would both encourage its own success and reflect creditably on the mother institution.

The new lecture room of the Smithsonian was the obvious venue for an opening ceremony; it was the only public meeting place of any size in antebellum Washington. Joseph Henry, the scientist who had ably administered the institution from the time it was chartered in 1846, was still supervising the building of its sandstone "castle" on the Mall, although he loathed James Renwick's design, condemning it as a mock-medieval "failure" totally unsuited to the scientific and practical needs of the nineteenth century. As soon as the east wing was completed in 1849, its lecture room was opened for business. But Henry still had to cope with crisis after crisis. The roof leaked, the heating system failed to work, a new upper floor caved in, and the sea of mud outside was such an impassable barrier that he was obliged to lay wooden planks around the building so that visitors could get in. The public didn't care; they came to every event in such crowds that Henry completely redesigned the lecture room in 1850 in order to seat, in his own precise words, "990 persons, of 16 inches to each."[61] By 1851, the Smithsonian was still four years short of completion, but already it was the most fashionable place in town for ceremonies of any scientific nature.

Whether or not it was Ryder who arranged the medical school's inauguration there, it is clear that the occasion was heralded and enhanced by his supreme talent—oratory. Georgetown's president was one of the most dazzling speakers of his day. He was so much in demand as a lecturer and preacher that he traveled constantly to cities as far away as Cincinnati, leaving the day-to-day management of the college to subordinates. In Washington, his talks attracted hundreds, including members of presidential administrations and the Congress.[62] If Ryder was to speak, a capacity audience of prominent citizens was guaranteed. And that is what happened on May 12, 1851. James Ryder may not have provided the new medical school with a chemistry professor or a single red cent, but he certainly launched it in style.

The contrast between the splendid setting of the Smithsonian, even in its unfinished state, and the humble rooms used for the medical school could not have been more stark. The new building on F Street had two sparsely furnished lecture rooms, an anatomy room for dissection work, and a small chemistry laboratory equipped with a few beakers, retorts, and basic chemicals. There was also a library of sorts for the faculty: copies of the *Boston Medical and Surgical Journal*, *Haye's Journal*, and the London *Lancet*; maybe even a book or two.[63]

In these surroundings, Georgetown's first medical students settled down to their lectures, in rooms lit by the shimmer of oil-lamps and candles.[64] The faculty minutes name four: Warwick Evans, Samuel Jacobs Radcliffe, and

Benjamin C. Riley, all from Washington, D.C.; and Henry Korwin Kalussowski, originally from Poland.[65] If there were others who dropped out, no record remains; but these four stayed the course.

They were embarking on slightly less than ten months of study, divided into two sessions that ran May to September and November to early March. For this they paid $160 for tuition ($70 for the first session; $90 for the second; $150 if both were paid in advance), $20 for the demonstrator's fee ($10 for each session), $5 for matriculation, and $25 for graduation—an outlay of $210 at most.[66] In return, the students received tickets for each professor's set of lectures, which they presented at the beginning of each class. Georgetown's annual medical tuition is now more than one hundred times that amount. Yet those fees, paltry as they seem today, were considerable in 1851. But they were not beyond the means of the kind of young men, mainly government clerks with some education, who were commonly attracted to train as physicians. In Washington in the 1850s, as the bureaucracy of a federal system was beginning to grow, such government posts offered attractive salaries averaging $1,200 a year (compared to an average $500 for grade-school teachers, for example).[67]

The Georgetown medical faculty seems to have modeled its operation to a large extent on the competition. Its fees duplicated those of the Columbian medical school; its two summer and winter courses were the same length; it distributed the same number of handbills (five hundred) and placed advertisements in the same newspapers.[68] There was, however, one significant difference between the two schools. Columbian's lectures were given during the day, Georgetown's in the evening. Many American medical schools in the second half of the nineteenth century operated only at night. The system was derided in later years as "sundown medicine," and its graduates as "sundown doctors." But in the context of the times, the arrangement made sense. A man in his early twenties had to have private means in order to study by day; whereas evening classes (beginning at 4:00 or 5:00 P.M. and continuing until 9:00 or 10:00 P.M.) gave opportunities to young men who had to earn their own living but were eager to improve their prospects. Sundown medicine, it can be argued, did for the American medical profession of the nineteenth century what the G.I. Bill did for veterans of World War II. The Georgetown professors were shrewd enough to exploit this market, and if they did so to gain a competitive edge over Columbian, it worked. Five years later Columbian was doing so badly that all lectures were suspended for the 1856–57 school year, and when they resumed in the fall of 1857 they too took place in the evening.[69]

No record has come down to us of the Georgetown professors' lectures to their first students. The faculty minutes for this period are sketchy, showing every sign that Flodoardo Howard, now styled the dean of the faculty while still serving as treasurer and secretary and running his private practice, was too busy to jot down more than a few notes on financial matters. The first mention of the students came in March 1852, when they presented themselves for oral examination by the entire faculty. These examinations took place at 8:00 P.M. and consisted solely of a few questions put to the candidates by each professor. We do not know what they were, but even Liebermann's interrogation is unlikely to have been more exacting than the single surgery question put to a Harvard medical degree aspirant in the 1850s: "Well, White, what would you do for a wart?"[70] At the end of a similar minimal ordeal the four candidates—Evans, Radcliffe, Riley, and Kalussowski—were each declared "entitled to the degree of M.D."[71]

The graduates had to wait four months for their diplomas, however, since it had been arranged that their degrees would be formally conferred at the Georgetown College Commencement. Duly, they showed up at Georgetown with their professors on the morning of July 20, 1852. The ceremonies began at 9:00 in the morning and lasted till 4:30 in the afternoon.[72] Sitting in the heat of a Washington high summer through more than seven hours of speeches, recitations and orations, some in Latin, with musical interludes only adding to the ordeal, must have been close to intolerable. But the medical men sat it out while diplomas were handed to seventeen college graduates. Then they waited for their own—in vain. The four medical graduates were ignored; their names were not even mentioned. Their diplomas, it turned out, had already been mailed to their homes.

The medical professors were outraged. After all they had overcome, all the sacrifices they had made—even after donating twenty-five dollars the faculty could ill afford to the college's annual Catholic Pilgrim's Day outing to St. Mary's City, Maryland[73]—they took the commencement fiasco as a deliberate snub. Joshua Ritchie went straight home afterwards and wrote an impassioned protest to the Jesuit who was Georgetown's vice president, Reverend Daniel Lynch. He wrote:

The unfriendly conduct of the college towards the medical department during the early part of the year, in its tacit abnegation of all connection with us, or interest in our success, prepared us for some mark of its disregard. . . . But the least indulgent among us could not have anticipated that you would have inflicted such an injury upon us, as was perpetuated by the omission of mention of the names of our medical graduates upon the occasion of your commencement today . . . and when all chances of remedying the evil by a public commencement of our own was denied us by your having already advanced to our students their diplomas . . .

After dispatching the letter to Lynch, Ritchie sent his draft to another faculty member—probably its president, Noble Young—asking him to show it to Howard and the others. He added wearily: "I am going to bed very sick."[74] It was the lowest point in the medical department's relationship with the college, all the more humiliating because it occurred at what should have been its first public show of success.

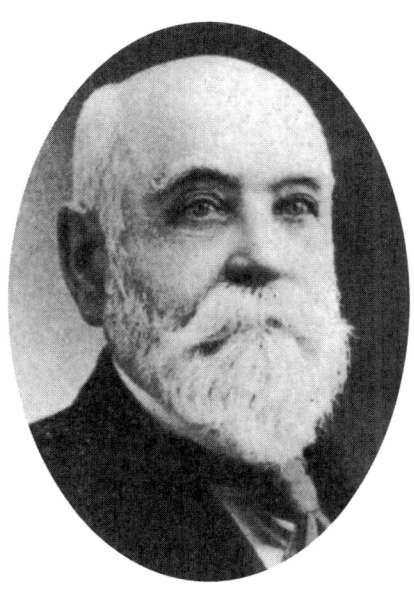

Warwick Evans, M.D., 1828–1915.
Courtesy of the Medical Society of the
District of Columbia.

Nevertheless, the department had graduated its first four alumni, and these now embarked on their careers. Warwick Evans (1828-1915), is considered Georgetown's first medical graduate because he was the first of the four to be examined. He was twenty-three years old at graduation, and he practiced medicine in Washington to the day of his death at age eighty-seven in 1915. Born in Portsmouth, New Hampshire, the son of Estwick Evans, a writer and explorer, Warwick had come to Washington as a three-year-old with his family in 1831. During his student days at the medical school his brother Edmund, who worked as President Millard Fillmore's secretary, was married in the White

House. Always well-disposed toward his alma mater, Warwick served as Georgetown's demonstrator of anatomy from 1865 to 1874 and afterwards became a professor of anatomy. His first wife, Mary, was an accomplished artist and prepared over five hundred anatomical charts for the school. In 1905, as a robust seventy-eight-year-old widower who had already fathered twelve children, Evans married his second wife, Emma Demming; their daughter, Virginia May, was born three years later. In 1989, Georgetown's medical awards ceremony was renamed Warwick Evans Night in his honor.[75]

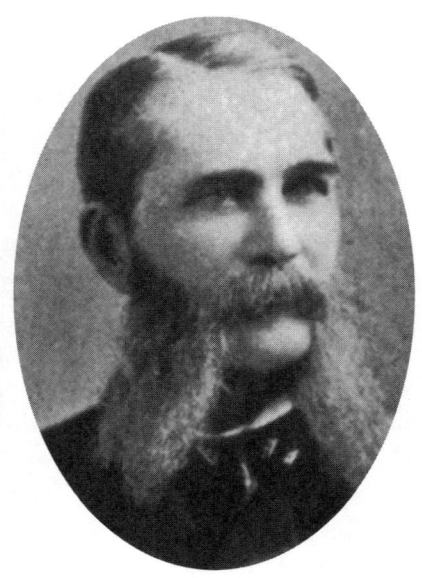

Samuel Jacobs Radcliffe, M.D., 1829–1903. Courtesy of the Medical Society of the District of Columbia.

Samuel Jacobs Radcliffe (1829-1903) was the son of a clerk in the District of Columbia's city government. He had been apprenticed to two local doctors, one of them being Flodoardo Howard, Georgetown's professor of obstetrics. After graduation, Radcliffe practiced in Washington until he moved to Baltimore in 1858. During the ensuing Civil War, he earned distinction as a Union army surgeon, rising to the rank of lieutenant-colonel as medical director of the 23rd Army Corps. He remained in the army, serving as assistant to the attending surgeon in Washington for many years.[76]

Of Benjamin C. Riley, we know nothing. He may have been related to Florence C. Riley, youngest daughter of a well-known local physician, Joshua, who lived and practiced on N Street in Georgetown.[77] Florence later married Benjamin's classmate Samuel Radcliffe.[78] In 1852 she was only sixteen years old[79], but it is gratifying to speculate that Benjamin introduced them then, thus sparking the medical school's first romance.

Of the four graduates, Henry Korwen Kalussowski (1806-1894) was by far the most extraordinary.[80] He was forty-five years old when he graduated—older than any of his professors—and already a great patriotic hero in his native Poland. Of aristocratic birth, he had begun studying medicine as a young man, but soon became a leader in one of the revolutionary armies that rose against Russia in 1830. In one battle, his troops held a whole Russian army at bay for seven days until a French ship arrived with reinforcements. After the Polish defeat in 1831, the twenty-five-year-old Kalussowski—decorated for bravery but suffering the effects of multiple wounds—fled to France. There he helped establish rebel Polish emigre organizations. Then he moved on to Belgium, where he married an Englishwoman, Anna Shea, and set up a publishing house devoted to works on Polish nationalism. In 1838, forced by financial problems to sell the business, he moved his family to London and then finally to the United States. Disaster struck soon after their arrival: his wife died, leaving him with three young children to raise. Kalussowski, who was reputed to speak eleven languages, made a precarious living as a teacher of French and Latin in New York and later in Washington. But Poland remained his passion. In 1842, he co-founded the Association of Poles in America. In 1848, he became an American citizen, but almost immediately left for Europe to take part in yet another Polish insurrection. On this occasion, he addressed the German parliament at Frankfurt on behalf of the Poles, was arrested by the Prussians, and was freed only after the American consul intervened—a fortunate consequence of his recent naturalization.

Returning to Washington in 1850, Kalussowski obtained a federal position as a clerk in the Land Office. Seeking to improve his prospects, though, he also enrolled in the first class of Georgetown medical school. (The link may have been Charles Liebermann, who as a Latvian patriot knew firsthand the hardships of Russian domination and had himself been briefly engaged in Poland's cause in the uprising of 1830.) Soon after the medical classes began in 1851, Kalussowski wrote to a friend:

> Just imagine that I am a regular medical student, I attend the course and in a year or eighteen months will take a doctor's degree if poverty or another misadventure does not finish me off. I study medicine to cease to be dependent on the whims and will of people or parties—the road back to my country is long, and even if it were short I am not needed there. People there can do without me, a fact of which I am more than certain. There are

two problems I have to face: one is my age, though that matters little as long as I am able to fulfill my plans, while the other—how to earn my living—is more difficult . . . I am busy from five in the morning till eight at night, earning my bread, going to the clinic or attending classes. However nothing can stop me from occasionally reading a newspaper or answering my friends' letters.[81]

During these hectic months Kalussowski found time to pen passionate letters in French to his fiancee, Mary Josephine Grimm, a Swiss woman twenty years his junior—and to write them out again in his copy book, now preserved in the national library of Poland. Occasionally the script falls into a jumble, suggesting he fell asleep at the task. The day after the medical school opened, he wrote to her: "Soon after you arrive, I will receive my degree of doctor of medicine, but I don't know if I could ever be a good doctor."[82] In late 1851, his beloved "Josee" crossed the Atlantic to marry him and in time bear him three more children. Perhaps because of his financial commitments, Kalussowski never practiced medicine, but instead climbed steadily up the federal government's career ladder, becoming director of the division for industrial and commercial affairs in the Secretariat of State. In 1867, the American government entrusted him with translating all the Russian documents involved in the purchase of Alaska. He never forgot Poland. During the Civil War, in which one of his sons fought on the Union side, he helped organize and equip the Polish Legion (later the 13th New York Infantry), at the same time sending aid to another war—the unsuccessful Polish insurrections of 1861 and 1863. Until the end of his life, he remained prominent in Polish American organizations, writing many publications for emigrés.

But Kalussowski never entirely gave up his dream of practicing medicine. In 1883, retired from government service and seventy-seven years old, he finally began advertising himself as a physician.[83] The attempt was shortlived, but his youngest son graduated in medicine and pharmacy and eventually became the dean of Columbian's School of Pharmacy.[84] Kalussowski died, aged eighty-eight, on December 23, 1894, and was buried in Rock Creek Cemetery, Washington. In 1964, a later generation of Polish-Americans met there to honor the seventieth anniversary of his death.[85] Kalussowski's connection with Georgetown—and, indeed, with medicine—was brief. Yet his story is classical, in that it describes the finest kind of American immigrants of this or any period: those who, escaping desperate conditions in their own lands, start over again across the ocean, constantly seeking self-improvement, and in doing so bring incomparable vigor to the New World.

What did they learn, these men who came from their daytime jobs, snatched a bite to eat, and then spent the rest of their waking hours studying medicine? By today's standards, of course, not much. All the theoretical knowledge qualifying them to go out into the world and practice as physicians and surgeons was fitted into four or five class hours each day, six days a week, for four months: probably less than five hundred hours in all. The second four-month course repeated the subject matter of the first.[86] Students listened to the same lectures delivered by the same professors, watched the same anatomical demonstrations, performed the same dissections, and made the same simple chemistry experiments during the winter session as they had in the summer. Again, in the context of the times, this was not as bizarre as it may now seem. These students had no textbooks, let alone computerized databases; repetition was the only effective way of ensuring that they thoroughly understood what they were being taught.

Six subjects were covered in these early years of the school: medicine, surgery, anatomy, chemistry, materia medica (medications), and obstetrics (comprising not only childbirth but the diseases of women and children, not yet known as gynecology and pediatrics). Even this degree of specialization was a pedagogical advance: in 1825, when Columbian's medical department had opened, its first professor of surgery had served also as professor of chemistry, mineralogy, and geology.[87] Specialties as we understand them today did not begin in Washington until the 1870s, starting with ophthalmology and laryngology. In 1851, doctors did not specialize even in the larger branches of medicine. All were family physicians in the widest sense, and this generality was reflected in medical education. It was not unusual in the 1850s for professors to switch chairs; a man who taught surgery one year might teach obstetrics the next. No one considered it odd; the body of medical knowledge was so small that they were expected to know it all.

This was a time when the diagnosis of disease was vague. A patient's appearance—dark or fair, ruddy or pale, fat or thin, brown or blue-eyed—was often still the main determinant of prescribed treatment. For want of a better explanation, many diseases were put down to heredity. "Cures" were limited to blood-letting, purgatives, fasting, alcoholic drinks, medicines of questionable value, and ancient herbal remedies.[88] Poisonous minerals and addictive drugs were regularly prescribed and administered. Pharmacists needed no license; and when control over the indiscriminate sale of drugs was proposed in the 1840s, Congress rejected the idea as an unconstitutional violation of civil liberties.[89] What we now know as conditions fundamental to health— fresh air, the cleanliness of a patient's body, bed, and sickroom—were often specifically forbidden for fear of the patient's "taking cold." Halfway through the nineteenth century, medicine, pharmacy, and nursing were still medieval.

So was surgery. Daring procedures had certainly been attempted in years past, sometimes even successfully. As early as 1718, a Boston surgeon performed mastectomy on a woman who survived a further thirty-nine years, possibly because her breast was not cancerous as diagnosed.[90] In 1736, a London surgeon excised the appendix of a patient who recovered.[91] And on Christmas Day 1809, the world's first successful ovariotomy was performed—not at the hands of any famous European surgeon, but by Ephraim McDowell, a country doctor working in the backwoods of Kentucky. He removed a seven-pound cyst from the ovary of forty-four-year-old Jane Crawford in a twenty-five-minute operation on his dining room table. Mrs. Crawford was up and about in five days, rode a horse sixty miles back to her home within a month, and lived until she was seventy-eight years old.[92]

But such heroic surgery was rare. It was attempted only in extreme emergency, usually as the last alternative to certain death—and then only by surgeons confident enough to try it on patients courageous enough to endure it. The pain of surgery was sometimes alleviated by administering alcohol, opium, or hypnosis to the patient, or occasionally by freezing a limb with packed ice, but more often by stoicism. Mrs. Crawford recited psalms. Most patients, held down by the surgeon's assistants, simply struggled and screamed; if they fainted from shock, it was a blessing to all concerned. Samuel Busey, recalling operations in the early 1840s, wrote: "Speed in execution and dexterity were important considerations, and a surgeon who combined both qualities seemed to occasion much less pain. The apparently complete absence of suffering in some cases was inexplicable."[93]

The use of anesthesia in surgery was publicly demonstrated for the first time on October 16, 1846, at Massachusetts General Hospital in Boston, during an operation to remove a neck tumor in front of the whole medical class of Harvard University. William T. G. Morton, a dentist who had previously used ether to extract teeth, administered it to the patient, and the surgeon John Collins Warren, then age seventy, performed the procedure. The patient felt no pain, and at the end Warren exclaimed: "Gentlemen, this is no humbug!" News of the breakthrough spread so rapidly that ether was being used in operations at other American and European hospitals within a few weeks. Chloroform quickly followed, first used operatively by James Young Simpson in Edinburgh in January 1847. The use of anesthesia did not merely lessen the suffering of patients; it also allowed surgeons to work in comparative calm, with less haste, more gentleness, and greater accuracy. Even so, it had an impact only on emergency surgery; elective surgery (operations chosen for non-life-threatening conditions) did not come into use until aseptic techniques became generally accepted several decades later.[94]

In the 1850s, an ordinary physician's surgical skills were employed most often in bloodletting. This was not only still used therapeutically for a wide range of conditions, but was also considered a useful tonic, commonly done twice-yearly, spring and fall. Samuel D. Gross, professor of surgery at Jefferson Medical College and the most famous American surgeon of his day, wrote that the quantity of blood drained at any one time varied from sixteen to twenty-four ounces: "Unless the loss was considerable," he added, "the patient did not consider that he had received an equivalent for his money."[95] Other routine surgical duties included bandaging, cleaning suppurating wounds, giving enemas and vaccinations, making and applying splints. Operative work was much less common, except in great hospitals like Bellevue in New York City where surgeons worked full-time in the surgical wards. In Washington, the typical physician-surgeon attended mainly to the repair of minor surface injuries or the removal of growths from the skin. More challenging surgery—dealing with gunshot wounds, compound fractures, or amputations—was undertaken by relatively few in the medical community. Those who did were the most experienced, most confident and, probably, the physically strongest doctors. It tended to be the swashbucklers among them, the "lions" of the profession, who attempted the most drastic surgery. Moreover, in the absence of antiseptic agents and aseptic procedures, surgery of any kind was commonly followed by infection, and infection frequently proved fatal.

Although the bacterial basis of contagion would not be scientifically established until 1878, several physicians had already begun by the 1840s to perceive a connection between dirt and the spread of disease. Some even washed their hands and cleaned their instruments before treating a patient. But the great majority of doctors saw no need to take even the simplest hygienic precautions, oblivious to the fact that they themselves were the principal vector of disease, particularly among women. "Neither surgeon, obstetrician, nor any other general practitioner hesitated to go direct from the dressing of a foul wound, a case of erysipelas or other infectious disease to a labor case," Busey recalled years later.[96]

During operations, the patient was laid on the table unwashed and usually in street clothes. If an instrument fell to the ground it was wiped on a rag or the surgeon's sleeve. Wounds were routinely swabbed with sponges that had been merely rinsed in water after use on other patients. Some surgeons donned aprons, but most operated in old frock coats encrusted with blood and pus from previous operations—stains worn proudly as badges of experience—and often kept sutures handily in pockets or dangling from buttonholes, or stuck ready-threaded needles into their lapels. Neither probes nor dressings, which usually consisted of torn-up bedsheets or other old rags, were sterilized. And the whole procedure was often attended by a crowd of students, the patient's relatives, or other curious spectators—who were rarely prevented from poking fingers into the wound. Even the most celebrated surgeons moistened sutures with their saliva before threading a surgical needle. Samuel Gross was frequently seen stropping the knife on his boot before making an incision. The high mortality rate that was the inevitable outcome of such practices was not confined to patients; some surgeons also died from infection that invaded insignificant abrasions on their hands through contact with a diseased patient, cadaver, or dressing.[97] Such was the state of surgery in the 1850s and for the several decades that followed.

The early medical students at Georgetown were fortunate to have Charles Liebermann as their professor of surgery. Whether or not he washed his hands preoperatively, Liebermann was highly admired by his

Washington peers for his intellect, surgical skills, and diagnostic acumen. Joseph M. Toner, one of the city's leading medical men and later president of the American Medical Association, said of Liebermann: "Washington had few physicians of more eminence." Another noted that he "often reached a correct diagnosis when others of his professional brethren had failed to do so."[98] Liebermann was brusque in manner and, Busey recalled, "when dealing with a refractory patient his remonstrance was not always couched in the choicest language." He made a point of never treating anyone who lived in his immediate neighborhood; and when one longstanding patient moved opposite his house and office on Thirteenth Street he flatly refused to continue as the man's doctor.[99] Liebermann's students, like his patients, must have been in awe of him.

But in October 1853, Liebermann abruptly resigned from the Georgetown medical faculty. So did Joshua Ritchie.[100] The likeliest explanation for their departure is frustration over the continuing absence of clinical facilities for the medical school. Its 1852–53 catalogue had boasted that "a large and commodious hospital is now in the course of erection, where students will have as ample an opportunity of clinical instruction as the metropolis can furnish."[101] But no such facility existed. In March 1853, the professors were still discussing less expensive ways to improve clinical instruction. They considered raising the roof and adding another story to the tiny, inadequate dispensary. They also explored a "plan for getting access for students to the Washington Asylum"—Saint Elizabeth's Hospital, the city's newly constructed institution for the insane, which was miles away on the banks of the Anacostia River.[102] In April, perhaps goaded by Liebermann, the faculty returned to the much more ambitious idea of pulling down the old dispensary and erecting a larger facility in its place. They opened negotiations with a local construction company for a building that would cost twenty-seven hundred dollars, to be paid for over three years from future profits of the medical school. At Liebermann's suggestion, they wrote to the Mother Superior of the Sisters of Charity, inviting the order to take charge of this new "infirmary." The best-trained nurses in the United States, these nuns already ran the Washington Infirmary for Columbian as well as many other hospitals; moreover, they did not require salaries. The letter was thus extremely respectful, pointing out that Saint Patrick's Catholic Church and the Washington Convent were just around the corner from the school.[103]

But within months, this plan was also abandoned, probably because most of the professors decided they could not afford it. They had each already invested several hundred dollars in the school and it was not yet making a profit. Twice they had voted themselves a modest dividend and both times were forced to reconsider.[104] So on financial grounds, the decision to do without a new clinic was justified.

But to Liebermann it was apparently the last straw. Years before, as a medical student in Berlin, he had attended the surgery demonstrations which were standard clinical instruction in Europe. There, in great and even beautiful amphitheaters such as the École de Chirurgie in Paris, where a huge skylight cast illumination from the apex of a decorated dome that would not have disgraced a cathedral, surgeons operated on patients in front of hundreds of students and anyone else who cared to witness the spectacle. They were splendid performances, second only in popularity to public executions; and the most famous surgeons operated with full theatrical flourish, often asking the audience to time them: William Fergusson of London, for example, could amputate at the thigh, close and dress the wound in three and a half minutes. Once finished, these star surgeons bowed to acknowledge applause. Bernhard Langenbeck, professor of surgery at the Ziegelstrasse Klinik in Berlin, carried out all his surgical duties for thirty-five years in the amphitheater—questioning, examining, and diagnosing patients publicly as well as operating on them there.[105]

By the mid-1850s, surgical amphitheaters had been established in several American cities, including Washington. To the frustration of the Georgetown faculty, the Washington Infirmary was completely remodeled in the fall of 1853 with a twenty-thousand-dollar grant from Congress. The new building provided more than a hundred rooms and a sizeable surgical amphitheater that seated three hundred people.[106] The following year, Noble Young once again leaped into the fray and led an organized attempt to separate the infirmary from Columbian's jurisdiction in order to make its facilities equally available to Georgetown students; once again he failed.[107] Georgetown—with funding from nowhere save the students' fees and the professors' pockets—remained a didactic proprietary school with few opportunities for clinical instruction.

The nearest Georgetown students came to practical surgery was in their anatomy classes. In a room on the upper floor of the medical school they dissected cadavers, a practice still clouded by public suspicion. Congress refused to make any legal provision for medical dissection in the District of Columbia, and in many states it was still a criminal offense. Grave-robbing was virtually the only means of procuring anatomical material, and many professors and demonstrators of anatomy in the medical schools (including Georgetown) were obliged to do it themselves, to save the expense of hiring a resurrectionist, as the professionals of this grisly trade were cynically called. The laws against grave-robbing were not generally enforced rigorously against doctors, but those who were caught were publicly denounced in the newspapers. In 1846, the parents of a nine-year-old girl whose body had been taken from her grave in Pittstown, New York, exacted their own peculiarly permanent revenge. They erected a new tombstone inscribed with the names of the resurrectionist, the physician-anatomist, and a verse:

Her body dissected by fiendish men;
Her bones anatomized;
Her soul, we trust, has risen to God,
Where few physicians rise.[108]

When grave-robbing scandals erupted from time to time, medical schools were inevitably the first to come under suspicion. So when a mutilated cadaver was found propped up outside the door of Georgetown medical school in January 1859, the professors treated the incident as more than a student prank. They reacted strongly and publicly, laying the matter before the grand jury and offering a fifty-dollar reward for the arrest and conviction of the culprit.[109] The students of Columbian speedily issued their own statement denying "any participation in or knowledge of the outrage."[110] The miscreant was never caught.

Charles Liebermann's successor as professor of surgery was John Marshall Snyder (1828-1863) who in 1853 was just two months short of his twenty-fifth birthday. Raised in Charlestown, Virginia, Snyder had served a one-year apprenticeship with Samuel Gross—who was then, before taking the chair at Jefferson Medical College, practicing in Louisville, Kentucky. Snyder received his medical degree from the City of New York University in 1850 and had been in practice for three years in Georgetown before his appointment to the medical faculty.[111] It is not clear how competent or reliable Snyder was as a teacher. (Some years later, the students demanded his removal because he had missed classes and skipped course material.[112]) But in 1857, Charles Liebermann returned as professor of surgery and Snyder was switched to the newly-vacant chair of obstetrics. The first incumbent of that chair, Flodoardo Howard, had decided to retire to his estate at Brookville, near Rockville, Maryland, and devote himself to farming.[113]

From 1852 through 1860, the medical school graduated fifty-nine students.[114] The total enrollment is not recorded, but it was probably not much higher. The best schools regularly failed 60 percent of their intake, but the Georgetown faculty minutes show each year that all students examined were immediately declared "entitled to the degree of M.D." In March 1860, two of that year's ten candidates were failed, "not having given satisfaction to the faculty." Three days later they took the examination again and were passed.[115]

Many of these early graduates, however, went on to notable medical careers. It was their own intellectual curiosity that enabled them to transcend the limitations of their formal training. Thus, in 1855 the alumni formed a Medico-Chirurgical Society. With Samuel Radcliffe and Warwick Evans as president and vice president, the group met quarterly to present essays and discuss medical matters; it was the forerunner of today's Medical Alumni Association.[116] The school was also used for weekly meetings of the Pathological Society of the District of Columbia. Most of the leading physicians of Washington were members, including all of the Georgetown professors. Pathological specimens were displayed, papers were read, and sometimes an unusual case was discussed in clinical detail.[117] These group meetings were social as well as scientific. In warm weather, their members, as well as the medical students, no doubt availed themselves of a new attraction just across the street from the medical school: Washington's first ice-cream parlor, only the second in the country, opened in 1856 by Jacob Fussell, a Baltimore milk dealer. And on the southwest corner of the F and Twelfth Streets intersection (today one of the entrances to the Metro Center, hub of the subway system), also stood the Great Falls Ice Company—making that intersection a haven of coolness in steamy Washington summers.[118]

By the end of the 1850s, Georgetown had established itself as Washington's second medical school, and its professors were prominent in the city's professional community. It now took sixteen months for students to graduate, but the course still consisted of only two four-month sessions: classes ran from November through February each year, the second year a repeat of the first, with degrees awarded at the end of the second session. The school's relationship with the college remained tenuous; after the fiasco of 1852, the medical department held its own separate commencements, usually at the Smithsonian, though the president of Georgetown College was always there to hand out the diplomas. But financially, the school still teetered on the brink of disaster.

When he returned to Georgetown in 1857, Charles Liebermann had taken over the duties of faculty treasurer. Each year the accounts were audited by other members and found "perfectly correct," and each year Liebermann was formally thanked for the "very able manner" in which he had kept them.[119] But there were problems with students who defaulted on their fees; although the faculty announced it would rigidly enforce the rule that "no student should be examined without having settled his indebtedness," it also allowed the treasurer "discretion" in settling with them.[120] In September 1860, this brought on a crisis. The auditors found that Liebermann had exercised his discretion a little too liberally: $420 owed by students had gone uncollected. The faculty ordered the dean, Johnson Eliot, to take over the treasurer's accounts and all funds in hand. Then a committee was appointed to retrieve the money owed.[121] There was no question that Liebermann was anything but scrupulously honest; but he was also a proud man. He resigned from Georgetown for the second time, and this time he never came back.

Liebermann's abrupt departure was a loss to the school, but it is easy to understand his colleagues' dismay over the uncollected $420. Expenses were always hard to meet; and rarely were there enough funds left over to pay faculty members any dividend on their investment. In 1857, the faculty had been obliged to allow new members the option of paying $50 a year "rent" for the privilege of a chair, in lieu of owning shares.[122] In 1859, money was so short that the faculty even sold a Georgetown medical diploma for $30 to a Welshman who wrote from Radnorshire asking for one, despite an angry letter from another Welshman, an authentic medical graduate of Georgetown, who knew the man and denounced him as a charlatan.[123] In retrospect, it is apparent that Washington could barely sustain two medical schools. Columbian's resources were equally stretched. In April 1856, just before suspending lectures for a year, its dean recorded "$8.25 in hand over all expenses to show for the winter's work."[124]

But Noble Young and his faculty struggled on, always emphasizing to students the high ideals of their chosen profession and the duty, through study and application, to keep pushing the limits of medical knowledge—"a progress to continue to the end of time," as Young put it in his 1857 valedictory address.[125] And he kept on trying to find ways to heal the festering sore of the school's clinical deficiencies. At the end of 1858, Young again petitioned Congress to establish a new general hospital in Washington.[126] The following March, he formed a committee "to take the first steps to the establishment of a free hospital," but three months later the faculty had to settle for reopening its old dispensary, which had long been closed, for two hours each Tuesday and Saturday morning.[127] Then in September 1859, another group began campaigning for a new general hospital, specifying that it should be staffed by local physicians but exclude "the faculties of the medical colleges at present in the District."[128] It was a bitter irony: the tactics Young had used ten years earlier against Columbian were now being used against Georgetown, but with far less cause. Only a few months earlier, Georgetown's want of clinical facilities had been captured in a pitiful faculty minute: "Dr. Liebermann was directed to ascertain on what terms Mr. Groux [a patient] would submit his malformation (cleft sternum) before the class."[129]

By the end of 1860, Georgetown's professors seemed no nearer to hospital privileges than they had been in 1849. They had no means of knowing that within a year or two they and their students would be up to their elbows in blood, struggling to cope with more clinical work than they could handle; that surgeons would be more urgently in demand than ever before in America; and that within five years there would be not one or two but sixty-five hospitals in Washington and neighboring Alexandria.[130] As the year ended and 1861 began, Washingtonians were fully aware that their country was accelerating down the slope towards civil war, but few foresaw the toll it would finally exact. The nation was about to enter a nightmare, an era in its history that would leave few families or institutions unscathed. Paradoxically, as is the way with war, there would be some whose fortunes it changed for the better. Georgetown medical school would be one of them.

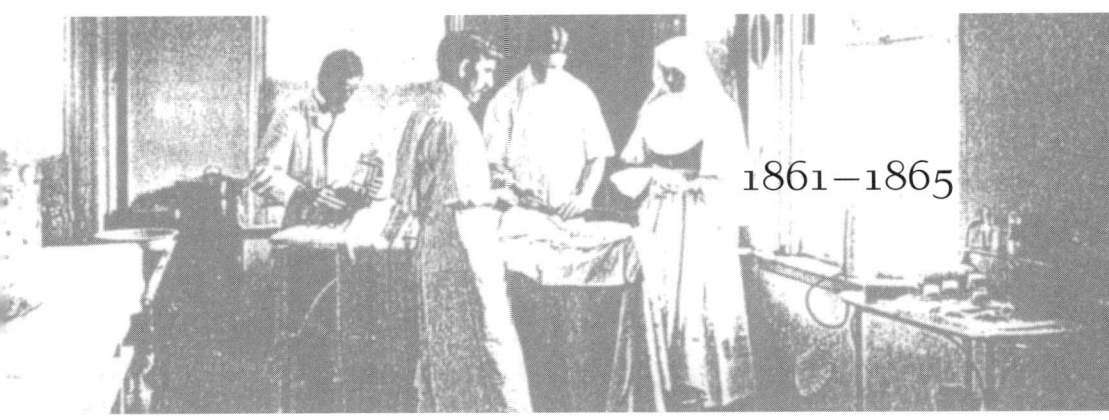

1861–1865

CHAPTER TWO

THE IMPACT OF THE CIVIL WAR

THE MEDICAL SCHOOL'S tenth commencement was held on Thursday, February 28, 1861, and for the first time since the traumatic commencement of 1852, it took place at Georgetown College. Relatives and friends crowded into the refectory to see eight graduates awarded their medical degrees. Afterwards, several young women in tight-waisted crinolines rushed forward to press bouquets on those they favored—their selection prompting one onlooker to remark: "We think the ladies might have been a little more impartial in their distribution."[1] It was an occasion they would ever after remember as a moment of normality before everything changed. Within months, at least six of the eight young men would be serving in opposing armies, one in Confederate gray and five in Union blue.[2]

This commencement was held a week or two earlier than usual. The following Monday, March 4, Abraham Lincoln was to be inaugurated as the first Republican president of a country no longer united, and Washington was tense. The gaunt mid-Westerner's election had already prompted seven Southern states to secede from the Union, and there were many who predicted he would not make it through inauguration day without being assassinated.[3]

In the event, the ceremonies passed off peacefully. But the citizens of Washington remained on edge, wondering whether the surrounding slave

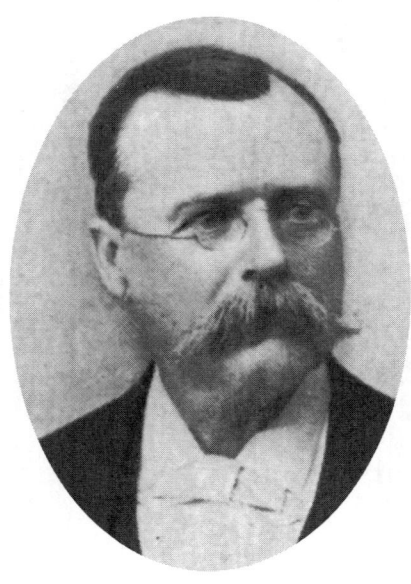

Reuban Cleary, M.D., 1835–98. Courtesy of the Medical Society of the District of Columbia.

states of Maryland and Virginia would secede and how Lincoln would react toward the newly-formed Confederacy. Whatever their sympathies for North or South, whatever their individual views on slavery and states' rights, Washingtonians who owned property or businesses worried that their city would not survive the secession crisis, no matter how it was resolved. If the country split into separate nations, neither side would want Washington as its capital. Yet if it came to civil war, the city would be in the front line and likely destroyed in the conflict. Already reflecting that dread prospect, business had slumped and real estate values collapsed. While rival factions defiantly wore the "secesh" cockade in their caps or retaliated by flaunting the stars and stripes, the city seethed with rumors of treason, Confederate spies, and plots to seize the Capitol.[4]

In this fevered atmosphere, the trial which opened at the Criminal Court in Washington's Judiciary Square on Saturday, March 9, attracted much attention. In the dock stood seven men accused of inciting a riot four months earlier on the night of Lincoln's election. Two were not only graduates of Georgetown medical school but currently employed there as its prosector and demonstrator of anatomy: Reuben Cleary, class of 1859, and John E. Willett, class of 1855.[5] They were local leaders of the National Volunteers, an organization that opposed "Black Republicanism" and championed Southern rights.[6]

Lincoln's election victory on November 6, 1860, though hardly unexpected, had sparked violence throughout the South that night. At the Democratic headquarters in Washington, where Cleary and his friends were drinking, feelings ran high. Shortly before midnight, witnesses heard

Cleary shout over the uproar "Let's take the Wigwam!" Then a crowd of about three hundred men tore into the dark streets to attack—and, some hoped, burn to the ground—the Republican Party headquarters on Indiana Avenue, known as the "Wigwam." In the ensuing mêlée, shots were fired, windows were stoned, and the mob broke into the building, driving the few Republicans who remained inside onto the roof. When police arrived, an officer heard Cleary give the order—"Fall in, Volunteers, we've done our duty!" They promptly arrested him.[7]

Reuben Cleary, a passionate defender of Southern rights, was no son of the plantation. Born in Alexandria in 1835 and raised in Washington, he was the second of ten children of a government bureaucrat.[8] After gradua-tion, Cleary and a classmate, Lucius Smith, shared a rented house on Four-and-a-half Street, just off Pennsylvania Avenue, and together strug-gled to build a medical practice. Athough Cleary advertised himself as a physician, in capital letters, in the 1860 Washington street directory, he was still working as a tax collector's clerk for the city council to pay the rent.[9] But he had friends. Several—including the mayor of Washington, James Berret, who a few months later would be jailed for refusing the oath of allegiance—spoke in his defense at the trial, describing him as a highly respectable citizen, "utterly incapable of embarking on disorderly proceedings." The jury was not impressed: it found Cleary and two others (though not his Georgetown colleague John Willett) guilty of causing an "affray." The verdict cost each a fifty-dollar fine; had they been convicted of inciting a riot, the judge said grimly, he would have been obliged "to impose a heavy imprisonment."[10] Within five weeks, Cleary left Washington forever. On April 22, five days before his twenty-sixth birthday, he joined the Confederate army in Alexandria and formed his own troop—calling it, with typical panache, Captain Reuben Cleary's Company of Washington Volunteers.[11]

By then, Confederate cannons had fired on the federal garrison at Fort Sumter, Lincoln had called for seventy-five thousand volunteer troops, Virginia had seceded from the Union, and the War between the States had begun.

On the April night in 1861 that Lincoln's call for volunteers went out over the telegraph wires, another young man—a twenty-two-year-old clerk named Charles Franklyn Rand—was drinking with friends at a tavern in the small town of Batavia in upstate New York and discussing the question uppermost in everyone's mind: how would Lincoln respond to the attack on Fort Sumter? They got their answer when the local telegraph operator burst in with the president's message. Amid the cheering, someone found paper to use as a makeshift muster roll and asked who would be first to enlist. Young Rand stepped forward and signed—less than ten minutes, it was said, after Lincoln put out the call. He later credited himself as the very first to volunteer for the Union army (an exaggeration since several units had mustered even before Sumter) in a force that eventually numbered more than 2.1 million men.[12] Rand, too, was eventually to become a Georgetown doctor. He enrolled in the medical school six years after the war.

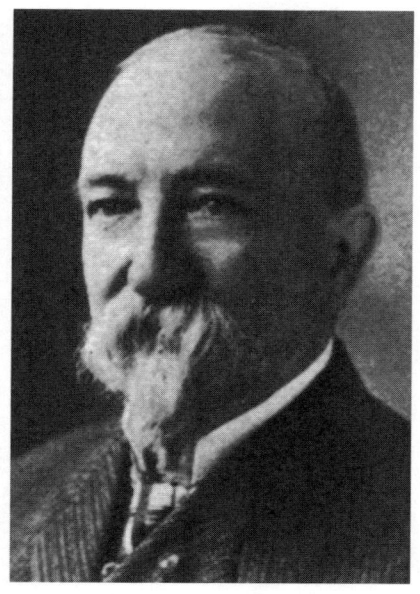

Charles Rand, M.D., 1839–1908. Courtesy of the Medical Society of the District of Columbia.

Rand was one of the fifty thousand troops, in volunteer regiments from all over the North, who flocked to the defense of Washington in the two months that followed, almost doubling the city's population. They were men of every type, from farm boys in rough homespun to patricians in elaborate uniforms with valets in tow, and they were quartered in every imaginable space—among the mahogany curio cases in the Patent Office, between the desks of the Treasury building and the stalls of the Center Market, even in the rotunda of the Capitol where, high above them, masons were beginning to erect the new marble dome.[13] Georgetown College was commandeered as a barracks for the 69th New York Regiment, composed of Irish-American Catholics, and later for the 79th, mainly American Scots. Most of the college students, overwhelmingly from the South, had already left; the few who remained on campus attempted their studies amid the clamor of rousing bugles, marching feet, shouted orders, and musket drill; they even had the thrill of a visit from

President Lincoln himself, who came to review the troops.[14]

In high summer, the Union army finally crossed the Long Bridge over the Potomac (where the Fourteenth Street Bridge now stands) into Virginia. The plan was to march on Richmond, seize the Confederate capital, and settle this pesky rebellion for good, so that one and all could go home and get on with their lives. On July 18, young Charles Rand was in a forward party in Virginia, some twenty-five miles southwest of Washington with six companies of his regiment, the 12th New York, which had been sent ahead to reconnoiter a narrow creek known as Bull Run. As they approached the creek at Blackburn's Ford, Confederate artillery and muskets opened fire from the woods that clustered thick on its banks. Within minutes the first casualties fell and the ill-trained New Yorkers, all five hundred of them, fled in panic. All, that is, except Rand and another youngster, Corporal James E. Cross, who obstinately stood their ground, reloading and aimlessly firing their antique muskets until, Rand said later, "the enemy refused to waste powder on us."[15] Rand's action was the first for which a Congressional Medal of Honor was awarded, making him the first acknowledged hero of the war.[16]

There is a wry twist to this episode. Reuben Cleary's troop, now more prosaically labeled Company H of the 7th Virginia Infantry regiment, was among those fighting in Colonel Jubal Early's brigade on the Confederate side of the creek. (Their musketry was as erratic as Rand's: their first enthusiastic volleys sprayed their own side, forcing Brigadier General James Longstreet to leap off his horse and lie on the ground.)[17] Thus these two young men, who never met but who at different times were taught medicine by the same professors, began their active service shooting at each other in the Battle of Blackburn's Ford.

The stories of Reuben Cleary and Charles Rand were minor incidents in America's most tragic struggle, but they illustrate a wider truth. Georgetown medical men were engaged on both sides in all the great events and battles of the Civil War, from Lincoln's election in 1860 to his assassination in 1865, from the first skirmish at Bull Run to the surrender at Appomattox.

It is impossible to say exactly how many of those who passed through the school as students or faculty served in the war. A search of many sources identifies 114 men *known* to have served—95 on the Union side and 19 for the Confederacy.[18] That tally includes those who graduated from, or taught at, the medical school before, during, and after the Civil War. But there were certainly many more: students who attended classes but never graduated; those who graduated and served but whose records are lost; and doctors who had graduated elsewhere but attended the special course on military surgery that Georgetown offered later in the war.

Of those known to have served, about half fought as soldiers in regular or volunteer regiments; one enlisted originally as a musician and another became a Confederate spy. The other half did put their medical training into practice in many different capacities. Some, still students, served in the lowliest roles as hospital stewards and dressers by day while attending medical school lectures by night. Many worked as "acting assistant surgeons" on contract to the army for limited periods. Most, including some who began on contract, were commissioned into the army as "assistant surgeons" or "surgeons" serving in the field or in military hospitals. A few rose higher, to positions as "surgeon-in-charge" of a military base hospital or as "medical director" of an army department with responsibility over the whole range of medical services in the field.

In all, twenty-one Georgetown men who were faculty members before, during, or after the war served in the conflict. With the exception of Charles Liebermann, these included every professor of surgery who taught at Georgetown over a period of forty years: John M. Snyder (1853–57), Johnson Eliot (1860–76), Thomas Antisell (military surgery, 1863–65), Robert Reyburn (clinical surgery, 1867–68), John Harry Thompson (clinical surgery, 1868–73 and 1874–76), Francis Asbury Ashford (1876–83), and John Brown Hamilton (1883–92). All served as surgeons except Ashford and Hamilton, who fought as soldiers before graduating in medicine. Ashford, who enlisted at age nineteen at the outbreak of war and saw action as an infantryman for the whole four years, was the only one of this group on the Confederate side.

For a school that had opened only ten years before the conflict began, Georgetown was conspicuously represented by both faculty and alumni. Whether they chose to wear the blue or the gray, all of them witnessed, and some directly experienced, the special horrors of disease, injury, and death that characterized the Civil War.

꿁

From the start, surgeons had a unique perspective on events. The rout of Union forces at the first battle of Bull Run (or, as Southerners called it, First Manassas) on Sunday, July 21—three days after the skirmish at Blackburn's Ford—came as a seismic shock to the North. Many reasons were given for the defeat, including the fact that Rose O'Neal Greenhow— a society lady of Washington and the Mata Hari of her time—had managed to smuggle a coded message to the Confederate commander, giving him the time and place of General Irvin McDowell's intended attack.[19] But a less romantic explanation was offered by William S. King, the veteran military surgeon who served at Bull Run as McDowell's medical director. He watched the Union troops as they rushed seven miles to the battlefield, marching at the double, even at a run, in full kit under scorching heat, and he predicted the outcome. "The weather was excessively hot," he reported, "and, as one of the causes of the Bull Run failure, I desire to record my belief that the exhaustion of our forces, by the long and forced march, contributed as much as anything else to the disasters of the day."[20]

The two armies sustained 3,574 casualties at Bull Run: 868 killed and 2,706 wounded.[21] King and his surgeons tended the Union wounded as best they could in the field—in one case King extracted a musket ball from the arm of a colonel while he remained on his horse, refusing to abandon command[22]—and then had them moved, with difficulty, back to Centreville. There, the church was emptied of its pews and every other large building was taken over for use as makeshift hospitals.[23] But the advancing Confederates soon overran Centreville and the Union surgeons had the choice of retreating with the army or staying with their patients. Several stayed and, contrary to the custom later in the war when captured surgeons were released swiftly or exchanged, these medics were to languish in Richmond as prisoners of war for more than a year.[24] The Confederate surgeons then moved *their* wounded, more than fifteen hundred men (one of them Douglass Cleary, Reuben's younger brother[25]) into Centreville too. So urgent was the need for medical hands that one young man who had just fought in the battle as a private in a

Confederate rifle company was instantly commissioned as an assistant surgeon. He was Arthur R. Barry, son of a Maryland plantation owner, and one of those who had laughingly accepted bouquets along with their degrees at Georgetown less than four months before.[26]

꿍

For physicians on both sides, Bull Run was their baptism into the medical horrors of a new kind of warfare. From a military perspective, the American Civil War was the first modern war, because it harnessed the new technologies of the nineteenth century. It was the first war to use railroads to move massed armies and the supplies they depended on; the first to use armored and turreted warships and even early versions of the submarine; the first to use remotely-detonated landmines; the first to use aerial reconnaissance (by balloon); the first to use telegraphy for the instant communication of orders and news; the first in which photography revealed the realities of the battlefield to shocked civilians; and, most crucially for medical men, the first to employ weapons of a range, rate of fire, and accuracy to inflict mass slaughter.

The tragedy is that, from a medical perspective, the Civil War was the last antiquated war. No new techniques were developed in time to cope with the devastating wounds caused by the increased firepower. And because it was fought just before antiseptic and aseptic measures became known, hundreds of thousands of lives were lost quite needlessly. Of more than three million men who fought, nearly six hundred thousand died from wounds or disease—more than the total number of American soldiers who have died in all other wars the United States has ever fought.[27]

The bayonet and the cannon on its caisson are the enduring images of the Civil War—standing to this day as icons on memorial battlefields. Yet neither was responsible for inflicting more than a fraction (altogether less than 6 percent) of injuries.[28] The real scourge was a conoidal, inch-long lead bullet invented by a French army officer, Claude-Étienne Minié. The minié ball, adopted by the U.S. Army in 1855, revolutionized the infantry by overcoming the old trade-off between firepower and accuracy. The smooth-bore musket was swift to load, but impossible to aim well. The spiral grooves of a rifle barrel gave its spinning bullet stability, and thus accuracy, in flight; but it was cumbersome

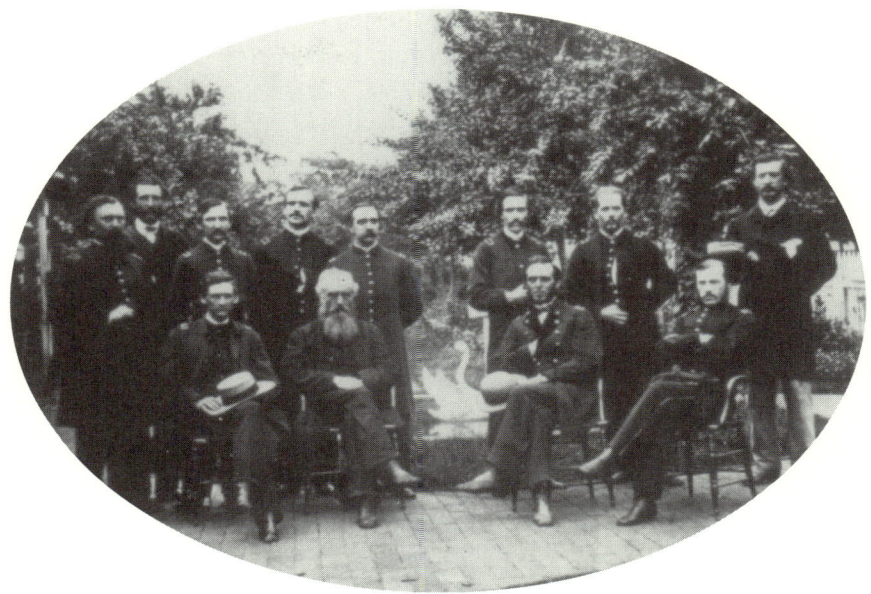

Among this group of surgeons who treated the
Union wounded at Armory Square Hospital,
a military facility erected on the Mall,
Washington, D.C., are Henry E. Woodbury
(a Georgetown University medical graduate,
1863) and D. W. Bliss (a Georgetown
medical professor after the war). Courtesy of
the National Library of Medicine.

to load. The new soft minié bullet, however, made a rifle as easy to load as a
musket ball; and it expanded on firing to fit the barrel's grooves, improving
both range and accuracy. A minié ball could fell a man half a mile away. But
its softness also caused horrifying wounds. On impact it flattened,
pulverising all bones in its path before lodging finally in the tissues.[29]

Such injuries would challenge surgeons of any era. But Civil War
surgeons were critically handicapped for a reason they never understood.
Time after time, they performed competent amputations and resections,
neatly extracted bullets or shell fragments, saw patients begin to recover and
then—inexplicably—die. Thousands of detailed reports of these operations
were collected and published in a multi-volume set after the war. As we
read them now, the puzzlement of the surgeons who wrote these reports is
plain. One such was written by Henry Elisha Woodbury, a Georgetown
medical graduate of 1863 who in the spring of 1865 was a volunteer

surgeon at Armory Square military hospital in Washington. He was treating a soldier with damage to the ulnar and median nerves from a shot through the arm. In severe pain, the soldier requested amputation, which was performed on April 10. "The patient seemed to be doing well until April 22 when he had a severe chill," Woodbury recorded. "From this time the symptoms of pyaemia were well marked. Sulphite of soda, iron and quinine were freely given, with stimulants [alcohol or narcotics], but the patient firmly believed he would die, and gradually sank until April 28 when he breathed his last."[30]

Today called septicemia and defined as blood poisoning caused by pus-producing bacteria, pyaemia was commonly given as the cause of death following amputation. It was the most dreaded of postoperative complications: the mortality rate was 97 percent.[31] But surgeons never recognized why it occurred. To them pyaemia described a range of symptoms: abscesses all over the body, sweating, fever, chills, and jaundice. Unaware of the real cause, and believing still that the suppuration of wounds—or "laudable pus" as they called it—was a sign of healthy healing, surgeons cast the blame on vague generalities. Thus "hospital disease," "bad air," "dietary deficiency" or, as Woodbury declared, the propensity of patients simply to give up the ghost, were all considered responsible for the high death rate. Throughout the war, surgeons disputed the relative merits of "flap" and "circular" methods of amputation; debated at length on the optimum time to amputate; argued over "conservative management" (leaving well alone); questioned whether resections were desirable; and studied the ever-mounting mortality figures for clues to the most successful methods[32]—yet never realizing that their constant use of nonsterile instruments, dressings, and treatments made all such intellectual effort irrelevant.

Just as in their antebellum civilian days, surgeons still wore aprons encrusted with the stains of previous operations, and on these they wiped their hands and knives. But now they often worked in conditions even less sanitary: on doors slung across trestles as makeshift operating tables; in barns only imperfectly cleared of animal manure; in camps where open trenches used as latrines by hundreds of men were only a few feet away; and sometimes in places where there was no water at all. The sheer volume of casualties that marked every battle left surgeons no time even for the care they might have employed in peacetime. After the carnage at Spotsylvania in May 1864, a surgeon described in a letter to his wife how he had operated virtually without rest for four days and two nights. "It does not seem as though I could take a knife in my hand today," he wrote, "yet there are a hundred cases of amputations waiting for me. . . . It is a scene of horror such as I never saw." War photographs showed severed arms and legs piled five feet high around the surgeons' tables.[31]

It seems extraordinary that anyone survived surgery in these conditions, yet the fact that thousands did survive obscured the realities of sepsis, merely reinforcing the surgeons' conviction that they were doing well. A few did raise the possibility that improved cleanliness might help, but they were ignored. Later in the war antiseptics—sodium hypochlorite, carbolic acid, and iodine, in the main—were introduced into military hospitals to cleanse the air, floors, and chamberpots to great effect, but only very rarely was their use extended to wounds—usually too late to do any good—and never to surgical instruments.[32]

Of course, there were advances. Before the war, few surgeons were skilled enough to ligate the great arteries; by its end, that procedure was routinely performed by thousands.[33] And of course there were spectacular successes. Edward Shippen, a surgeon with the U.S. Volunteers, performed an amputation at the hip joint in April 1863—one of only five attempted during the Civil War—and received a cheerful letter from the patient the following November: "I can run all over on my crutches . . . and I can go as well as most any other person on them."[34] But almost certainly such triumphs were rarer than apparently miraculous recoveries where no surgery had been attempted at all. One such was recorded in 1863, again by Henry Woodbury, then in attendance at a military hospital housed in a former girls' school in Georgetown. The patient, a twenty-two-year-old lieutenant wounded at Chancellorsville, had been shot in the abdomen just below the umbilicus. Abdominal gunshot wounds were nearly always fatal, so surgeons generally left them untouched.[35] The lieutenant had already endured a gruelling three-day journey to Georgetown and arrived in a weak condition; but two days later the minié ball passed into his intestine and was excreted. The man recovered, returned to his regiment, and was wounded six more times—once suffering yet another minié ball in the abdomen which, like the first, he excreted and survived.[36] Stamina and luck, it seems, were often more successful than surgery.

Only rarely, and then by accident, were any real medical discoveries made. The most remarkable concerned maggots. When badly injured soldiers were left untended on the battlefield, sometimes for three days or more in broiling heat and covered with flies, maggots would multiply in their wounds, wriggling around in a way that disgusted both victims and the medical attendants when they finally reached hospital. Maggots were a visible "infection" that surgeons could see and destroy, which they did most effectively with injections of chloroform. But there came a time when Confederate surgeons at Chattanooga, bereft of medical supplies, had to leave the gangrenous wounds of their patients unbandaged and maggoty. To their astonishment the wounds healed perfectly: the maggots ate away the diseased tissue, leaving the rest clean and healthy. Thereafter, and with great success, many Confederate surgeons encouraged the appetites of maggots, while their Unionist colleagues continued to kill their patients along with the parasites. (In World War I this simple, if distasteful, remedy was revived and maggots were specially bred to treat osteomyelitis. In the 1990s, maggots were brought back again in Europe for the successful treatment of wounds which modern antibiotics had failed to heal.)[37]

Years later, when surgeons at last grasped the reason for their failures, they were appalled. Robert Reyburn, who served as a surgeon in the Union army throughout the war and afterwards became professor of clinical surgery and dean of the medical school, was one of the few Georgetown physicians to leave a personal record of wartime experiences. Writing in 1906, he described the treatment of the wounded in Alexandria in 1862:

> Cold water dressing was the universal way of treating gunshot wounds in those days. In the hospitals could be seen long rows of iron bedsteads occupied by the wounded soldiers, and above, suspended from the ceiling, were perforated tin vessels containing water which was allowed to gradually trickle on the wounded limbs. . . . It was not known that by use of nonsterilized fluids, fresh sources of infection were being added to the already infected wound. Had it been known in those days what now is known of methods of preventing infection, the writer verily believes that 100,000 lives could have been saved . . . The results of the treatment of gunshot wounds . . . were simply dreadful and make one shudder to recall it.[38]

Located in the heart of Washington, Georgetown medical school became part of the war machine, not only in the sense of turning out army surgeons but also in helping to provide care to the tens of thousands of sick and wounded in the city's many military hospitals. Having endured a decade with minimal clinical facilities, the school found itself by July 1862 within four blocks of ten temporary hospitals crammed into several local churches, Odd Fellowes Hall, and the Patent Office, and not far from dozens more.39 Washington had become the principal emergency ward of the North.

In April 1861, utterly unprepared for war, the city still had only one general hospital, the Washington Infirmary. Immediately, the government took it over for military use. Thus, ironically, Columbian medical school abruptly lost both the clinical facilities that Georgetown had long coveted and even the roof over its head. For two years, the Columbian faculty moved from one rented building to another until it was reduced to teaching a handful of students in an abandoned church. The school closed early in 1863.40

The three-hundred-bed infirmary was pitifully inadequate to cope with even the earliest casualties of Bull Run. Three months later, a freak fire burned it to the ground, leaving the city with no proper hospital at all.41 Instead, the sick and wounded were cared for in private homes and churches, colleges and schools, theaters, government buildings of all kinds, and vast camps of tents that filled the city's vacant lots and sprawled over Capitol Hill. The government was not slow to seize houses vacated by Southern sympathizers. The banker William Corcoran, for example, had prudently moved to Europe for the duration; Harewood, his country estate just north of the city, was converted into one of the Union's largest military hospitals.42

At the end of 1862, some of the more ramshackle arrangements began to be replaced by purpose-built military hospitals erected by the government. The wooden huts were barrack-like, but they were arranged around spacious compounds in the new pavilion style that allowed free circulation of air and, to an extent, the segregation of different medical conditions.43 They were sorely needed, for it had quickly become apparent that twice as many troops were dying from disease as from wounds. Men who had lived healthy lives on farms, and were confidently expected to make the strongest soldiers, quickly succumbed to the everyday infections of life in close confines with others. Men who had never cooked their own food or washed their own clothes now fell victim to poor diet and personal squalor. Army camps were

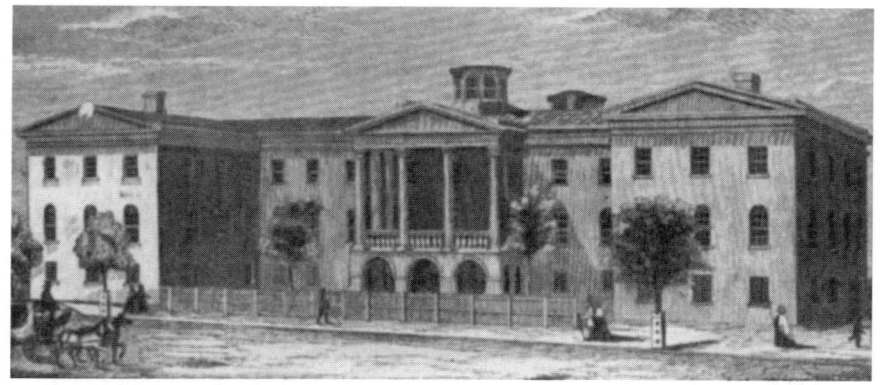

*The Washington Infirmary as it looked before the Civil War.
Courtesy of the Library of Congress.*

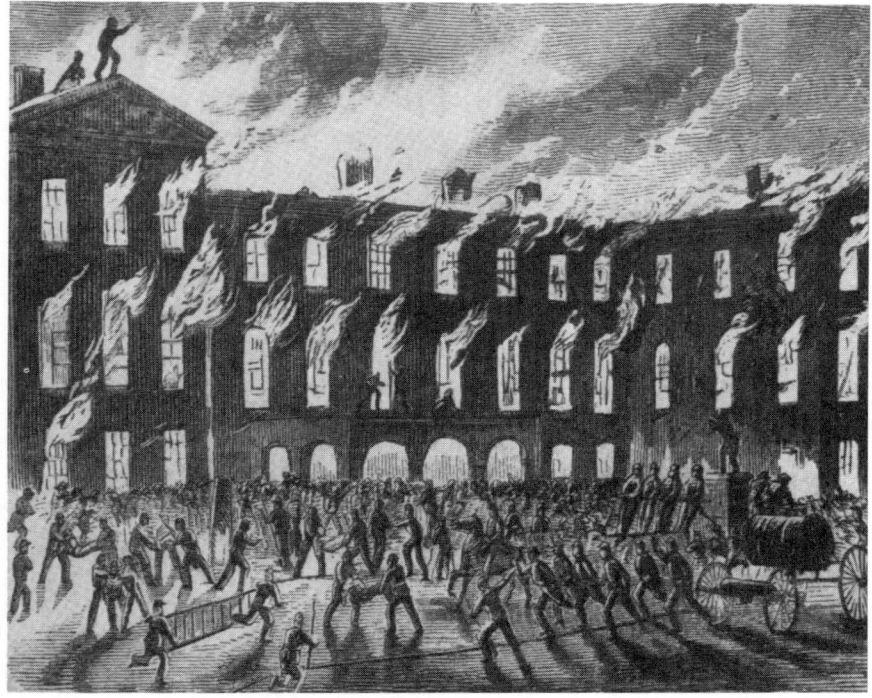

*A freak fire destroyed the Infirmary, Washington's only
hospital, on the night of November 3, 1861. Reproduced from
Harper's Weekly, November 23, 1861. Courtesy of the
Library of Congress.*

breeding grounds for viruses and bacteria; the hospitals filled with cases of typhus, dysentery, malaria, measles, mumps, and nearly-universal diarrhea. Union surgeons dealt with more than four hundred thousand wounds in the Civil War; but they treated some six million cases of disease.[44]

No one who lived in Washington could ignore what Walt Whitman immortalized as "the great army of the wounded." Daily, they poured into the city by railroad car and river steamer after long and agonizing journeys from the front lines, weakened by exposure and hunger as well as by injury and sickness. Washington newspapers regularly published lists of patients in each hospital; but the confusion was so great that people arriving from far away to find wounded relatives might search for days in vain. At the peak, the District of Columbia had fifty hospitals housing fifty thousand men.[45]

So the Georgetown medical students of this era, unlike their predecessors, were both surrounded by opportunities for clinical experience and had it thrust upon them. Every hand, skilled or not, was needed. Students who in peacetime would have worked as clerks while pursuing their studies now served as stewards in the hospitals. The job was less menial than might be supposed: stewards dispensed drugs, applied bandages and changed dressings, performed "minor" surgical tasks such as extracting teeth, and supervised cooking services.[46] No system of examination tested the competence of stewards before 1864.[47] Under pressure of war, some men were even promoted to more exacting duties while still students. Daniel Roberts Brower, in later life a leading neurologist and psychiatrist in Chicago, passed his army medical board examination and was appointed an acting assistant surgeon two months before receiving his Georgetown degree in March 1864.[48] And as early as December 1862, Alonzo Boothby was the first of several students to request early examination by the faculty "to enable him to embrace an advantageous offer at one of the Government hospitals of Washington."[49]

Georgetown's professors were familiar faces in the military hospitals. Of the eight who were faculty members at the beginning of the war, all but two served the Union army as surgeons. (The exceptions were Noble Young, who at age fifty-three was still president of the faculty and professor of medicine, and Montgomery Johns, who had joined the school as professor of anatomy in 1861.) Four served as acting assistant surgeons on contract to the army, working part-time or for limited periods in the hospitals: John Snyder, professor of obstetrics; Silas Loomis, a Georgetown graduate of 1857 who had become adjunct professor of chemistry and physics; Richard Croggan, an 1860 graduate who was demonstrator of anatomy; and Johnson Eliot, who had succeeded Liebermann as professor of surgery.

The mild-mannered Eliot, the only one of the school's founders to serve in the Civil War, worked in the hospitals and at the front. After the Union army had again suffered a costly defeat at the second battle of Bull Run (Manassas) in August 1862, he was one of hundreds of physicians who answered the urgent call for medical volunteers. More than twenty thousand troops had been killed or wounded; but amid scenes of utter confusion, it was discovered that many surgeons, medical supplies, and ambulances had been abandoned on the Peninsula, southeast of Richmond, where Robert E. Lee's forces had driven back McClellan's. In Washington, the volunteers hastily packed bags of instruments and left by every possible conveyance, from jammed railroad cars to hire-cabs commandeered at saber point from indignant drivers and paying passengers.[50] By the time the medics reached the battlefields, some of the wounded had been lying for three days where they had fallen; thousands had bled to death. Clara Barton, the future founder of the American Red Cross, was there as a nurse: "The men were brought down from the field . . . till they covered acres," she wrote.[51] In this landscape of slaughter, Eliot set up his operating room in an abandoned house at Chantilly and worked nonstop through that night and the next day, tending both Confederate and Union wounded. The battle rolled on around him. Not far away, Stonewall Jackson's troops fought those of John Pope in a violent thunderstorm. Eliot did not stop work even when told that Confederate cavalry had surrounded his makeshift hospital. He was taken prisoner, but soon released on Jackson's personal order.[52] Then the forty-seven-year-old professor of surgery walked the twenty miles from Chantilly back to the comparative sanity of Washington.[53]

The fifth faculty member serving in the Union army was James Ethelbert Morgan, who had taught at Georgetown since 1852 and was now professor of materia medica. At the outbreak of war, he organized the 4th Regiment of D.C. Volunteers and served as its first colonel; but he soon stepped down to become its surgeon, and in 1862 he was appointed surgeon to the Quartermaster's Hospital in Washington. He was also, for the duration, surgeon-in-charge of the Soldiers' Rest, where troops laid over on their way to the front or convalesced on the way back.[54]

The Georgetown professor who rose highest in the wartime military medical service was Thomas Antisell, who had joined the faculty in 1858 and now held the multiple chair of medical chemistry, toxicology, and physiology. Antisell was one of the all-time stars of the medical school—a man who, though primarily a surgeon, achieved distinction in so many fields that his story is worth telling.

Like Liebermann before him, Antisell was an immigrant who had been a political revolutionary in his own country. He was an Irishman of Huguenot ancestry, born in Dublin in 1817, the son of a distinguished barrister.[55] Following in the footsteps of his maternal grandfather, a noted Irish surgeon, Antisell graduated in turn from the Dublin School of Medicine, the Irish Apothecaries' Hall, and the Royal College of Surgeons in London. In 1844, he toured Europe to study with several great medical teachers; one, Jean Dumas, was the celebrated chemist whose lectures at the Sorbonne in Paris were at the same time inspiring the young Louis Pasteur.[56] Returning to Dublin in 1845, Antisell practiced medicine there for the next three years, published books on agricultural chemistry and the geology of Ireland, and became involved in patriotic politics.

The 1840s were the worst years in Ireland's history: the decade of potato famines that caused both massive migration to the United States and a new wave of rebellion against repressive British rule. Antisell joined the Young Ireland Party, a nationalist organization of men who, like himself, were members of Dublin's Anglo-Irish elite. As such, they posed more of a threat to the government than starving peasants ever did. So the British arrested Antisell and sentenced him to imprisonment and exile. In the fall of 1848, he left Ireland forever, working his passage as a surgeon on a ship bound for New York.

There, over the next five years, Antisell built a new medical practice, ran his own chemistry laboratory, and was a visiting lecturer at medical schools in Massachusetts and Vermont. Then, in 1854, he embarked on one of the great adventures of his life, as the geologist attached to the Pacific Railroad Survey on the 32nd Parallel. This expedition, led by army topographical engineer Lieutenant John G. Parke, was one of several commissioned by Congress to find the best route for a transcontinental railway. At the same time these surveys provided unprecedented opportunities for scientists to explore the central and western parts of the largely unexplored continent. Antisell, as geologist to the most southerly proposed

route, identified many rock forma-
tions in California and the Arizona
Territory along the way, and was the
first to find deposits of bitumen (oil)
in southern California. (Fifty years
later those rich oil fields were yielding
81 million barrels a year.) That significant study was the last of Antisell's
exploits in practical geology in the
United States, although in the 1870s,
by then a chemist of international
repute and an expert on the manufacture of bituminous oils, he spent six
years advising on the development of
resources in the northern islands of
Japan at the invitation of the emperor,
who in gratitude later awarded him
the Order of the Rising Sun of Meiji.
The former Irish revolutionary was
thus decreed an honorary Japanese
nobleman, with the right to carry two
swords.

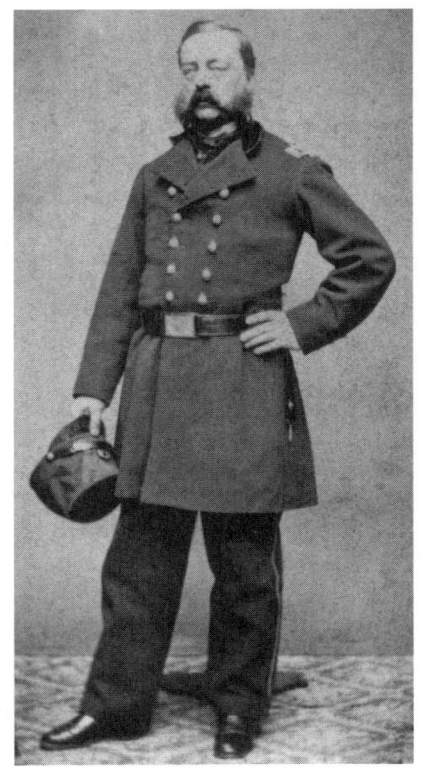

*Thomas Antisell, M.D., 1817–93, in his
Civil War uniform. Courtesy of the
National Library of Medicine.*

Antisell arrived in Washington
in 1856 to take up a government post
as chief examiner in charge of the
chemistry department of the U.S.
Patent Office. Two years later, he also accepted the chair of chemistry and
physiology at Georgetown medical school.[57] By now he had married for the
second time and was raising the first five of his eight children.[58] Antisell
chose to live not in Washington but across the Potomac on the Virginia
shore, where he bought an estate close by the southern end of the Long
Bridge. It meant a daily ride on horseback to his job at the Patent Office and,
during the winter months of teaching evening classes at the medical school,
a journey home after dark, but Antisell obviously thought it worthwhile.
Surrounded by woodland and orchards, the house commanded a fine view
of the Capitol directly across the river. It was a lovely spot, but, as events

turned out, an unfortunate choice. Immediately after Virginia seceded from the Union in April 1861, President Lincoln ordered the army to secure the land on that side of the Potomac, as part of the defenses of Washington. Troops under Colonel (later General) Samuel Heintzleman crossed the Long Bridge and commandeered Antisell's house and land. Antisell was obliged to move out and find a new home in Washington, while the soldiers cut down his trees to build Fort Albany.[59]

All of Antisell's energy, experience, and extraordinary stamina were put to the test during the Civil War. He quickly returned to surgery. Although now almost forty-five years old, the upper age limit for army service, he was appointed surgeon with the rank of major in the U.S. Volunteers on October 2, 1861, and served continuously in ever more demanding roles until mustered out as a lieutenant-colonel, brevetted for "faithful and meritorious service," on October 7, 1865.

"Noted for his reckless disregard of personal dangers," as a colleague reported,[60] Antisell throughout those four years tended wounded soldiers in the field as a brigade surgeon in General Banks' division of the Army of the Potomac; supervised the entire range of medical services in the field as medical director of the Department of the Shenandoah and later of the 12th Army Corps; served at Second Manassas, Antietam, and other battles; ran Washington's largest military medical facility as surgeon-in-charge of the three thousand-bed Harewood Hospital; served as president of the Army Medical Board, which examined the competence of doctors entering the service; and finally was attending surgeon to sick and wounded volunteer officers in Washington. The only time he took leave was after hostilities ceased, while waiting to be mustered out.[61]

Antisell's meteoric wartime career almost exactly reflected the rapid development of the Union army's medical service from a small and anti-quated unit to a huge logistical operation that by 1865 had become the model for armies worldwide. Civil War surgery may not have been cause for much pride; but the development of ambulance teams and the organization of field hospitals were innovations that gave the wounded more chance of survival than in any previous wars.

These new measures were the work of two particularly brilliant young men: William Alexander Hammond, appointed surgeon general of the Army Medical Corps in April 1862 at the age of thirty-three; and thirty-eight-year-old Jonathan Letterman, who became medical director of the Army of the Potomac two months later. To the fury of regular officers of vastly greater seniority, both were elevated to these positions from the lowest commissioned medical rank of assistant surgeon. Thereafter they consistently cut through red tape and introduced reforms that, over time, had profound consequences. Some took effect at once: accurate "care cards" were now attached to the wounded sent to the rear, for example; and the examinations for men applying to be army surgeons were made more stringent. Arguably, as we shall see, their most significant innovations were two which, at the time, overworked field surgeons must have cursed. The surgeons were now ordered to compile detailed reports of every procedure they performed; and also to preserve and send to Washington interesting surgical specimens that would eventually go on display in a projected medical museum.[62]

The only innovation suggested by Hammond that was not implemented—not, that is, until the end of the century—was to set up an army graduate medical school to train doctors in the techniques of military medicine. But this idea of special instruction to convert both medical students and qualified physicians into effective military surgeons—an urgent wartime need—was seized upon and promoted by Thomas Antisell.

On February 2, 1863, the Georgetown medical faculty minutes recorded: "Dr. Antisell proposed the establishing of a new chair in accordance with the suggestion of the Surgeon General USA, to be styled Chair of Military Surgery, Physiology and Hygiene." It was the first such chair in the nation and, naturally, Antisell was appointed its professor.[63] By this time he had served more than twelve months in the field and was just beginning his eight months as surgeon in charge of Harewood Hospital. When the course on military surgery began the next October, Antisell left Harewood for a less demanding role as examiner, and later president, of the Army Medical Board. Throughout the war he was able to juggle his military and teaching duties so well that, except for the winter of 1861–62, he was always in Washington from October to March, the length of the annual course.[64]

No record of Antisell's lectures on military surgery has survived; it is unlikely that he ever wrote them down. "He was an able man and excellent lecturer, very practical and seldom used notes," one of his students recalled.[65] But a similar course was taught at Bellevue Medical College in New York by Frank Hastings Hamilton, a celebrated professor of surgery who had entered the war as a brigade surgeon at the same time as Antisell. Hamilton described in an 1865 textbook the very different demands of military surgery and the difficulties in teaching it to men unaccustomed to wartime imperatives.

With the advent of anesthesia, he wrote, surgeons had become used to taking their time on refinements during operations; but in dealing with vast numbers of wounded men "maximum speed" was once again of the essence: "It will not do to let one man die of haemorrhage from the femoral artery because you wish to apply a ligature very methodically to the ulnar artery of another; nor to amputate a limb by circular incision when by oval incision it can be done in half the time." Students had now to be taught that they would not be operating in ideal conditions; that ingenuity and improvisation must make up for want of resources—fashioning splints from fence posts, styptic from green persimmon juice, tenaculums from bent knitting needles, bandages from torn tent cloths. The challenge, Hamilton said, was to convey all this in such a way that students, especially the inattentive, would not confuse the desperate expedient with "the general law." If his students saw military surgeons as battlefield heroes who wielded scalpels rather than swords, Hamilton's lectures must have quickly disillusioned them. Actual surgery, he stressed, was the smallest part of a surgeon's duties: "The fact is that neither tactics nor strategy will serve an army of invalids." The surgeon's main concern was to keep the troops fit for combat: supervising their diet, dress, and personal hygiene, organizing sanitation in camp and trying to ensure that camps were set up in healthy surroundings.[66]

This, in the conditions of the Civil War, was a recipe for frustration. Soldiers routinely ignored requests to use the "sinks" (latrines), instead of relieving themselves anywhere they pleased, just as their commanders resisted recommendations not to bivouac in swamps or sites without water.[67] (Medical officers had little real authority within a regiment; before 1865 they were allowed no rank higher than major.[68]) In his own lectures, too, Antisell undoubtedly laid great emphasis on military hygiene. Years earlier he had published a book on ways to improve city sanitation in Dublin[69]; his reports as medical director of the army in the Shenandoah in the summer of 1862 were peppered with tart observations on noisome conditions. Called to one corps encampment where soldiers were falling sick in unusual numbers, he found "the regiments lay so close alongside that the sinks of one regiment were not farther than thirty feet from the company tents of another. . . . The offal, and other remains of the cattle slaughtered by regiments, lay unburied and decomposing on the grass in the rear of each, and thus two fertile sources of disease were apparent."[70]

Whether a soldier was "fit for duty" was not always easy to decide, of course, as Hamilton pointed out. It was not simply a matter of distinguishing between, say, a cold and a fever. "Feigned diseases need to be studied," he wrote, to teach a surgeon the "ingenious dissimulations practiced by soldiers to relieve themselves from duty, or to obtain a discharge or a pension."[71] Some were ingenious indeed. One surgeon in an Ohio infantry regiment described his bafflement at the number of men who reported at morning sick call complaining of headaches and displaying heavily-coated tongues. Finally someone revealed the trick: "The camp was surrounded by rose-bushes in bloom, and a liberal chewing of rose-leaves a little before sick call produced the effect I saw on the tongue."[72] Men who had truly had enough of war often went much further. Self-mutilations—in particular shot-off trigger fingers—were common.[73]

With their practical experience in the field, men like Antisell and Hamilton were ideally suited to teach courses on military surgery, but there were many aspects of wartime medicine that were difficult to convey theoretically. Hamilton listed, in addition to the topics above, the special diseases and injuries of war, construction of field hospitals, transportation of the sick and wounded from the field of battle—and lastly, he added with bleak humor, "a thorough knowledge of geography, climatology, meteorology, geology and botany, with many other kindred subjects belonging to the natural sciences."[74]

It is doubtful whether these courses, which began when the war was more than half over, benefited more than a relative handful of graduates. But anything to improve competence in the field helped. As the war raged on, newspapers regularly published stories of surgeons too drunk to tie a ligature, of newly graduated doctors overly eager to amputate "for the experience," of men hastily promoted to "surgeon" who had never held a scalpel. At the beginning of the war, the Army Medical Board did conduct examinations that were reasonably rigorous, and it did fail a fair percentage of applicants. But the board had no control over volunteer regiments raised by the states. The surgeons in these were appointed by state governors or commanding officers; some states insisted on strict examinations, others held none. As the war continued and physicians became harder to recruit—they were not subject to the draft and were finding their civilian practices more lucrative now that so many competitors were in the army—recruitment and promotion grew more lax.[75] Georgetown had direct evidence of this when William F. Tibbals, a nephew of Flodoardo Howard, applied to enter the medical school in January of 1865. Before the war, Tibbals wrote, he had worked in a country drug store, and subsequently served the 5th Ohio Volunteer Infantry as a hospital steward until May 1862. Then, he noted, "I was promoted to assistant surgeon without solicitation and unbeknownst to myself until the Colonel handed me my commission. I served in this capacity until October last."[76]

In so large a force of medical volunteers, there were bound to be many whose formal training was less than ideal, and some who were incompetent or even charlatans. Yet the overall impression gained from thousands of day-to-day reports filed by the surgeons at the time is of sound professional skill and devotion to duty. Many had given up comfortable careers for a life of hardship and a wage of $165 or less per month, out of which they paid for their own food, accoutrements, and horse.[77] And those who served in field positions risked more than a rough billet and long hours.

In theory, surgeons were neutral. They wore green sashes to denote their noncombatant status, and all field hospitals and ambulances flew yellow flags edged in green.[78] These gave little protection. "It is not an uncommon belief that medical officers are seldom exposed to the fire of the enemy," wrote Jonathan Letterman, medical director of the Army of the Potomac. "My observation and experience since I have been connected to this army, especially, has shown me that they are almost as much exposed as officers of the line."[79] When Surgeon General Hammond and his successor

Joseph K. Barnes demanded higher pay and rank for the medical corps, their most pressing argument was that army surgeons were more vulnerable to danger than any other category of noncombatant staff officers.[80]

Statistics prove that point. By the end of the war, 42 surgeons in the Union army had been killed or died of wounds received in action; 290 died from disease or accident incurred in the line of duty; and four died in Confederate prisons—336 medical men lost in all. A further 73 were wounded in action, and countless more suffered severe sickness and disabilities.[81]

Of the tens of thousands of books written on the Civil War, very few focus on the vital role of medical officers and most give it no mention. Thus, many of the deeds of courage of these men as they went about their rescue work under remorseless fire are now lost to history. It is, however, a matter of record that the first Union medical officer to be killed in the Civil War was a Georgetown man.[82] Samuel W. Everett was one of the earliest faculty members: he had been hired for the school in October 1850, seven months before it actually opened, and served first as demonstrator and later as adjunct professor of anatomy. Born in London in 1820, he was a highly educated man and a talented artist who had traveled extensively in Europe; some of his delightful ink drawings of London and Paris are preserved in the Georgetown University Archives. Everett joined the Union army at the outbreak as surgeon to the 10th Illinois Volunteers. In late 1861, he was promoted to medical director, Department of Missouri; later he was posted to Tennessee.

Everett was one of those surgeons who did not hesitate in crises to charge into action. That is how he died at Shiloh, the first great slaughter of the war, where both armies lost a total of more than three thousand dead and sixteen thousand wounded. The American Medical Association recorded:

> On the battlefield of Shiloh, April 6, 1862, at about 8:00 A.M., he fell, pierced by two bullets, one through the forehead and the other through the body; the wounds were instantly fatal. He had been actively engaged in his surgical duties from the commencement of the action, when General [Benjamin] Prentiss saw him stop men who were retreating and induce them to return to the front. A short time afterward he was seen to rally fifty men and lead them personally into the fight, during one of the

most critical periods of the engagement. It was at this time, when in near proximity to the enemy, and between the opposing lines, that he was shot dead from his horse.[83]

So far as is known, Georgetown medical school lost only two others in the war (whereas Georgetown College lost at least 114 of its alumni[84]). Both had been classmates of Reuben Cleary, graduating with him in 1859. The first, George W. Hill of Ohio, serving in the Union army as a captain in the 12th Kentucky Infantry, was killed in action in the siege of Atlanta, Georgia, on August 6, 1864.[85] The other, Dent Burroughs of Maryland, who served in a Confederate artillery battalion and fought in General Hood's division at Gettysburg, was killed in the defense of Richmond on February 12, 1865.[86]

Many more Georgetown men, of course, saw action in battle after battle—far too many to mention here. At Gettysburg, the deadliest battle of the war, which in the first three days of July 1863 cost more than fifty thousand casualties and changed the fortunes of the Union, at least eleven Georgetown medical school men were there as soldiers or surgeons. Seven were Confederates; four were Unionists.[87] Reuben Cleary was with the 7th Virginia, which took part in Pickett's famous charge at Cemetery Ridge and was one of the units most devastated by the Unionists' withering fire. His regiment suffered ninety-four casualties and saw its commander, Colonel Waller T. Patton (great-uncle of the World War II general), killed by a shot through the jaw.[88] Francis Ashford, future professor of surgery, was with the 17th Virginia and also fought in Pickett's brigade.[89] Arthur Barry, by this time a seasoned surgeon with the 9th Virginia, was one of those who coped with the carnage on the Confederate side; Ralph Walsh, George Sylvester, and Abraham B. Shekell, who had all graduated from Georgetown only four months earlier, were acting assistant surgeons doing the best they could for the equally terrible casualties on the Union side.[90]

Medical director Jonathan Letterman, in his report on Gettysburg, said that 650 Union medical officers were on duty in the battle, giving immediate treatment to more than twenty thousand wounded soldiers, of whom over six thousand were captured Confederates. "The labor performed by these officers was immense," he wrote. "Some of them fainted from exhaustion induced by over exertion, and others became ill from the same cause. [Their] skill and devotion . . . could not be surpassed." Thirteen, he added, were wounded and one died from wounds.[91] All eleven Georgetown men known to have been at Gettysburg survived—although one of those in gray, Wilfred McLeod, was captured during Lee's retreat and confined at Fort Delaware; he escaped and by September was back in action with his Maryland cavalry regiment.[92]

For sheer courage, one other Georgetown man deserves special mention. John Harry Thompson, who became clinical professor of surgery after the war, was one of only nine Civil War surgeons to be awarded the Congressional Medal of Honor.[93] On March 14, 1862, as brigade surgeon to the 43rd New York Volunteers, he was at the battle of New Berne, where Unionist troops under Major General Ambrose Burnside captured a foothold on the coast of North Carolina. Thick fog that morning obscured the location and strength of the Confederate defenses; and Thompson, having no wounded to tend yet, volunteered to go out alone and reconnoiter. "When he had got some distance the dense mist suddenly lifted and revealed him standing alone and unprotected in plain view and easy range of long lines of the enemy formed in order of battle as if awaiting an attack," one account reported. "They opened fire on him and he ran for cover. He was not harmed before reaching the woods, and when he got behind a tree made a sketch of the enemy's position and returned to camp."[94] As the battle raged, Thompson continued to relay orders from his commanding officer, Major General John Gray Foster, to deployed units "under the hottest fire."[95] Then he resumed his surgical duties on the battlefield.[96]

Thompson was a highly experienced surgeon. Born in England in 1824, he had degrees from the Royal College of Surgeons in London and the College of Physicians and Surgeons in New York. He had already, in the service of the East India Company in the 1850s, seen action during the Sepoy Rebellion in India.[97] He certainly appears to have had confidence in his own abilities. Within a month of New Berne, General Burnside had him dismissed from the army for "alarmism," apparently because Thompson had roused the troops from their sleep in the face of some perceived danger that turned out to be groundless. Burnside later "cheerfully" recommended Thompson's reinstatement—with the dry proviso that "he will not permit himself to interfere with military matters not pertaining to his profession."[98]

Thompson subsequently became brigade surgeon to the 139th New York Volunteers until poor health forced his resignation in December, 1863. For the rest of the war, he worked as a contract surgeon in the military hospital at Judiciary Square in Washington.[99]

It was while he was serving as Georgetown's clinical professor of surgery after the war that Thompson was awarded his Medal of Honor in November 1870.[100] Two years later, among the incoming students of the class of 1873 who attended his operative demonstrations was Charles Rand, Georgetown medical school's other Medal of Honor recipient. Out of more than 2.1 million troops and medics on the Union side in the Civil War, Medals of Honor were awarded to 1,519 men and one woman (also a surgeon).[101] Given the relatively small number of Georgetown medical alumni and faculty who served, it is the more remarkable that two were awarded the highest honor their country could bestow.

⟶☉

By March 1865, the Confederacy was running out of men, supplies, and hope. Desperate to save Richmond, Robert E. Lee's Army of Northern Virginia had been entrenched at Petersburg through the winter, but its defensive lines were increasingly stretched, and on April 1 they broke under relentless bombardment by the Union forces. As Jefferson Davis and the Confederate government evacuated Richmond, Lee retreated westward, pursued by Sheridan and Grant.

Five days later a portion of Lee's straggling forces was cut off at Sayler's Creek; surrounded and outnumbered, nearly eight thousand men surrendered to Sheridan.[102] Francis Ashford was one of them.[103] The remnants of Reuben Cleary's regiment, which had already lost half its men in the final battle at Petersburg, surrendered too. But Cleary was not among them. A month earlier he had been detached for "temporary" duty with a corps of artillery; so with the rest of Lee's exhausted army, Cleary marched onward to Appomattox.[104]

There on Palm Sunday, April 9, Lee surrendered to Grant. Arthur Barry, who had served without break as a hospital and field surgeon almost since his graduation in 1861, was among those who surrendered.[105] So was Carl Kleinschmidt, a Prussian who had graduated from Georgetown in

1862 and had immediately chosen to go South, serving as an assistant surgeon with the 3rd Arkansas Infantry in most of the battles of northern Virginia, at Gettysburg, and the Wilderness. Unlike Barry, who was imprisoned at Fortress Monroe for several weeks, Kleinschmidt received his parole the next day. He then walked two hundred miles back to his home in Georgetown—beginning a journey that led eventually to a professorship at the medical school and the presidency of the Medical Society of D.C.[106] Reuben Cleary, however, did not surrender at Appomattox, though how he managed to escape is not known. There were many Confederates who, stunned by defeat, vowed never to surrender; perhaps Cleary was one of them. In any event, he was finally captured at Fairfax Court House two weeks later on April 22, four years to the day after he had enlisted in the Confederate Army.[107]

The surrender of Lee was not quite the end, of course. Nevertheless, Washington went wild: victory guns boomed over the city, gaslight and candles shone in every window, fireworks rained brilliant sparks on streets full of bunting and flags. Throngs of cheering people hung around the White House, and the returning hero General Ulysses S. Grant, thinking to report to the War Department on foot, was mobbed by well-wishers and had to be rescued by police.[108] It all came to an abrupt halt on Good Friday, April 14. President Lincoln reluctantly agreed to venture out into the chill, foggy evening to attend a performance of an English farce, *Our American Cousin*, at Ford's Theater on Tenth Street. He took his seat in a box near the stage.

Once again, a Georgetown man was there. This time it was a medical student, Samuel Read Ward, who had come to the performance because the man of the moment, General Grant, was expected to attend. Disappointingly, Grant did not appear. Instead, at 10:15 P.M., Ward was eye-witness to one of the most dramatic scenes in history: he heard a shot and then saw a man who looked like an actor, "a bright shiny dagger in his hand," leap from the presidential box to the stage and cry "*Sic semper tyrannis!*" as though declaiming a line from a great tragedy. Then came Mrs. Lincoln's scream—"*He has killed the president!*"—and the hushed theater erupted in pandemonium.[109]

Lincoln was still alive, but barely. Not wanting him to die in a "godless theater" on Good Friday, attendants carried him to a house across the street

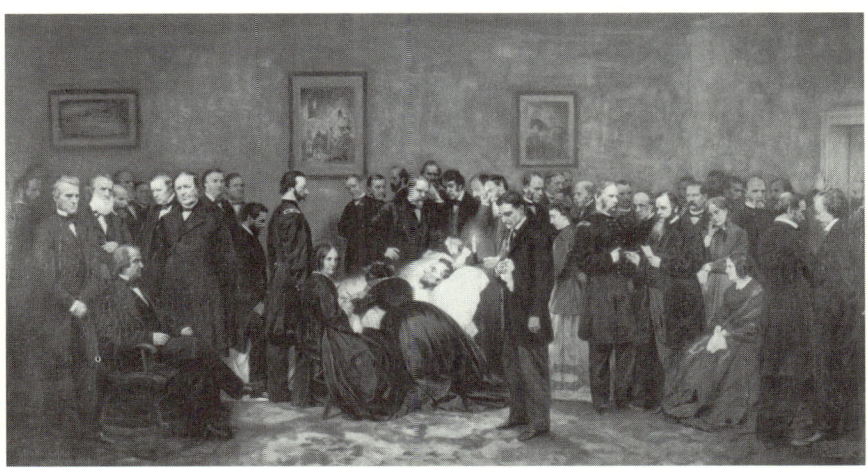

Alonzo Chappell's 1866 painting of the people who attended the death of Abraham Lincoln is a romantic composite; the room where Lincoln actually died was tiny. Charles Liebermann is placed seventh from the left on the back row. Courtesy of Brown University.

and leading physicians were urgently summoned. The ball from John Wilkes Booth's pistol had entered the rear of the president's skull on the left side, passed diagonally across the brain and lodged immediately behind the right eye, so that the eyeball protruded.[110] That was why one of the doctors called was Charles Liebermann, then president of the Medical Society of D.C., and still the city's foremost ophthalmic surgeon. Liebermann cut a little of Lincoln's hair from around the entry wound, the better to examine it.[111] But he could do nothing; no one could. Abraham Lincoln died at 7:22 the next morning.

The night of the assassination passed in alarm and anguish for the citizens of Washington. Robert Reyburn was summoned around 11:00 P.M. by his commander, the one-armed General Martin D. Hardin, who was in charge of the defenses of Washington. Reyburn wrote:

> Dreary was the time we passed at headquarters that night. The spirit of murder seemed to be in the very air and the wildest rumors were prevalent. At one time we heard that Vice President Johnson, Secretary Stanton and General Grant had been murdered. Then rumors came that

other members of the Cabinet had been attacked, followed by the news, which we speedily authenticated, of the wounding of Secretary Seward and members of his household. Men looked at each other in dismay, wondering what dreadful news we would next hear. The troops in the city of Washington were all under arms that night, no one knowing what military exigency might arise requiring their services.

Lincoln's body was moved the next day from the house on Tenth Street to the north room on the second story of the White House. General Hardin, Robert Reyburn, and two other staff officers mounted guard there, for a twenty-four-hour detail beginning at 6:00 P.M. on Sunday, April 16. The four men conducted members of the cabinet, the Senate, and their wives, to view the dead president. "It was a most affecting and painful scene," Reyburn recorded. "During the evening of our watch, and the whole of the day following, there was a continuous stream of mourning visitors to the room. These included almost all the eminent statesmen and politicians of that famous era in the history of our republic."

On guard at the open coffin, Reyburn could study what he called the "massive grandeur" of Lincoln's head; and he was seized with an urge to possess a lock of the president's hair. In the fashion of the time, many had been cut that day for Lincoln's family, but Hardin had flatly refused Reyburn the same privilege. When everyone had gone for the night, however, the general turned to him: "Doctor, I can't give you any of the president's hair," he said, "but I see a lock of it has dropped upon the floor and if you capture it I shall make no objection." Reyburn, writing years later in the classical third-person style he favored, recalled his delight: "You may be sure that the writer seized upon the precious relic at once. And if he committed larceny on that occasion, it is one sin that has never burdened his conscience."[112]

Washington thirsted to avenge the murder of a president whom many, like Walt Whitman, called "father." Booth was hunted down and shot dead on April 26, and his nine accomplices were arrested and brought to trial. Just as after the assassination of another president nearly one hundred years later, conspiracy theories abounded; this time it was the "Catholic connection." To Georgetown College's vast embarrassment, three alumni were convicted of involvement in the murder of Lincoln and the attempt on

Seward. David Herold was hanged; Samuel Arnold and Dr. Samuel Mudd were sentenced to hard labor for life at Dry Tortugas, a grim military prison on a waterless island off Key West, Florida.[113] Mudd, who had set the leg that Booth broke in his leap from the presidential box, was not a graduate of the medical school, but in prison at Dry Tortugas he met someone who was: Joseph Sim Smith (class of 1857), the garrison's physician. Two years later, in August 1867, Smith died in a yellow fever epidemic, together with the garrison commander and forty officers and inmates. Though still a prisoner, Mudd took over as physician and, in effect, as post commander too. For this act he was released by order of President Andrew Johnson on February 8, 1869. Mudd's grandson Richard D. Mudd, a doctor who graduated from Georgetown in 1926, spent his life trying to prove that in treating Booth's fractured leg, his grandfather had done no more than his professional duty, and to clear the family name—long perpetuated in the derogatory phrase: "his name is mud"—from its notorious involvement in the assassination of Lincoln.[114]

The war was over and, as the era of reconstruction began, people tried to put their lives back in order. Many bore the scars of that devastating conflict, physical and emotional, for the rest of their lives.

Charles Rand's remaining years were dominated by a terrible wound he had received at the battle of Gaine's Mill on June 27, 1862, a year after his stand at Blackburn's Ford. Lieutenant John B. Foote, who was present at both battles and was the officer whose testimony finally won Rand his Medal of Honor, described what happened:

> By my side at Gaine's Mill he fell, a musket ball crushing through his body, mashing his right shoulder to jelly. I saw him rise to his feet, the lifeblood spurting into his eyes and ears. I saw him seize a clod of earth and cram it into his wound, trying to staunch the flow. . . . He was later taken to Savage Station, where his right shoulder joint and six inches of the shaft of the arm were removed. Portions of shattered shoulder bone and fragments of his clothing were taken out through his back, the bullet having passed through his lung.

While Rand was on the operating table, the field hospital was captured by Confederates; that night he lay in a hospital tent alongside a Confederate major, also severely wounded. They quickly struck up a friendship. The next day, the battle of Savage Station was fought around them. Too weak to walk, the pair dragged themselves out of their tent and, propped up against a hardtack box, they watched the bombardment and cavalry charges as spectators together, each cheering on his own side. It was the Unionists, under McClellan, who won; but the excitement nearly killed Rand. As he tried to crawl back into the tent, he began hemorrhaging. The surgeon, no doubt vexed, had to remove all the silver wires suturing the six-inch wound; with great skill he sewed Rand up again and saved his life.[115]

Despite his disability, Rand stayed in the army after the war, took his medical degree at Georgetown (1873), and established a successful practice, first in his hometown of Batavia, New York, and later in Washington. But the wound never ceased to trouble him and in 1893 "unremitting pain" forced him to abandon his professional work. It was only then that he thought to apply for a Medal of Honor. However, he became so obsessed with exacting his due that even years after getting it he was still arguing with the War Department about the precise wording of the citation. The thick file of papers on his case shows that the authorities regarded Rand as a nuisance and a braggart, and that he himself had no clear memory of just what had happened in those moments of terror at Blackburn's Ford.[116] Yet there is no doubting Rand's bravery later in the war. Perhaps, as often happens, Rand became brave *after* the heroic accident of that stand defined his life as a defier of death, first as a warrior and later as a physician. He died on October 13, 1908, and was buried with full military honors at Arlington Cemetery.[117]

Thomas Antisell also suffered during his final years. After a lifetime of vigorous pursuits that had taken him on adventures around the world, he was paralyzed by a stroke in the fall of 1890 and forced to give up work. His intellectual brilliance had evidently brought him little long-term financial success, because he now began pressing the government for compensation. On September 23, 1890, he filed for an invalidity pension, claiming a "disease of the nervous system" incurred during his service in the Civil War. The army doctor who examined the seventy-three-year-old Antisell judged his condition to be "general senile paralysis" and offered no evidence that it had resulted from his war service. Nevertheless, he was granted a small pension of twelve dollars a month.[118]

Next, Antisell sought restitution for the loss of his home beside the Potomac; during its years as a Union garrison, the estate had been ruined and the house destroyed. A private bill to support his claim for ten thousand dollars was introduced in Congress in 1892. The claims committee ruled that he was entitled to nothing for the loss of his estate, but did allow twenty-five hundred dollars for "the value of the orchard, the forest trees and the fencing used for military purposes by the Army."[119] Whether Antisell ever received this is unclear for he died soon afterwards, on June 14, 1893, at his home on Q Street. Some of the foremost medical and military men of Washington mourned at his funeral; the pallbearers included Arthur Snyder and Charles Liebermann, the sons of his former surgery colleagues at Georgetown. As a mark of respect by his adopted city, Thomas Antisell was buried in Congressional Cemetery.[120]

And what of Reuben Cleary, the young man who had ridden off to Virginia in 1861, so full of dash and hope? He had survived Williamsburg, Gettysburg, Petersburg, and many other battles; but he never recovered from the death of the Confederacy. Rather than endure a federal ascendancy, he chose exile. Arriving in Brazil on August 10, 1865, he made his home at Lages in a remote region five hundred miles south of Rio de Janeiro. There he settled down at last to practice medicine and in 1870 married the daughter of one of the many German immigrant families in the area. But his life among a native population so backward that their favorite medicine, he wrote, "was a tea made of dog turds that they call jasmine," was one of constant frustration.

In 1885, by now fifty years old, he wrote a memoir of his experiences in Brazil. The manuscript, in a fine steady hand, reveals that even twenty years after the end of the Civil War, Reuben Cleary had lost none of his passion for the rights of the South, nor any of his bitterness at the outcome. Previous books on Brazil, he said, had lured "many a poor Confederate exile . . . to seek an 'eldorado' in this land of promise," only to suffer "just such bitter disappointment as they had found in their own country when they put their faith in law as established, and immutable justice, yet were deprived of their political rights by more brutal forces." Slavery was still the principal economic system in Brazil. "That slavery is a curse I know very well,"

Cleary wrote, "but to employ wicked means and false assurances to extin-guish it, and sacrifice thousands of precious lives, as well as ruin many thousands more of innocent people, I consider a greater crime." With all the scorn of his Irish ancestry, Cleary blamed the English for perpetrating slavery on America and then, when it ceased to be profitable, hypocritically leading the campaign to abolish it—thus "causing hundreds of thousands of deaths for which they return sanctimonious thanks to an insulted Deity."[121]

Cleary died in Rio de Janeiro on February 12, 1898, at age sixty-two.[122] His book was never published, but ten years later Dr. Joseph Theophilus Howard donated the draft manuscript to the Library of Congress.[123] Howard had graduated from Georgetown with Cleary in 1859 and served the Union in the war as a contract surgeon in the military hospitals of Washington.[124] Somehow, despite the political and geographical gulfs between them, the two classmates had stayed in touch for nearly forty years.

In absolute contrast to the shattered lives of so many individuals, Georgetown medical school emerged from the maelstrom in flourishing condition, well placed to face the postwar years with confidence. The wartime demand for doctors had driven its enrollment of students from 29 in the 1861–62 session to 127 in session of 1864–65.[125] In the last year of the war, a second five-month session was introduced from March to July, in part to enable students to complete the two required courses in one year rather than two.[126] It also eased the crowding in the cramped old building on F Street, no larger now than when enrollment was barely in double figures.

The school had graduated a total of seventy students during the war—more than in the decade before it—with half of those getting their degrees in the final year.[127] Two commencements were held in 1865. Twenty students were graduated on March 2 at Ford's Theater. The theater was booked for the second ceremony in July, when fifteen more students were to be given their degrees; but by then the site of Lincoln's assassination had closed in shame, not to be used for public events for another hundred years.[128]

Georgetown was fortunate. Its faculty had remained remarkably stable through the war. Only John Snyder had gone. He had died at his home in August 1863, aged thirty-three, after falling from an oak tree he had scaled to saw off a high branch.[129] The familiar figure of Flodoardo Howard then

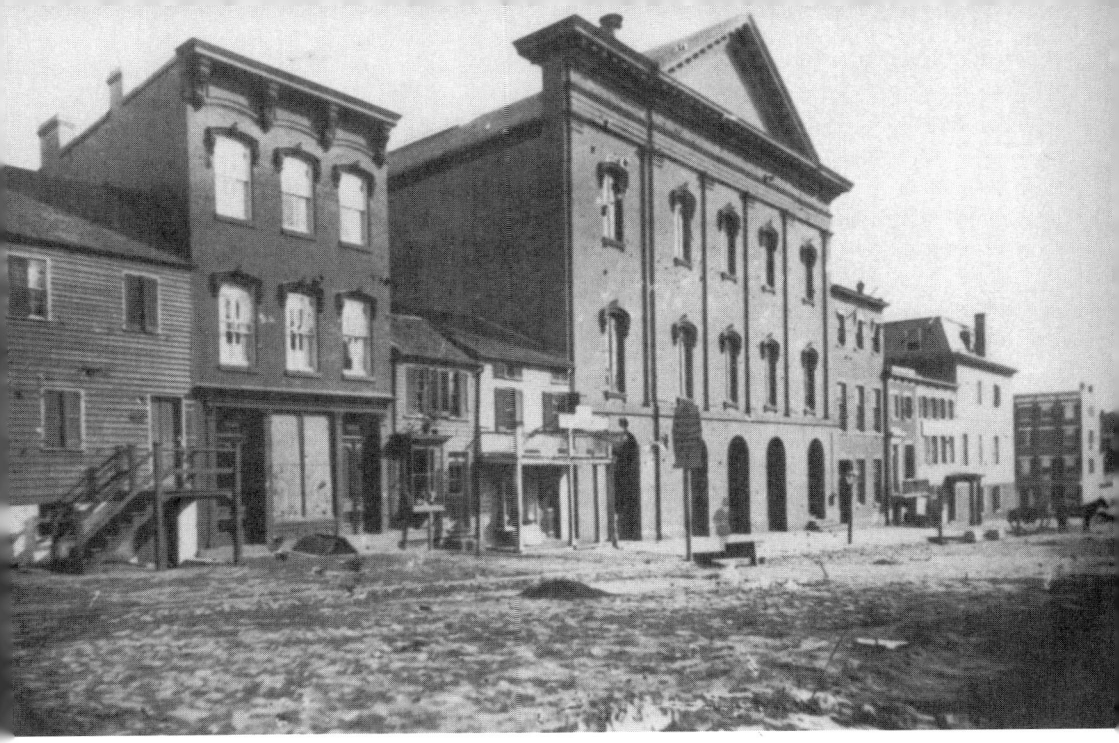

The large brick building in the center of this early photograph of Tenth Street, taken circa 1861 by Matthew Brady, is Ford's Theater, where Abraham Lincoln was shot in 1865, seven weeks after Georgetown medical school held its March commencement there.

The school's second building, into which it moved in 1868, can be seen four doors down from the theater. The muddy street was typical of downtown Washington's lack of pavement before the 1870s. Courtesy of the Library of Congress.

returned from rural retirement to take over again as professor of obstetrics.[130] Columbian medical school had fared less well. At the outbreak of war its professor of medicine, Alexander Garnett, left Washington to serve the cause of his native Virginia, becoming personal physician to both Jefferson Davis and Robert E. Lee. Later, the rest of the faculty was in constant flux. This upheaval, worsened by its wanderings through a succession of temporary homes after the loss of the infirmary, finally forced Columbian's closing in 1863.[131]

By the end of the war, therefore, Georgetown had only one competitor south of Baltimore. Miraculously, the Medical College of Virginia in Richmond had survived the invasion and burning of the city in 1865. Richmond had turned out four hundred surgeons for the Confederacy, shortening its sessions to four months and graduating two classes a year. All other medical schools in the South, including the oldest and most prestigious in Charleston and in New Orleans, had closed early in the war.[132]

The Civil War brought no breakthroughs in medical or surgical practice; but it did bring three advances in medical education. First and foremost, it had given a generation of doctors clinical experience on a scale unimaginable in peacetime. "At the close of the war," one nineteenth-century historian noted, "hundreds of young doctors returned to their homes, better physicians and surgeons than they could otherwise have hoped to become."[133] Secondly, all those specimens that Surgeon General Hammond had ordered collected in the field were used to establish the Army Medical Museum, which became the world's largest display of every kind of surgical disease and injury (and as such was to play an important role in Georgetown's instruction after the war). The third advance was that, again thanks to Hammond, the war had been documented. For the first time in any war, surgeons had been obliged to write reports on the procedures they performed. Compiled later by George Otis and Joseph Woodward into twelve thick volumes, these reports became a priceless archive—unique not only as a historical chronicle but, more important, as a systematic record of what had been, in essence, a huge clinical trial.[134]

Thomas Antisell, addressing the first postwar class of Georgetown medical students, anticipated the result:

> When the medical history of this war comes to be fully written; when the statistics in the hands of the Surgical Bureau of the War Department, under the care of surgeons Otis and Woodward, shall have been published; when ordinary gunshot injuries can be classified by the thousand, and the rarer forms of injury, as of joints, by the hundred, is it too much to say that surgery will become a more exact science, and that modes of operation will no longer be left to the choice of the surgeon, but that those which result in greater safety to life will only be adopted, no matter what may be the peculiar views of the operator?[135]

Antisell was right, though for a reason he could not foresee: surgery was indeed about to become a more exact science. Even as Antisell spoke, in October 1865, a professor of surgery in Glasgow, Scotland, was experimenting with carbolic acid to sterilize open wounds.[136] Joseph Lister's pioneering work on antisepsis, building on Louis Pasteur's early research into the bacterial basis of pus formation, came just too late to save the hundreds of thousands of lives and limbs sacrificed in the Civil War. But it laid the foundation of modern surgical practice.

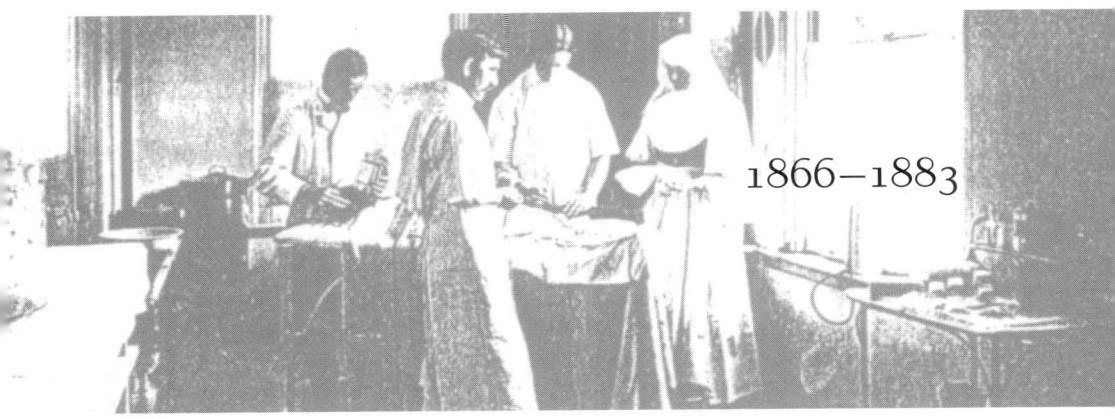

1866–1883

CHAPTER THREE

RECONSTRUCTION, RIVALRY, & REFORM

THE END OF the war could not, of course, bring about a ceasefire of feeling. As former Confederates returned to Washington, rejoining many Southern sympathizers who had never left, the city seethed with partisan animosities and sometimes violent recriminations. The medical students enrolled at Georgetown in 1866–67 were fairly evenly drawn from North and South. Inevitably there were outbursts.

One occurred in the class of Thomas Antisell, the geologist/chemist and military surgeon who was now teaching physiology. Lecturing one day on racial differences, he spoke disparagingly of the anatomy and intellect of Africans. One student recalled:

> This called forth violent hissing from the Yankee element in the class and vociferous cheering from the Southerners. The din increased until perfect bedlam prevailed and Dr. Antisell merely stood with his arms folded . . . When the men had quieted sufficiently he said, "Gentlemen, what I've stated has no political significance, but is fact. Truth is mighty and will prevail." He then walked out of the room. When the full import of his final statement sunk into the minds of the students, chaos reigned supreme and actual physical violence was narrowly escaped.[1]

71

Despite these tensions, the medical school had emerged strengthened from the war. Noble Young, always the most tenacious in fighting for Georgetown's advancement, was more than anyone conscious of the gains it had made during its first fifteen years. "We have struggled against opposition of the most formidable character," he told the graduating class in March 1866. "We have sought from our public authorities an equal participation in advantages bestowed on others . . . but all in vain. We have been left to struggle alone and unaided in our enterprise . . . But we are beginning to receive our reward."[2]

They were indeed. The following October, 124 students enrolled in the school, only 3 less than the peak of 1864−65, and for the next three years numbers remained high.[3] Profits were robust in consequence. In March 1867, after operating costs had been paid, each professor received for his five months of winter teaching a dividend of $1,267.24, and the following year only a little less[4]—not a bad part-time income when Washington was caught in a postwar recession and unemployment was hitting doctors' fees.

By the spring of 1868, the faculty felt prosperous enough to consider moving out of the cramped building on F Street. More spacious premises were urgently needed. Indeed, it is difficult to understand how so many students could have fitted into only two floors of the old building: the ground floor had been let out to commercial businesses since the days of low enrollment before the war.[5] But the move was necessary for reasons of competitive prestige as well as space, because Columbian medical school was now back in business, after a stroke of luck that must have made Noble Young grind his teeth. Columbian had acquired a large, impressive building on H Street—an outright gift from William Corcoran, the banker who had returned to Washington after sitting out the war in Europe.[6] Georgetown had no such benefactor; as usual, the Georgetown professors had to pay their own way.

The building they chose was on the corner of Tenth and E Streets in the center of Washington. Ironically, it had housed Columbian's first medical school from 1825 to 1844, but for that reason suited their purpose. Washington citizens had long called it "the Old Medical College" and within the profession it was known as "the cradle of medical education" in the city. Even so, the faculty only narrowly voted to go ahead with the move, mainly because the asked-for rent of fourteen hundred dollars a year was "deemed exorbitant." But toward the end of March, 1868, they managed to beat this down to thirteen hundred dollars and signed a five-year lease.[7]

As spring turned into early summer, the outlook for the medical school seemed rosy. The core faculty was an uncommonly cohesive and loyal group. Three of its founders—Noble Young (medicine), Johnson Eliot (surgery), and Flodoardo Howard (obstetrics)—were still in place; James Ethelbert Morgan (materia medica) had been on the faculty since 1852, Thomas Antisell (physiology, hygiene, and medical chemistry) since 1858, and Silas Loomis (general chemistry and toxicology) and Montgomery Johns (anatomy) since 1861. Even the demonstrator of anatomy had long-time connections to the school: he was Warwick Evans, its first graduate, now age forty.[8]

The war had brutally taught the need to equip doctors with practical skills; so a return to the old classroom-dominated curriculum was unthinkable. "Practical medicine and surgery" were the new priorities in medical education, and the faculty did its best to ensure that good clinical instruction would be part of the new course. Antisell, indeed, insisted upon it. Back in 1864—against opposition from others on the faculty—he had pushed through a resolution that "hereafter, hospital clinical instruction will be required from students *before* graduation."[9] To this end, between March 1865 and January 1867, Georgetown arranged such training for its students at all three of the civilian hospitals remaining in Washington now that the military facilities had closed down. The faculty contrived this by appointing the physicians in charge of medicine or surgery at these hospitals as "clinical professors" of the school: Daniel R. Hagner in clinical medicine at Providence Hospital; John Harry Thompson in clinical obstetric medicine and surgery at the Columbia Hospital for Women; and Robert Reyburn in clinical surgery at the Freedmen's Hospital.[10]

It was a coup for Georgetown, because these physicians wielded considerable power; it was entirely up to them whether students would be admitted to their hospitals for instruction. In Thompson's case, he had founded the Columbia Hospital for Women himself—even securing, with the help of Secretary of War Stanton, annual grants from Congress of ten thousand dollars to help pay operating costs. The fifty-bed facility opened in March of 1866, in a building that had earlier housed a military hospital and was now chartered to provide medical services to women free of charge. The hospital (still flourishing today) was the first in Washington to offer specialized care for obstetrics and gynecology. In its first six years, more than seven hundred operations were performed there. Thompson thus became one of the city's earliest specialists, in a practice that could hardly have been more distant from his recent experiences in the Civil War.[11]

Those first clinical professors were not paid by Georgetown—at least, not until 1870 when Thompson negotiated a fee of ten dollars for every student graduated—and they were permitted no say in the running of the school.[12] But the prestige of a medical school position, at a time when physicians competed to collect as many "appointments" as possible, was sufficient to persuade them to teach for free on Saturday afternoons and Sunday mornings—the only times when the students, who worked week-days and went to class at night, could attend clinics.[13] Robert Reyburn did not even wait to be invited; he volunteered his services to Georgetown and was appointed immediately.[14]

All three recruits were able men, but Reyburn was a star. At age thirty-five, he had already made a name as a surgeon of stature. Born in Scotland in 1833, he had crossed the Atlantic with his widowed mother at the age of ten and settled in Philadelphia, where, in 1856, he received his medical degree from the city's College of Medicine and Surgery. By the time he joined the Union army six years later, his skills in operative surgery were so well regarded that he rose like a rocket through the ranks of "acting" assistant surgeon and "commissioned" assistant surgeon to "full" surgeon in just five weeks. Reyburn was a highly accomplished man—a writer and poet, a devout Episcopalian, and a dedicated Republican activist, as well as a first-class physician—but the driving force in his life was humanitarianism, expressed most keenly in his work on behalf of the "freedmen," the slaves emancipated by Lincoln's proclamation of 1863. At the end of the war, brevetted a lieutenant colonel, Reyburn was appointed to the Freedmen's Bureau, which had been set up by the federal government under the command of General Oliver O. Howard to provide food, clothing, and medical care to hundreds of thousands of former slaves. Most were in a pitiful condition: between 1865 and 1872, the bureau treated more than 430,000 black patients at 104 hospitals and dispensaries throughout the South. Reyburn became the bureau's chief medical officer and also surgeon in charge of the largest of its facilities, the Freedmen's Hospital in Washington. It was the start of Reconstruction and, for Reyburn, the start of a life-long crusade for civil rights, a stance that would bring him both opprobrium and honor— and cause mayhem within the local medical community a few years later.[15]

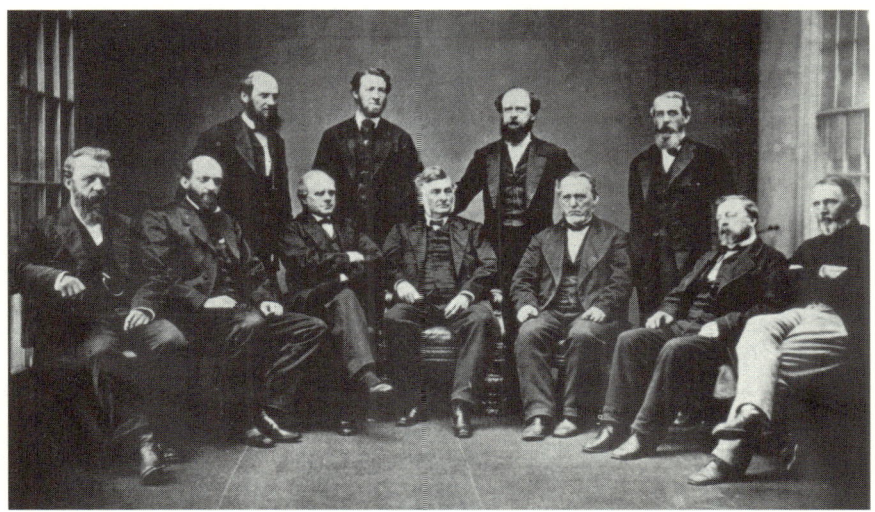

The entire Georgetown medical school faculty in 1868. Seated, left to right: Silas Loomis, James Ethelbert Morgan, Johnson Eliot, Noble Young, Flodoardo Howard, Thomas Antisell, Montgomery Johns. Standing, left to right: Daniel Hagner, Robert Reyburn, John Harry Thompson, and Warwick Evans. The photograph, commissioned by the class of 1868, was taken by Alexander Gardner. Courtesy of Georgetown University Archives.

Reyburn's appointment to Georgetown in January 1867 was a major gain for the faculty, not only because of his standing but because he brought such unrivalled opportunities for instruction in clinical surgery. In its opening year, 1866–67, the Freedmen's Hospital treated more than twenty-three thousand patients, making it by far the largest medical facility in Washington.[16] The faculty recognized Reyburn's value: in March 1868 he was promoted to a full professorship in a specially-created chair that encompassed operative surgery, histology, and microscopic and pathological anatomy.[17]

Between them, the eleven Georgetown faculty members offered students classroom instruction and a range of clinical opportunities superior to the majority of the nation's medical schools at this time. And the students must have known it. In gratitude, the graduating class of March 1868 paid tribute by commissioning a photograph of the eleven posed in a formal group. It was taken by Alexander Gardner, the famous Civil War photographer who had trained under Matthew Brady and ran his Washington studio. The photograph so pleased the faculty that they decided to have it framed and presented to the president of Georgetown College.[18] It signified the success and solidity of the medical school at a time of civic and national disarray; it showed confidence in the future.

But on the horizon was a tiny cloud, and by September it had swelled to a storm. The first rumble was recorded at the faculty meeting of August 7, 1868: "Dr. Young was delegated by the Faculty to confer with Dr. Loomis in regard to his connection with another Medical Faculty."[19] The phrasing was understated. Silas Loomis, professor of general chemistry, had more than a "connection" with the third medical school now being established in Washington. He was its founder. The school was at Howard University; and, since January 1867, Loomis had been organizing it along the same principles as the new university being set up by General Howard: namely, to provide higher education to anyone, regardless of sex, color, or race.[20] This was a novel idea in Washington. Women and black students had graduated from a few other medical schools in the United States (the first in 1849 and 1822 respectively[21]); but neither Georgetown nor Columbian admitted them. By the summer of 1868, when the Georgetown faculty took notice, Howard's medical faculty had already been appointed, with Loomis elected to the chair of chemistry, but financing was still uncertain and it was not clear whether the new school would open, as planned, in the fall.

Loomis said as much to Noble Young, who reported the conversation indignantly to the Georgetown faculty on August 19: "Dr. Loomis states that he has been appointed a professor in another medical institution but has not accepted the appointment; said institution is not yet in full operation; that when such full operation shall occur and the institution offers such inducements as shall be sufficient in the estimation of Dr. Loomis, the said Loomis will then feel himself justified in deciding as to which institution he will attach himself." Loomis, reasonably enough from his point of view, was hedging his bets; perhaps he felt that as a graduate of the medical school in 1857, a faculty member since 1861, and the protégé and friend of Thomas Antisell, his position at Georgetown was secure. The faculty's response, however, was swift and unequivocal. The five professors present at that meeting (Young, Eliot, Howard, Morgan, and Johns) resolved unanimously "that the present Chair of Chemistry be hereby declared abolished, and that the resignation of Dr. Loomis will be agreeable to the Faculty."[22]

But a far worse problem now confronted them. Silas Loomis was not the only Georgetown professor "connected" with Howard. Robert Reyburn had been elected its first professor of surgery. In fact, the first meeting of the embryonic Howard faculty had been held in his office on I Street the previous May.[23] Certainly the Georgetown faculty did not want to lose Reyburn, but they did need to know where he stood. Unfortunately, Reyburn was away in the South on his work for the Freedmen's Bureau. Johnson Eliot, still dean of the faculty, went to great lengths to contact him with letters sent via "General Howard's dispatches"; but by September 16—two weeks before the start of the new session—he still had received no reply from Reyburn.[24]

This was a tense time for the faculty. Having at last gained ascendancy over Columbian, which now had 60 students enrolled compared to Georgetown's 113, they perceived the emergence of a third medical school as a major threat—not least because, in the era of reconstruction, it was likely to receive federal funding. As they waited for Reyburn's return, their anxiety is revealed in an agitated letter written on September 7 by Joseph Taber Johnson, who had graduated from Georgetown in 1865 and was now, at twenty-three, the professor-elect of obstetrics at Howard medical school. Writing in haste to General Howard, Johnson warned him of the mood at Georgetown:

> ... Dr. Loomis has already been expelled from [Georgetown] on account of his connection with the Howard University or, as they put it, a "rival college," and in conversation with one of the professors of the Old College last week he told me that they only awaited an expression from Dr. Reyburn to do the same by him.

> Reyburn is away now, and will not be back for about a week, and his Faculty are anxiously waiting his return. They all like him as a man, and as a professor, and are hoping to secure him for their school. One of the officers of the Faculty told me earnestly this morning that he regarded the Med. Department of Howard University as a much more dangerous rival

than the Med. Dept. of Columbian College, and said he knew that [Howard] would, in a few years, have more endowments and more students than they would . . .

He says Reyburn is [Howard's] best man—that he has the largest hospital in the city and can afford the college he is connected with more advantages for clinical instruction than any man in the city, and that they are going to get him away from [Howard]. He says it would be a staggering blow in the eyes of the community for Reyburn, who has become known to all the colored men in the city who have had anything to do with doctors, and is also known generally to have been elected to a professorship, to withdraw [from Howard] and permanently join [Georgetown], and I think so too. They are confident they will secure him. They fear . . . the growth of [Howard] if Reyburn who is so popular in theirs withdraws from them and comes to ours. They will do their best to make him renounce [Howard] for ever or turn him out [of Georgetown] the day he gets back.[25]

Reyburn finally showed up to face the Georgetown faculty on September 23. It was true, he said, that he had been elected professor of surgery at Howard; but he had not accepted, believing that it would never get under way. However, that had changed and "much to his regret," the faculty minutes paraphrased, "he now felt compelled to accept the appointment" because of his position with the Freedmen's Bureau and his close association with General Howard. He assured the faculty of his strong feelings for Georgetown but offered to resign "if it was deemed necessary for him to do so."

Reyburn's explanation was more tactful but essentially the same as Loomis had given; though Loomis had gotten shorter shrift. Clearly Reyburn was hoping that Georgetown would allow him to hold chairs at both schools, and to encourage that aim he played a strong card: he offered to continue to make the clinical facilities of Freedmen's Hospital available to Georgetown students. It did not work. The Georgetown elders—Young, Eliot, and Howard—conferred privately for a few minutes and then asked for Reyburn's resignation. Reyburn went round the room expressing a "kind and cordial sentiment" to each faculty member and then left.[26]

Four weeks later Howard medical school began its first session with eight students and six faculty members, each of the latter on a salary of one thousand dollars a year. Silas Loomis was their president and Joseph Taber Johnson their secretary. And the next year Robert Reyburn masterminded the transfer of Freedmen's Hospital to a custom-built brick building next to the medical school on the Howard campus, making it in effect the university hospital.[27] Georgetown students no longer attended clinical lectures there.

The departures of Loomis and Reyburn brought yet another blow to Georgetown. After Loomis' expulsion, Thomas Antisell, who for ten years had played a leading role in shaping the school's policies, most recently in its emphasis on clinical instruction, abruptly ceased to attend faculty meetings. No hint of discord is recorded in the minutes, but it is not hard to deduce his reason. The two men were close friends with many common interests, both polymaths with a shared passion for chemistry, invention, and a range of scientific pursuits, and it was Antisell who had nominated Loomis to the Georgetown faculty seven years earlier.[28] Antisell greatly admired Reyburn too. In fact, the previous May he had nominated Reyburn to run against Johnson Eliot for dean of the faculty Eliot won, but it was the first time in the school's history that the election of an officer had been contested.[29] Through the winter of 1868–69, Antisell delivered his lectures, but rumors began to circulate that he intended resigning at the end of the session. Receiving no definite explanation from Antisell on this crucial point, the faculty finally informed him in March that he was "no longer a professor" at Georgetown. The move brought a strong protest from the students, who revered Antisell.[30] Nevertheless, he departed in the spring of 1869 to become professor of chemistry at Maryland Agricultural College.[31] Georgetown was left without three of the esteemed professors who had sat so proudly for that faculty photograph less than twelve months before.

Amidst this internal strife, the medical school moved into its second home on the northeast corner of Tenth and E Streets, where it was to remain for the next eighteen years. Much more spacious than the F Street building, its dissecting and lecture rooms were large, airy, and well lit; and it even had its own amphitheater, warmed by a coal-burning stove. The first lecture was given there on October 1, 1868, shortly after John Harry Thompson had been hastily transferred to Reyburn's chair of operative surgery, and an elderly chemist, Edward Foreman, had been appointed to replace Loomis.[32]

One advantage of the new location was its fortuitous proximity to the Army Medical Museum, which a year earlier had moved into the former Ford's Theater, just four doors up on Tenth Street. Surgeon General Hammond's 1862 order that every type of specimen be collected from surgeons' tables in military base and field hospitals had been obeyed to the letter. The specimens arrived in Washington by the wagon-load, there to be sorted, preserved, mounted, and labeled. According to Ralph Walsh, a Georgetown medical graduate (1863) who helped with this work in its early days, some of the alcohol used to preserve moist surgical specimens was contraband liquor seized during the war from women attempting to smuggle it across the Long Bridge to sell at great profit in the South. "Frequently women were arrested with belts under their skirts, to which were attached tin sectional cans holding from a quart to a gallon and, in a number of cases, false breasts, each holding a quart or more," Walsh recalled.[33]

Specimen collection continued long after the war and many Washington surgeons, including the Georgetown professors, contributed. By far the most prolific donor over the next half-century was another Georgetown graduate, Daniel Smith Lamb. He had worked at the museum from 1865 to 1867 as a medical student, and continued his professional association with it until he retired at the age of eighty in 1923. From the mid-1870s Lamb was the city's leading pathologist and the more unusual results of his autopsies went straight to the museum. Its collection was "largely the result of his untiring zeal and devotion," one tribute noted; and its first history, published in 1917, was also chronicled by Lamb.[34]

As soon as the museum opened in the spring of 1867, already with several thousand specimens on display, the Georgetown professors began urging their students to make use of it. "[Here] are accumulated preparations of every variety and shade of injury that man can sustain," Johnson Eliot told the class. "All the remarkable and interesting cases of wounds and injuries which occurred during the war and all the remarkable morbid specimens from our numerous hospitals are here arranged for inspection and study. It is indeed the most valuable collection in the world and attracts to this city medical gentlemen from all parts of the country."[35] Housed in the

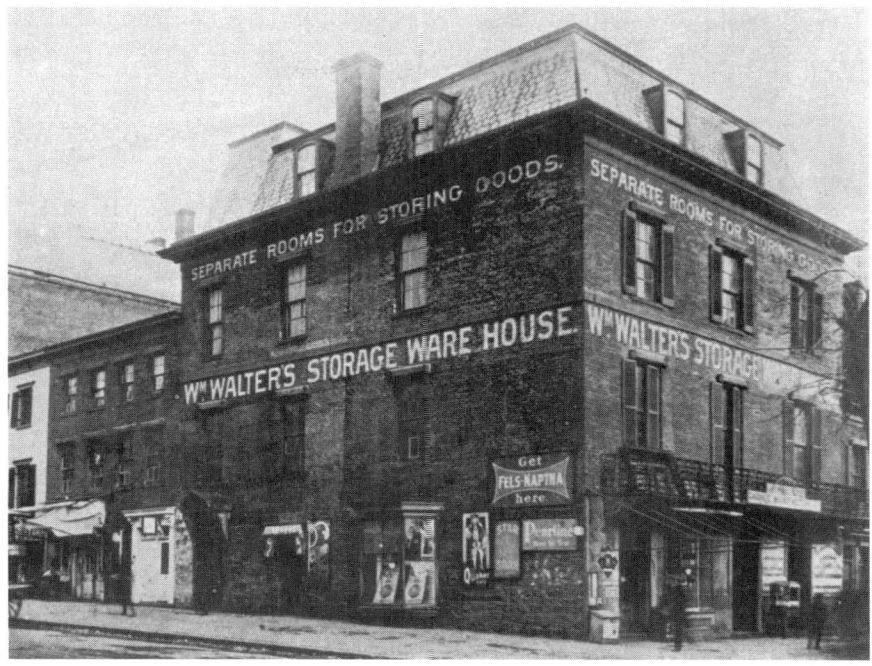

The building occupied by Georgetown
University medical school from 1868 to 1886
stood at the northeast corner of Tenth and E
Streets, Washington, D.C. This is a later
photograph, probably taken around 1900.
Courtesy of Georgetown University Archives.

same building—to be precise, in the former dress circle of the old theater—
was the Surgeon General's Library, which formed the basis of the later
National Library of Medicine. Between 1868 and 1874, under the guidance
of John Shaw Billings, its collection grew from ten thousand to more than
fifty thousand volumes. These were freely available for study by anyone.
Even readers from outside Washington could borrow books by leaving a
fifty dollar deposit. (Among the leading physicians who availed themselves
of this service were William Osler, William Halsted, and Walter Reed.)[36]
Together, the museum and the library provided unparalleled opportunities
for study, and the medical school advertised the fact prominently, indeed
almost proprietorially, in its brochures.

Eliot continued to combine his duties as dean with teaching "the principles and practice of surgery," as he had during the war. Daniel Roberts

Brower, one of his wartime students, recalled him as a good teacher: "No one could leave this school without being well grounded in the surgery of those days."[37] But now, able at last to go beyond Eliot's classroom instruction, the students walked the wards with their clinical professors and observed surgical operations in progress. John Harry Thompson's clinics at the Columbia Hospital for Women, which included some general surgery as well as gynecological procedures, were especially popular with the class. Daniel Lamb, one of his early students, remembered Thompson as "a very fluent speaker, a very resourceful man. . . . I recall that one time he brought before the class a woman with a tumor on the scalp, which, after handling a little, he said was a *fatty* tumor, and proceeded to operate. At the first puncture some fluid squirted out and he promptly said: 'Gentlemen, as I told you, we have here a *cystic* tumor.'" [38] Described by one of his most eminent peers as "a surgeon of great intelligence and a very accurate observer,"[39] Thompson laid unusual emphasis on the science of surgery, as well as its techniques. Surgeons, he declared, should "not content themselves with the mere eclat of practical surgery in the ward or theater, surrounded by an admiring class of students and associate practitioners, but carefully record and digest the history of all important cases, and publish them for the benefit of the medical public and the advancement of scientific truth."[40] More than most surgeons of his time, Thompson published case reports, illustrated often by accomplished drawings. He appears to have been highly regarded in Washington. Eventually, though, under suspicion of malpractice and mismanagement, he left the United States in 1877 and settled in Italy.[41]

With the new emphasis on clinical instruction, Georgetown students were now getting a better education for their money than they had done, which perhaps justified the substantial rise in fees in 1868. During the school's first eleven years, the cost of tuition of each annual course had remained at $90; in 1863 it had gone to $105. In March 1868, however, Georgetown and Columbian formed a joint consultative committee to discuss "matters of common interest," and their first act of cooperation was to increase fees. Both schools agreed to charge $135 a year for the full course or $20 a ticket for any one set of lectures.[42]

It had taken nearly two decades, and the common threat posed by Howard, for the two medical schools to bury their antagonism. The new spirit of relative amity was reinforced the following year when the new Providence Hospital opened. The old hospital had been founded in a private house in 1861 by a celebrated local physician, Joseph M. Toner, to provide care for civilians after the military had taken over the Washington Infirmary. The new building, privately funded and purpose built, was Washington's only general hospital in the postwar period; and whereas Columbian's faculty and students had monopolized the old infirmary before the war, Toner made it clear that no single group would have exclusive claim on Providence. "All the physicians in the District will have an equality of privileges in the institution; consequently, any physician who may send a patient to the hospital can attend the same if he wishes to do so," newspaper advertisements announced. In the circumstances, it must have been highly gratifying for three of Georgetown's founders—Liebermann, Howard, and Eliot; although, oddly, not Young, who over the years had been the principal agitator for equal privileges—to be appointed to the advisory and consulting board of the new Providence Hospital.43

The Georgetown-Columbian consultative committee soon confronted a challenge greater than fixing fees. In the dark early hours of Sunday, January 10, 1869, the police chased and stopped a horse-drawn hackney carriage travelling at full speed towards the Capitol. "It was found," the *Star* reported laconically, "that the passengers consisted of Thomas Carr and Harry Clark, two live white men, and two dead bodies of females (both nude)." Before daybreak it became known that the women had been buried the previous day in the cemetery of the Washington almshouse, and a hostile crowd a thousand strong gathered outside the precinct station.44 Grave-robbing was in the news again.

The two culprits, Carr and Clark, were neither criminals like the notorious Burke and Hare—whose method of procuring bodies for medical schools in Scotland forty years earlier was to murder people—nor entrepreneurial middlemen. They were the demonstrators of anatomy at Columbian medical school. The Columbian faculty promptly paid their fines of sixty dollars each plus costs, and were no doubt relieved that press coverage of the affair did not mention Columbian by name—even though no reader was left in doubt of the convicted men's intent. "The bodies are now in the dead house of the almshouse where [they will remain] until they can be of no use to doctors," the *Star* said. Columbian's professors were acutely embarrassed. They privately reminded Carr and Clark of their duty to observe "more caution and entire secrecy in the manner of supplying the College with anatomical material" and made it clear that if the "misadventure" were repeated, next time they would pay their own fines.[45]

The Georgetown medical faculty took a there-but-for-the-grace-of-God attitude to the scandal. After all, it might easily have been their own demonstrator, Warwick Evans, who had been caught. Or even their professor of anatomy, Montgomery Johns. He lived miles away in College Park, Maryland, where he taught by day at the Agricultural College. Every afternoon he rode into Washington to deliver evening lectures in the dissecting room and, according to Daniel Lamb, "slept there through the night, except when stealing cadavers from graveyards, and returned to the Park in the morning."[46]

The topic was discussed at the next joint meeting with Columbian, which resulted in a proposal adopted by each school: "The committee recommends to the Demonstrators of the two colleges to employ a Resurrectionist for both institutions, and to act in concert in procuring material; and also not to permit students to accompany the Resurrectionist."[47] How Warwick Evans reacted to this edict is not recorded. He had repeatedly, for more than two years, urged the faculty "to discuss the price of cadavers." When he asked them to raise the price to twenty dollars a body, "after much discussion" they set it at fifteen dollars.[48] Evidently this was remuneration for his own illegal midnight activities; grave-robbing was the main duty of a "demonstrator of anatomy."

Procuring dissecting material was a constant headache for medical schools. The new emphasis on clinical instruction meant only that the students got to watch their professors at work; they did not actually lay hands on any patients. In peacetime, at least, it was only through dissection that students learned the rudiments of surgery, so cadavers had to be obtained. Some states, led by Massachusetts in 1831, had already introduced laws permitting dissection.[49] But in most areas it remained a crime—with the result, James Morgan complained in an address to the

Georgetown students in 1869, that "the physician is compelled in many states of our Union to risk his reputation, his liberty, and even his life in order to obtain a knowledge of our profession." If caught, he said, the physician at the very least "is denounced in the public prints as a 'body-snatcher' and held up to detestation by the whole world."[50]

Congress still refused to pass any statute to make anatomical material available legally in the District of Columbia. The arrest of Carr and Clark prompted local doctors to renew their lobbying efforts, and the Medical Society of D.C. publicly drew attention to the laws of Europe, where the bodies of executed criminals or suicides or, in some countries, of people who had died in poorhouses, could legally be handed over to medical schools.[51] All their arguments were in vain: not until 1902 did Congress pass an act that set up an Anatomical Board for D.C. and made unclaimed cadavers legally available for medical use.[52]

In the meantime, resurrectionists flourished in Washington. The most notorious of them, a man named Janssen, once sold a body to one of the city's medical schools, then stole it back from the dissecting room the following night to sell it to another. He also set himself up as a lecturer on the fine art of body snatching and gave public demonstrations using a fake corpse. In the end, Janssen was attracting so much adverse publicity, which of course rebounded on the medical schools, that the Georgetown and Columbian faculties jointly paid him to leave town.[53]

Physicians always distinguished the deeds of professional resurrectionists, whom they regarded as criminal riffraff, from their own identical activities, which they saw as a necessary means to a nobler end. Ordinary citizens, however, rarely perceived the difference. As late as 1884, Johnson Eliot's son, Llewellyn, resigned his post as demonstrator of anatomy at Georgetown because grave-robbing had become too personally risky. Llewellyn, who had graduated from Georgetown a decade earlier, had just inherited his father's extensive private practice; and, as he wrote in a frank letter to the faculty: "Since the death of my father, attention to my own interests prevents my running any unnecessary risk of being apprehended as a resurrectionist, to say nothing of the exposure consequent upon such works." His father, in fact, as a young man had been Columbian's demonstrator and later Georgetown's first professor of anatomy—and, as such, had probably snatched more than a few bodies himself. Clearly Johnson

Eliot had understood the burdens of a demonstrator's position. Shortly before his death, he advised Llewellyn "to go out no more."[54]

᠀

Washington in 1869 was superficially the same town it had been before the war. Most of its streets were still unpaved, muddy, and infested with animals; the Washington monument was still a half-built stump; citizens and visitors alike complained about inadequate transportation and the absence of a sewerage system. When Washingtonians became enthusiastic about the notion of hosting a world fair, and even managed to raise subscriptions of $2 million towards financing it, Congress flatly refused. One Senator described Washington as "the ugliest city in the whole country," and scoffed that "the idea of inviting the world to see this town" was "altogether out of the question." Philadelphia was chosen instead.[55]

Yet the city was changing. By 1867, the population of the District of Columbia was almost 60 percent larger than it had been in 1860. Nearly 127,000 people now lived in the district, and nearly one-third of them were black. Contrary to all expectations, the nation's capital had not been invaded by Confederate forces during the war, but it had been inundated by former slaves who had fled the plantations of the South to seek refuge in the nearest Northern city. After 1862, when Congress passed laws to free both those fugitives and the 3,100 slaves still owned in the District of Columbia, tens of thousands more poured in. The inability of most of these refugees to fend for themselves after lives spent in slavery as legal and social dependents caused immense problems for the municipal government. The Freedmen's Bureau dispensed food, clothing, and medical care, but these freed people were not free of misery. Mostly unskilled and illiterate, they lived in crowded, disease-ridden shanties that sprang up in alleyways and vacant lots throughout the city.[56]

Yet for a few years after the end of the Civil War there was a brief but real honeymoon with civil rights in Washington, the like of which would not be seen again for a hundred years. In 1866, after months of stormy debate, Congress gave the vote to all men in the District of Columbia, irrespective of color—an act passed nineteen months before the ratification of the Fourteenth Amendment similarly allowed male suffrage nationwide, and four years before the Fifteenth Amendment specifically forebade any attempt to deny the right to vote on grounds of race or color. Statutes enacted by the new and self-governing Washington City Council in 1869 and 1870 forbade racial discrimination in restaurants, bars, hotels, theaters, and other places of public entertainment, and proprietors who broke the laws were fined.[57] For the first time, blacks were allowed to ride the street-cars with whites.[58] A Washington judge insisted on appointing black jurors to the criminal court in 1869,[59] by which time a number of middle-class blacks were working in government positions and two had been elected to the city council. The honeymoon spirit was so strong that one of those councillors actually voted at first against the anti-discrimination reforms of 1869–70 on the grounds that they were now unnecessary.[60]

These rapid developments were watched with interest, even incredulity, by the rest of the nation, particularly by the South, where new and ingenious forms of discrimination were being imposed every day. Opposition from whites—overt opposition, at any rate—in Washington was less than might be supposed, because an early form of political correctness was in play. In the Civil War, liberality towards blacks had become equated with loyalty to the Union; so those who publicly criticized the new measures risked being branded as "hidden rebels." This sentiment was most pointedly voiced by Representative George Julian of Indiana in a speech during the House debate on black suffrage: "Nor shall I stop to inquire very critically whether the negroes are *fit* to vote," he said. "As between themselves and white rebels, who deserve to be hung, they are eminently fit."[61] Nevertheless, prejudice was never far below the surface. Blacks were excluded from many labor unions and from most churches, and whites protested about their receiving equal treatment in the workplace.[62] Moreover, black suffrage and other privileges came to an abrupt end on February 21, 1871, when Congress took back control of the District of Columbia and all its citizens lost the right to vote.[63] Washington was still, after all, a southern town at heart.

Into these troubled waters a rock was thrown that was to raise tidal waves of bitterness in the medical community for years to come. Two black physicians, Alexander T. Augusta and Charles B. Purvis, applied early in June 1869 to become members of the Medical Society of the District of Columbia. Both were leaders of Washington's small but growing black

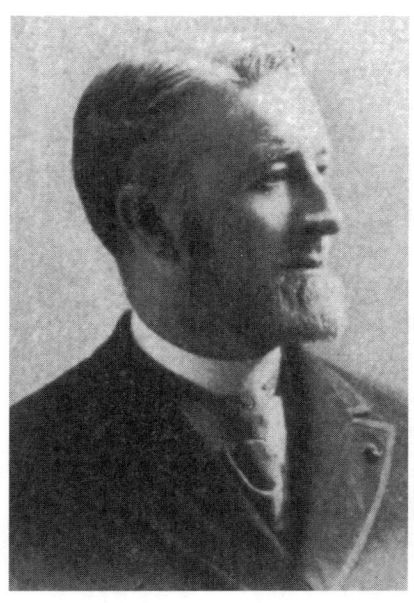

Robert Reyburn, M.D., 1833–1909.
Courtesy of the Medical Society of the
District of Columbia.

middle class, which included men like Frederick Douglass, editor of the nation's first black newspaper, the *New Era*, and John Mercer Langston, a lawyer who would later become Virginia's first black representative in Congress.[64] The two doctors were well qualified: they possessed respectable medical degrees, were licensed by the society to practice in the city, and had served with distinction as army surgeons during the Civil War.[65] But on the evening of Wednesday June 16, 1869, their applications were voted down by an overwhelming majority at a brief meeting of the society that was attended by far more members than usual.[66]

There the matter might have rested, had it not been for Georgetown's former professor of clinical surgery, Robert Reyburn. By birth a Glaswegian Scot, Reyburn had inherited at least one of his countrymen's most notable attributes: he was a born fighter. Refusing to accept the Medical Society's rejection of Augusta and Purvis, he went straight for the jugular. He petitioned Congress to repeal the society's charter. The bill was introduced in the Senate on December 9 by Senator Charles Sumner who said, in explanation, that the society's exclusion of the black physicians harmed them in two ways: because its rules barred members from consulting professionally with nonmembers, and because its meetings provided the only forum in Washington for scientific discussions that benefited the continuing education of doctors. The action of the society's members "degrades a long suffering and deeply injured race," he said, "but it also degrades themselves. Nobody can do such a meanness without degradation."[67]

This move stunned the society. Its immediate response, on January 5, 1870, was to revise its rules regarding the election of members. Among other changes, the majority needed to approve a new member was raised from two-thirds to three-fourths.[68] In the debate on these revisions, Reyburn was allowed to read out a resolution that encapsulated the principle on which he stood: "That no physician who is otherwise eligible should be excluded from membership in this society on account of race or color." He elaborated at length, arguing that the clerical, legal, and other professions had opened their doors to blacks, and that, as the medical profession would eventually have to do the same, the society might as well submit gracefully sooner rather than later. One physician inquired if that meant allowing "colored physicians" to attend meetings and "mix in generally." Reyburn replied: "Unquestionably so." His resolution was not allowed to be put to a vote.[69]

The Medical Society of D.C., founded in 1817, was at this time fifty-two years old and thriving. Most of the successful physicians in the District of Columbia—and those who aspired to be—were members. In an age of blatant charlatanism, they felt proud of the importance they enjoyed as upholders of professional standards. So almost all of them—even some who were basically sympathetic to the black physicians' cause—were outraged by Reyburn's attack, particularly as he, and the few who supported him, were members themselves.[70] In a published explanation of its position— "An Appeal to Congress," January 12, 1870, written in part by two former Georgetown professors, Charles Liebermann and James Lovejoy—the society pointed out that it did not deny licenses to properly qualified black physicians; but it insisted that membership in the society was "not a right they could demand but a benefit which it was optional for the Society to bestow."[71] The Senate committee heard testimony and concluded in its report on February 8 that the society had refused Augusta and Purvis its privileges "solely on account of color." If the society's defense meant that it had become essentially a social club, rather than a scientific body, the report declared, it was no longer "worthy of congressional care." Despite this plain language, the Sumner bill was passed over four times, and although it was revived twice more over the following ten years, nothing came of it.[72]

But Reyburn did not wait on Congress. He developed a new strategy that escalated the controversy still further. He founded a new medical association, grandly named the National Medical Society, which offered "equal rights and privileges to regular practitioners of medicine and surgery" in the district, regardless of color.[73] He then took his crusade to the floor of the annual convention of the American Medical Association, which that year happened to be meeting in Washington, D.C.

The AMA convention, the medical profession's most prestigious event of the year, was held at Lincoln Hall in the first week of May 1870. More than four hundred delegates attended the four-day event, many from the Southern states who were returning for the first time since 1860. In a speech that opened the proceedings, Thomas Antisell specifically welcomed them—to much applause. The agenda scheduled daytime sessions of scientific papers and debate on medical issues, with evenings to be spent convivially at receptions given by the president of the United States, the surgeon general, and the mayor of Washington. But one issue dominated the proceedings: would the AMA recognize five new organizations from Washington that were seeking to be accredited as delegates that year—four of which included black physicians?[74]

It quickly became clear to the delegates from the rest of the nation that a new civil war was being waged between the Washington factions in Lincoln Hall; only this time it was the rebels who were championing black rights. The proceedings were so rowdy—with each camp publicly hurling accusations at each other, or being hissed and booed, or not allowed to speak—that even on the first day a motion was made, amid laughter, "that the opposing delegations from the District of Columbia be permitted to go out and in some convenient place fight out their difficulty and settle it."[75]

The opening salvo was fired by the Medical Society of D.C., led by Samuel Busey (who had been, and would soon be again, a Georgetown professor). Race was not mentioned. Busey simply asked the AMA to exclude, for "ethical" reasons, "any delegate who is a member of the so-called National Medical Society of D.C." plus "any faculty" or "any hospital" that employed its members, on the grounds that this society had been "formed in contempt of the organized Medical Society and [had] attempted, through legislative influence, to break down the Medical Society of D.C." Worded this way, the demand effectively excluded not only Reyburn's new association but also Howard medical school, the Freedmen's Hospital, the Smallpox Hospital, and all the black delegates.

Reyburn himself could not be excluded. He was an officer of the AMA that year, serving as its librarian and also, ironically, as chairman of the credentials committee which had to decide the issue. He counter-attacked by demanding, also on "ethical" grounds, the exclusion of all thirty delegates who were members of the Medical Society. But in the end, after days of wrangling, those thirty were allowed to vote on the question of who should be recognized, whereas Reyburn's colleagues were not. Thus, the society carried the day. If all the Washington delegates had been prevented from voting on that point, which one delegate proposed as being the only fair way to handle the issue, Reyburn's bid for recognition would have passed by a single vote.[76]

Robert Reyburn had lost his great gamble. The outcome was racial segregation in the medical community for the next eighty-two years. His new society continued, eventually becoming the Medico-Chirurgical Society of the District of Columbia. Reyburn was its first president, and for many years the same small group of liberal whites who had fought the AMA battle of 1870 continued as its members. When the last of them died, it became a wholly black organization.[77] Not until 1952 did the Medical Society of D.C. accept black members.[78]

The events of 1869–70 were so traumatic for Washington physicians that forty years later, when the first history of the Medical Society came to be written, its authors observed that "the story, even now, is painful to tell, although the intense partisanship of that time has long faded away."[79] The Georgetown professors were personally caught up in the controversy and as divided as the rest of the community in their views. Noble Young and Johnson Eliot, Georgetown's delegates to the AMA convention, were solidly behind the Medical Society; although Eliot remained a close friend of Robert Reyburn, they never saw eye to eye on what the *Star* habitually called "the colored question."[80] But Flodoardo Howard, John Harry Thompson, and the professor of anatomy, John Holston, all sympathized sufficiently with Reyburn's cause to take office as vice presidents of his renegade society two years later.[81] Of the new generation of faculty, Louis Mackall, the professor of clinical medicine, was vice president of the Medical Society when Reyburn launched his attempt to repeal its charter.[82] But two other new and distinguished faculty members were among Reyburn's most vociferous supporters.[83] One was Christopher C. Cox, a physician and lawyer. He had been the surgeon general of Maryland in 1862, vice president of the AMA in 1863, and lieutenant governor of

Maryland in 1864, and he was now Georgetown's professor of medical jurisprudence and hygiene.[84] The other was the professor of urinary pathology and therapeutics, Dr. Doctor Willard Bliss. (He was always referred to as "D.W." to avoid his confusing given names, bestowed by his parents in honor of some New York physician—probably the one who assisted at his birth in 1825.)[85]

Animosities lingered. In 1871, Cox and Bliss were appointed president and secretary of the newly-formed D.C. Board of Health, which was tasked with clearing the streets of marauding livestock, improving city hygiene, and introducing a system for the reporting of contagious diseases. At once the Medical Society of D.C. rose in wrath, not only because it opposed the latter measure as "an onerous and almost impossible task" to impose on the medical profession, but also because it objected to the board's officers.[86] Cox had been denied membership in the society, probably because of his support for Reyburn. Bliss had been expelled from the society after deliberately breaching its rule that members could not consult professionally with nonmembers. Provocatively, he had called in both Cox and Augusta while treating an important patient, the vice president of the United States.[87] The medical war of 1869–70 was being waged on new fronts.

Another Board of Health member was the lawyer John Mercer Langston. Though legally black, he was lighter-skinned than his good friend Bliss, a man of swarthy complexion and huge sideburns. Once, on a trip to New England, the two were conversing with the Boston Board of Health when its president remarked: "I believe you have a colored member on your board?" Langston replied blithely: "Yes, we have. He is a man of great ability. . . . Of rare scholarly attainments, he is a sanitarian that it would be difficult to match anywhere in our country. And it is not certain that he has an equal in Europe . . . Mr. President, our colored member is here; and I have now the honor to present to you my distinguished friend, Dr. D. W. Bliss!" Bliss, chuckling, said: "Gentlemen, it is true we have a colored member; and it is true that he is here. But it has not yet been determined whether my friend Langston or myself is that person. I am darker than he; but his hair curls more than mine."[88]

Such easy camaraderie between black and white was not common in the Washington of the 1870s. It took courage and conviction for a white to stand up for civil rights, particularly within the close-knit medical community where conservative ideals and conformity of opinion were something of a requirement in the constant struggle to maintain and strengthen professional standards. At a time wher most of the black population were illiterate, black doctors were still regarded as suspect in spite of the proven intellectual strengths of men like Augusta and Purvis. White doctors who championed their cause were treated by colleagues with attitudes ranging from puzzlement through skepticism to open hostility. Of the few who took that brave stand, most were Georgetown men: Reyburn, Loomis, Cox, Bliss, Joseph Taber Johnson, and Daniel Lamb. All were physicians of distinction, yet all met derision and ostracism. In some cases their careers were seriously affected. Bliss, the most prosperous physician in Washington at the time of his expulsion from the Medical Society in 1871, saw his practice decline therafter until he was unable to support his family; by 1876 he was forced to apologize to the society and seek re-election.[89]

Immediately after the contentious AMA conference of 1870, Reyburn and Johnson had both resigned from the Medical Society.[90] Much of their time was devoted thereafter to building up the new Howard medical school. But in June 1873, the Howard trustees, who had already cut the professors' salaries from $1,000 to $833 a year, decided to lower its medical tuition fees to $40 (nearly $100 less than Georgetown and Columbian were charging) and announced that the professors' remuneration would henceforth be paid from those fees, "divided pro rata." Reyburn was supporting a large family, and Johnson had just married; both opted not to continue with the faculty on those terms.[91] In Washington and across the nation, 1873 was a year of acute economic depression and hardship, and it is significant that by October both men, like Bliss, found it expedient to seek re-election to the Medical Society.[92] After that, their careers picked up again. Reyburn returned to Georgetown as professor of histology, microscopy, and clinical surgery in 1874, and the following year Johnson joined the faculty as lecturer in obstetrics and the clinical diseases of women.[93] Johnson, who in time became Washington's most distinguished gynecologist, remained a professor at Georgetown for nearly four decades. Reyburn stayed four years, serving two years as dean. Then he returned to his beloved cause of educating medical students at Howard, where he remained a professor, and for the last seven years served as dean, until his death in 1909. The week after he died, the Medical Society of the District of Columbia met formally and in strength to eulogize the life of its erstwhile most rebellious member.94

❧

While this early civil rights movement waxed and waned, a man of mixed race—of part European and part African ancestry—was appointed prefect of studies (1867), then vice president (1869), and finally president (1874) of Georgetown College. In an era when radical new ideas were being promoted on what a "real university" should be, Patrick Healy's intellect, energy, and high standards made him the man for the times.

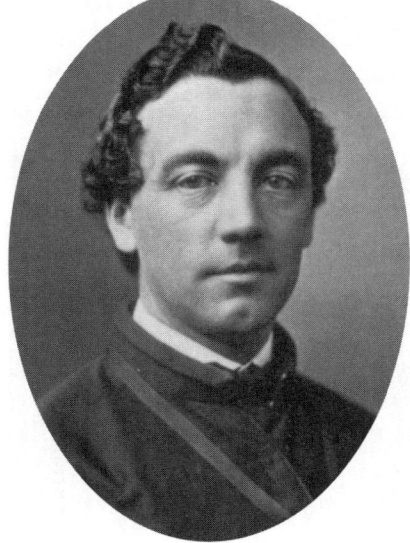

Reverend Patrick Healy, S.J., president of Georgetown University, 1873–82. Courtesy of Georgetown University Archives.

He was the son of Michael Healy, an immigrant Irish plantation owner who farmed cotton and corn near what is now Macon, Georgia, and one of his mulatto slaves, Eliza. Because of the antimiscegenation laws then strictly enforced, the couple could never marry legally, but they had ten children. Under Georgia law, the children were all counted as slaves. But by the time Michael died in August 1850, three months after his beloved Eliza, he had sent all of them to be educated at Catholic schools in the North— where de facto, they lived free. They were a remarkable clan. One son became the bishop of Portland, Maine; another, vicar general of the archdiocese of Boston; the three daughters became nuns, one rising to mother superior. Another son, Michael, sought a very different life. Having escaped from school by anchoring a rope to a statue of the Virgin Mary to climb over the wall, he ran away to sea and eventually became a captain of a cutter in the Revenue-Marine, forerunner of the U.S. Coast Guard. Known as "Hell-Roaring Mike" for his hard drinking and explosive temper, he was a brilliant seaman whose exploits patrolling the vast and dangerous waters off Alaska brought him national fame both as a heroic rescuer of shipwrecked sailors and as defendant in a notorious courtmartial.[95]

Patrick Healy lacked none of his family's ambition and flair; and, to their credit, his Jesuit superiors recognized his worth. Under his guidance, Georgetown College changed more nearly into a university as we understand the term today. He modernized its undergraduate curriculum, placing more emphasis on science and mathematics; he introduced new courses and raised standards of examination; he begged, borrowed, and ran the knife-edge of near-bankruptcy in order to erect the splendid Romanesque building which now bears his name. He also introduced a postgraduate program, and he correctly foresaw the roles of the medical school and the new law school, opened in 1870, as crucial to Georgetown's ultimate stature.[96]

The medical faculty was itself moving in the direction of reform. As early as March 1868, Noble Young had initiated discussion at faculty meetings on "the necessity of an early reorganization" and various attempts were begun to broaden and strengthen the curriculum.[97] Over the years that followed, new professors and lecturers were appointed to teach a wider range of subjects, such as the study of bones and tissues, and diseases of the eye and ear. In 1871, a "school of pharmacy"—actually not much more than a chair—was created; but it lasted only three years and graduated only nine students. And throughout the 1870s, supplementary courses held in the summer months signalled the growing trend toward specialization; among the topics covered were diseases of "the head and abdomen," "the throat, heart, and lungs," "the respiratory organs and laryngoscopy."[98]

In 1876, these piecemeal efforts to broaden the course gave way to a more dramatic change. After lengthy discussions with Healy, the medical faculty was sweepingly reorganized, and the curricular reforms which quickly followed brought the school to the highest ranks of nineteenth century medical education.

Georgetown's elder statesmen—Noble Young, now age sixty-eight; Flodoardo Howard, sixty-two; Johnson Eliot, sixty-one; and James Morgan, fifty-two—became professors emeriti, ceding their chairs to a

dynamic group of younger men.99 The new leadership included physicians who were already among the most celebrated in Washington and
others who would become so. Samuel Busey, who had been a professor at
the school in 1853–58, now returned at age forty-eight to occupy Young's
chair of medicine. A graduate of the University of Pennsylvania medical
school, he had practiced in Washington since 1848, sharing lodgings in
those early days with the young Abraham Lincoln. Later he served seven
terms as president of the Medical Society of D.C. and co-founded two city
hospitals. At the national level, he served as vice president of the AMA
(1877) and co-founded the American Gynecological Society, the American
Dermatological Association, the American Pediatric Society, and the
Association of American Physicians. A prolific writer, he was the leading
chronicler of the city's medical activities up to his death in 1901.[100] Busey
was now also elected vice president of the faculty, Young having retained
the presidency. As a faculty officer, he worked closely with the new dean,
none other than his recent adversary, Robert Reyburn, now professor of
anatomy. Reyburn's principal supporter in the AMA controversy of 1870,
Joseph Taber Johnson, succeeded Flodoardo Howard as professor of obstetrics and the diseases of women and children. And the former Confederate
soldier Francis Asbury Ashford was appointed to Johnson Eliot's long-
held chair as professor of surgery.

But it was another old Confederate, now the new professor of physiology, who led the crusade for curriculum reform at the school. Like so
many remarkable Georgetown professors, Carl Hermann Anton
Kleinschmidt was an immigrant. Born in Prussia and educated in
Westphalia, he arrived in the United States in 1857 at age eighteen, settled
with his parents in Georgetown, helped in their small store, learned
English, and began studying theology. But then, persuaded by
Georgetown's former professor of surgery John Snyder, he enrolled in the
medical school, graduating in 1862. Kleinschmidt was the young man who
chose the Southern cause, served three hard years as an assistant surgeon,
surrendered at Appomattox, and walked the two hundred miles back
home. He then left the country to further his study of medicine at the
University of Berlin.[101] That experience, like Liebermann's at the same
university thirty years earlier, radically influenced Kleinschmidt's thinking
on medical education.

In European medical schools, he wrote, the student "is not admitted to a final examination until after a curriculum from 3 to 7 years, and during all this period his studies are carefully graded, taking him from the lower to the higher branches. Moreover, in order to be promoted from a lower to a higher class, he must undergo a rigid examination. It is almost superfluous to add that clinical instruction and work in the chemical and physiological laboratories go hand in hand with didactic lectures." By contrast, in most American medical schools "as a rule we find a requirement of about 10 months of actual instruction, spread over a period of two years and of a pupillage of three years under some

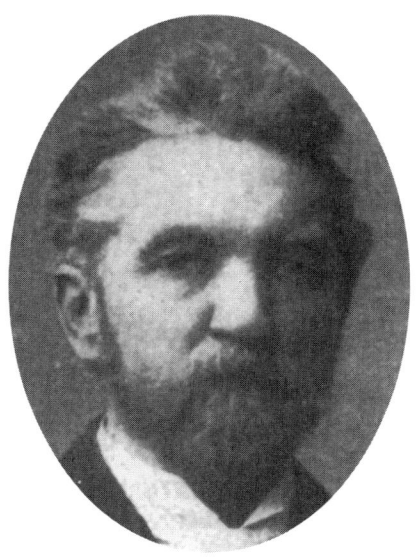

Carl Kleinschmidt, M.D., 1839–1905. Courtesy of the Medical Society of the District of Columbia.

practitioner in good standing; the latter, however, by no means insisted upon and generally only nominal." Scathingly, he inquired: "Would you confide the repairing of a valuable watch to the tender mercies of an apprentice of 10 months' experience in his calling?"

Compared to most schools, Georgetown's curriculum was reasonably progressive even before the reforms of 1876–78. Even so, it clearly fitted Kleinschmidt's blunt description of what was fundamentally wrong with American medical education:

> A student enters college, takes out his tickets and attends lectures; he may be utterly ignorant of anatomy and physiology, yet he is instructed in medicine, surgery and obstetrics, all of them presupposing a thorough knowledge of the structure and working of the organism. Whilst being initiated in the very A, B and C of the fundamental branches . . . his professor of medicine might be expounding on the etiology, pathology and treatment of the diseases of the heart, his professor of surgery the theory of

inflammation and the migration of the colorless corpuscles, and his professor of obstetrics the signs and symptoms of pregnancy. In other words, we have had no grading of subjects and the result has been that the student has yearly listened to the same lectures, his second course representing a "twice-told tale." Nothing can be less calculated to instruct, nothing can be more apt to bewilder the brain of the student, than this ruinous mode of lecturing to a mixed class upon all branches at once. . . . Yet this repetitional system has, with us, become the order of the day, and we have taken heed of neither proficiency nor deficiency in the student, but have seemingly been intent upon the one thing, the manufacture of physicians in the shortest possible time. . . . Our medical institutions have rested content with the status of over 50 years ago and some of them have actually lowered the standard. Medicine has widened its field and scope, and our college curricula have been contracted, thus presenting an anomalous condition not seen elsewhere in the civilized world.

Strong words. They come from Kleinschmidt's paper "The Necessity for a Higher Standard of Medical Education," which was published after he delivered it as the introductory address at the opening of the medical school's 1878–79 session.[102] Clearly it expressed Kleinschmidt's own deep convictions. Much more, however, was it the public justification of a daring policy that the faculty, with the full backing of Patrick Healy, had decided upon. Georgetown now made it obligatory for its medical students to take a three-year course. Two months were added to each winter session, and an optional two-month summer course was offered, so that a total of nine months' instruction was available each year. The course was carefully graded; students were required to undergo regular tests; and to advance they had to pass, by an aggregate score of 65 percent, an annual written examination of three hours in each branch (with the same questions now asked of each candidate). Daily lectures were reduced from four or five to two or three, to give students more time to absorb what they had heard and for private study in the textbooks that were now abundant. More emphasis was laid on practical anatomy, experiments, and clinical instruction, to "teach the student," Kleinschmidt explained, "not only to *know*, but also to render him capable to *do*."[103]

This sudden raising of standards was an extraordinarily courageous step for Georgetown to take—and a risky one. Very few American medical schools had yet adopted a three-year course: Chicago had pioneered it in 1859, though only as an option, and only a minority of students chose it over the standard two-year course; Harvard had followed in 1871, Pennsylvania in 1877.[104] The immediate result at Harvard, as Kleinschmidt pointed out, had been "a heavy monetary loss . . . simply because students found it less troublesome to matriculate at schools where the old plan was still in force." Pennsylvania, indeed, had gone ahead only when "generous friends of the institution" agreed to underwrite its losses if enrollment temporarily fell. The outlook for Georgetown, a school without endowments or rich benefactors, was far bleaker.

Enrollments had already fallen, dropping from 113 in 1868–69 to 35 in 1876–77, the year when the decision to reform was made.[105] To ease the inevitable blow, the faculty made two concessions: it stopped short of requiring students to take a preliminary examination before matriculation— an omission, Kleinschmidt said, the faculty intended to rectify "at no distant day"—and in 1880 it cut the annual tuition fees to their pre–Civil War level of one hundred dollars.[106] Despite this, numbers sank to a low of 26 in 1882–83 and rose no higher than 47 until nearly the end of the 1880s. For years, Georgetown had to compete with schools that still awarded medical degrees to students who had completed less demanding work in only ten months of study. When the newly-established Association of American Medical Colleges passed a resolution in 1880 requiring each of its members to establish the three-year graded course, several schools withdrew from the association rather than comply.[107] Even by 1890 only 26 out of 127 schools nationwide had done so.[108]

They were difficult times, and the faculty frequently dipped into their own pockets to keep the school running. They could expect no financial help from the university, which itself was in dire straits. In April 1879, while Patrick Healy was crossing the country in search of donations to fund the new building, his deputy wrote desperately: "There is no money. I have borrowed from friends for short intervals. . . . I have spent all the money received for tuition."[109] Healy could give the medical professors only moral support; but this he did, backing their brave endeavor with the strength of his own reforming zeal. He proudly paid public tribute to "their strenuous efforts for the advancement of medical education [which] I have not suggested, but approved; not guided, but seconded." He publicly commended them for having acted "out of regard for their profession, casting aside all thought of emoluments . . . paying, in fact, where they should have received," and for having "stepped unhesitatingly into the advanced ranks and marched abreast with the oldest and best medical institutions in the country."[110]

⋘⊙

Although Johnson Eliot relinquished the chair of surgery in 1876 after sixteen years' tenure, he ceased neither clinical teaching nor his demanding medical practice. In the twenty-five years since the opening of the medical school, he had raised six children with his wife, Mary, had generated a large income which he lavished on charitable causes, and had risen high in the esteem of his peers. His operations at Providence and several other Washington hospitals drew large crowds of colleagues and students.

George Kober, who had learned surgery from Eliot at Georgetown in the years 1871–73, and followed in his footsteps to become dean of the medical school, described him as "a thorough anatomist, a bold and deliberate operator" and one of the pioneers of ovariotomy in Washington. Eliot's "brilliant operations," as Kober called them, included three cases of removal of the superior maxilla, two cases of amputation at the hip joint, one of the early successful excisions of the head of the humerus, two cases of removal of palatopharyngeal sarcoma, ligation of the subclavian artery, and simultaneous amputation of both legs.[111] But the operation for which Eliot was most admired was a procedure rarely attempted before: the simultaneous ligation of the carotid and subclavian arteries for aneurism of the innominate artery.

He performed it on Sunday morning, October 12, 1876, at Providence Hospital, on a forty-one-year-old black man whose condition—a pulsating tumor "the size of a man's fist" on his neck—was clearly hopeless. Eliot was assisted by his successor at Georgetown, Francis Ashford, and by Robert Reyburn. The throng of spectators included Carl Kleinschmidt and Joseph Taber Johnson; Surgeon General Philip Wales of the U.S. Navy; Army Surgeon George Otis, editor of the great *Medical and Surgical History of the Civil War*; Eliot's son, Llewellyn; and a visiting professor of surgery from "Warsaw Medical College, Russia."

Johnson Eliot's own published account of this operation reveals a great deal about both surgical practice of the time and the way surgeons then wrote "scientific" papers. The details were vague: "About seven or eight cases," Eliot began, "have been reported up to the present time." The style was dramatic and self-serving: the patient "begged earnestly for relief, and expressed his willingness to undergo any mode of treatment that afforded the slightest hope of prolonging his life." References to previous attempts were brief and imprecise: "Rossi's case died in six days; Heath's recovered . . ." with no effort to explain who these surgeons were. The operation itself, performed with an unspecified anesthetic, warranted a single sentence: "I proceeded to ligate the primitive carotid in its upper cervical region, and immediately afterwards tied the subclavian in the third surgical division."

The rest of the paper described in detail the postoperative care and steadily deteriorating condition of the patient through the twenty-five days before he died. To a modern reader, the observations clearly document the progress of infection and fever to the point of delirium—and incidentally suggest that Eliot either cut or tied the patient's right recurrent laryngeal nerve and paralysed his right vocal cord, which would explain his reported difficulty in swallowing and breathing. But Eliot—rejecting, or perhaps still not even aware of, the existence of bacteria—could not read the symptoms correctly. He concluded, albeit with reservations, that death was due to blood loss. "There can be no question as to the cause of the poor fellow's death," he began confidently, but then had to admit that "losing 36 or 38 ounces in the course of 25 days . . . was not thought sufficient to have caused his death." The learned professor Thomas Antisell suggested a way out of the difficulty: the clot of the aneurism itself, he calculated, "would be equal to 5 pounds 13 ounces which, with the hemorrhages, about 38 ounces, would represent a total loss of blood to the system of 8 pounds 3 ounces . . . [leaving] only 1 pound 13 ounces at the time of death."[112]

So the patient died and the case contributed nothing to medical knowledge. But the operation was celebrated in Washington and much enhanced Eliot's reputation. In these last years of old-style surgery, before germ theory and aseptic principles ushered in a new era, experienced surgeons who attempted difficult procedures with confidence and steady hands were held in awe as masters of the profession. And the operations themselves, with the surgeon the focus of fascinated attention in the amphitheater, provided excellent publicity. Compared to many surgeons of his day, Eliot was not a vain or self-promoting man. But it was probably no accident that he performed that simultaneous ligation on a Sunday, three days after admitting his patient to the hospital. All but the most urgent operations in the amphitheaters were done on weekends, when students, other physicians, and the public had the time to attend.[113]

Francis Asbury Ashford succeeded Eliot in 1876 as Georgetown's new professor of surgery. He was thirty-five, he had graduated from Columbian only nine years earlier, and his meteoric career marks him as a young man in a hurry, eager to catch up after four years sacrificed to war. Born on September 14, 1841, on his grandfather's farm in Fairfax County, Virginia, but reared mainly in Washington, Ashford had returned to the farm and was running it, as a youth of nineteen, when the Civil War began. Enlisting at once, he served throughout the conflict in the Confederate Army of Northern Virginia, fighting every battle and rising to second, then first, lieutenant. He was, a contemporary noted, "often specially detailed for the execution of orders of the most delicate character and requiring the exercise of unflinching bravery and coolness of judgment."[114] Those same qualities would make him a fine surgeon.

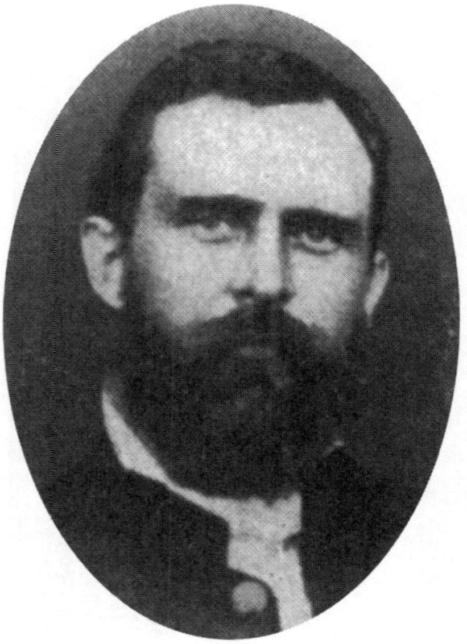

Francis Asbury Ashford, M.D., 1841–83. Courtesy of the Medical Society of the District of Columbia.

Ashford was a handsome man whose "powerful and attractive personality" quickly won him friends in the Washington medical community as it had in the army. Released on oath of allegiance to the Union in June, 1865, after two months' imprisonment at Johnson's Island, he began studying medicine with one of Washington's most prominent physicians, Thomas Miller, who came to regard him as a second son. Miller's house on F Street had been known during the war as the city's headquarters for Southern sympathizers, and afterwards he often entertained former Confederate officers, including the generals Lee, Beauregard, and Longstreet. Jefferson Davis's wife even stayed there while her husband was a prisoner at Fort Monroe.[115] Ashford also took the medical course at Columbian, graduating in 1867. He immediately secured a position as John Harry Thompson's assistant in surgery at the Columbia Hospital for Women, and began to build a practice, sharing an office at 1731 Pennsylvania Avenue with Samuel Busey. Three years later they founded Children's Hospital together.

A tiny structure compared to its modern counterpart, the original Children's Hospital was one block away from the medical school on E Street and had only twelve beds and a small outpatient dispensary.[116] But it made Ashford's name. "With the admission of the first patient to the hospital, February 11, 1871, who was suffering from hip-joint disease, he began his practical studies of the joint afflictions of children," Busey recalled. "During the 12 succeeding years he devoted himself to this branch of surgery. . . . The records of the hospital attest the brilliant results he had attained in this special department, as well as in the wider field of general surgery, and the surgical ward will ever remain a monument to his skill, good judgment and operative dexterity."[117]

By 1872, Ashford was prospering enough to marry Isabella Kelly and start a family. Thereafter he earned success in obstetrics and gynecology— being specially admired for his surgery on women's pelvic organs—as well as the diseases of children. In Washington winters, his sleigh was a familiar sight as he drove through the snow to visit patients at home and in hospital. In 1874, the Georgetown faculty invited him to deliver a course of lectures on orthopedic surgery at Children's.[118] and then, in the reorganization of 1876, appointed him to the chair of surgery. Ashford was popular among the students. One passing reference to him, by a self-styled "disciple" in Georgetown's *College Journal*, suggests that he even allowed seniors to operate under his supervision, decades before any kind of residency system was introduced in the United States: "In operative surgery, he not only himself performed the various operations from the simplest to the most capital, but even had the members of the graduating class, in turn, repeat the same at the weekly rehearsals."[119]

In another way, too, Ashford proved himself a progressive: he was among the first in Washington—and, indeed, in the world—to own a telephone. Using Alexander Graham's Bell's revolutionary apparatus, he could speak remotely to Samuel Busey and Children's Hospital, two more of the city's original 188 telephone subscribers in 1878.[120]

Ashford's election as dean of the Georgetown faculty in 1878 sealed his local reputation. But he was not one to rest content on past success. Having helped found one hospital, he now became determined to organize another. For over twenty years, Washington physicians had tried without success to establish a general hospital—defined as one that gave comprehensive treatment to the poor free of charge. Of the hospitals then in the District of Columbia, Providence offered general care but mainly for paying patients; the Central Dispensary and Emergency Hospital (originally set up next to Georgetown's school in 1871 by some of its professors[121]) treated the poor, but only on an outpatient or emergency basis; Columbia was exclusively for the diseases of women; Children's offered pediatric care; the Freedmen's was for black patients; and the old Alms House, according to a protest petition signed by over eighty local doctors, accommodated "about 150 patients, in which the vicious, criminal, vagrant and a few deserving paupers are promiscuously commingled as one class." In May 1874, Carl Kleinschmidt and a colleague had opened a general hospital in Georgetown, but less than two years later a lack of financial support forced them to close it. The crusade for a general hospital, one contemporary noted, "was never successful until Ashford took the helm" in 1877.[122]

Even Ashford's driving energy failed to ignite public feelings, however, until an event occurred that horrified Washington and the nation. At 9:30 on the morning of July 2, 1881, President James Garfield was shot by Charles Guiteau at the Baltimore and Potomac railroad station in Washington. A bullet entered Garfield's back, near the spine. The wounded president lingered for eleven weeks, and his death brought scenes of mourning vividly reminiscent of Lincoln's assassination only sixteen years before. Amid the anger and grief, one Lewis J. Davis wrote a letter to the *Washington Evening Star* proposing that a hospital in Garfield's memory be erected at the railroad station where he had been shot. Ashford immediately contacted Davis, and as a result of their efforts the idea caught on.[123] Subscriptions poured in, and on May 18, 1882, the charter for the Garfield Memorial Hospital (although not at the site of the assassination) was approved by Congress.

❧

As never before, the shooting of President Garfield focused the nation's attention on surgery. Newspapers reported his wounds, medical treatment, and death in such detail that, one biographer noted in 1892, "many surgical methods and many technical terms, which hitherto had been the exclusive property of the profession, became perfectly familiar with all."[124] The national debate centered on one question: was the wound mortal, or could the physicians have saved Garfield's life?

Altogether, thirteen doctors attended the wounded president or were called in for consultation. The best known was David Hayes Agnew, professor of surgery at the University of Pennsylvania, whose journey from Philadelphia to Washington on the night of the shooting set a new train speed record.[125] But the two who cared daily for Garfield from the first examination in an upstairs room at the railroad depot, through two months at the White House, to his death in New Jersey on September 19, were his personal physician D. W. Bliss (now restored to eminence after making his peace with the Medical Society) and Robert Reyburn.

Reyburn was summoned to the depot by Bliss about fifteen minutes after the shooting. "Hastening upstairs on my arrival," he wrote later, "I saw President Garfield lying on a mattress on the floor . . . I asked him, 'Mr. President, are you badly hurt?' He answered, 'I'm afraid I am.' The President was deathly pale, almost pulseless and apparently dying from internal hemorrhage." To everyone's surprise, since the bullet eluded probes and remained lodged deep in his body, Garfield survived both the journey to the White House and the night, and after a few days seemed to recover. Bliss continued as surgeon-in-charge and appointed three assistants: Surgeon General Joseph Barnes, who came twice a day to consult; and also Reyburn and army surgeon Joseph Woodward, who attended three times a day to make routine checks on temperature and pulse, took notes and issued bulletins, and slept alternate nights at the White House.

No surgery was performed; treatment was limited to changing the patient's dressings. To prevent bedsores, the paralyzed president, a man over six feet tall and weighing two hundred pounds, had to be turned in bed "fifty, sixty, sometimes 100 times a day" in summer heat exceeding ninety degrees. But, though tedious, his care was politically delicate. Out of Garfield's hearing, there were disagreements over the wording of the medical bulletins. Bliss wanted no mention of unfavorable symptoms or developments because the president always read the newspapers. "We were placed in a very embarrassing position," Reyburn wrote, implying that he and Woodward favored more truthful bulletins.

Mail poured into the White House by the bushel, bringing not only good wishes from Queen Victoria and all the other crowned heads of Europe but quantities of unsolicited advice. "Every crank and vendor of patent medicines in the country seemed to think himself called upon to offer to cure the President. One man gravely suggested that the President's body should be inverted for some hours in order that the bullet might gravitate downward and thus aid its removal," Reyburn recalled. Another sent a sketch of a machine designed to draw out the bullet by suction. In fact, the team of physicians did very little, but they did it meticulously well. At a time when Listerian practices were still not fully accepted, Garfield's wound was dressed antiseptically throughout the long weeks he lingered, according to Reyburn. "The most scrupulous cleanliness of the instruments and surgical appliances was observed, and also of the antiseptic solutions used for the daily washing out of the wound, and every effort was made to make them as aseptic as possible. The carbolic spray was also invariably used during the dressing of the wound."

After Garfield died, the physicians faced a blitz of criticism expressed through the newspapers for allowing him to journey to New Jersey to convalesce (which in fact they had vehemently resisted) and for not attempting heroic surgery. Had they done so, though, Garfield would probably not have lasted as long as he did. Long afterwards, Reyburn remained convinced that:

> . . . the President was mortally wounded when he received the fatal shot.
> . . . The immediate cause of his death was the spontaneous rupture of a traumatic aneurism formed on the splenic artery, probably as a result of

the abrasion of the outer coats of this blood vessel by the bullet at the time of shooting. This was a complication that could neither be foreseen nor prevented . . . The proximate cause of his death (and one that would have inevitably soon terminated his life, even had the bursting of the aneurism not taken place) was the profound condition of septic poisoning which existed in the case of the President for a considerable time previous to his death.[126]

﹏

Garfield's death was seen as a national tragedy. But Georgetown medical school was more profoundly affected by four other losses that afflicted them over the next two years. In February 1882, Patrick Healy, stricken down by increasing ill health, resigned the presidency of Georgetown University. To the medical faculty, he wrote: "I desire that my last official act should be this expression of my gratitude towards those who so ably cooperated with me in the cause of education."[127] Healy survived, a sick man, for another thirty years, twice the time he had served at Georgetown.[128] But during his tenure he had transformed the university and established, more than any of his predecessors, a close relationship of mutual regard with the medical school.

A year after Healy left Georgetown, the first of the medical school's founders died. Noble Young, thought to be the oldest physician then practicing in Washington, died at age seventy-four on April 11, 1883, while visiting his married daughter at Sacketts Harbor, New York. Brought back to the city, his coffin was followed to Congressional Cemetery by a huge crowd of colleagues, civic dignitaries, former students, and patients.[129] Eight months later, the school lost another founder, Johnson Eliot, who had been working right up to the time he contracted pneumonia a week before his death on December 30, 1883, at the age of sixty-eight.[130] Of the remaining founders, Charles Liebermann survived another three years, beyond his seventy-second birthday, to March 26, 1886; he was buried in Rock Creek Cemetery, his grave marked by a granite monument twelve feet high.[131] Flodoardo Howard outlived them all; widowed in 1883, he married again two years later at age seventy-one, signing a prenuptial agreement which, on his death in January 1888, conveyed to his new wife both his

Washington house and his Rockville estate—to the dismay, presumably, of his four grown children.[132]

But one death shocked the medical faculty more than the others. Francis Ashford succumbed to a heart attack at his home on New York Avenue on May 19, 1883. He was forty-one years old. He had fallen ill a week earlier and summoned his colleagues to the house to resign his position as dean of the faculty and to transfer its accounts and records to his successor. The other professors offered to cover his busy medical practice between them, "so that its emoluments [will be] secured to you during this period of temporary retirement," Busey confirmed in a letter to Ashford the same day.[133] But on the evening of May 18, as Busey and others were at a meeting of the Washington Obstetric and Gynecological Society (which Ashford had co-founded a year earlier), word came that he was dying.[134]

Ashford's untimely death left his widow with a one-month-old daughter and four young sons—the eldest of whom, Bailey K. Ashford, was destined to become one of Georgetown medical school's most distinguished graduates as an internationally-famous pioneer in tropical diseases. Bailey, not quite ten years old at his father's death, wrote much later that Ashford had been not only a brilliant and remarkably energetic man, but one much loved by colleagues, students, and patients alike; a man of means who daily treated poor patients free of charge.[135] That was more than filial piety. Every Washington institution Ashford had helped establish or been involved with in his truncated career went into deep mourning; Children's Hospital draped swathes of black crepe over the pictures and statuary in its lobby.[136] And the Georgetown medical faculty, stunned by its loss, set about trying to find a new professor of surgery.

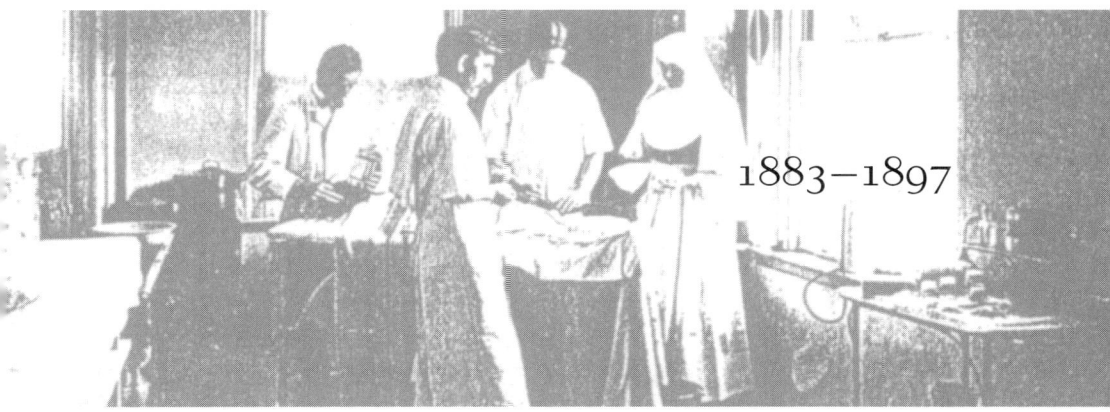

CHAPTER FOUR

ASEPTIC SURGERY, SPECIALIZATION, & THE END OF "SUNDOWN MEDICINE"

THE MAN CHOSEN to be Georgetown's fifth professor of surgery was very different from the unassuming Eliot or the beloved Ashford. John Brown Hamilton was a man of overwhelming presence—a forceful, aggressive egocentric who relished political and intellectual combat and cared little if he made enemies in the process. He was also an excellent surgeon and an able administrator who delighted in juggling several demanding appointments simultaneously.

Hamilton was already nationally known—having become, in 1879, the second surgeon general of the United States Marine Hospital Service (MHS). This organization was the first federal agency to coordinate any kind of health activities nationwide. A uniformed service modeled on the military structures of the U.S. Army and Navy medical corps (each of which had its own surgeon general), the MHS then mainly provided medical care for merchant seamen. Later, in part due to Hamilton's efforts, it evolved into the U.S. Public Health Service.

Born on an Illinois farm in 1847, Hamilton had served as a seventeen-year-old Unionist soldier in the last year of the Civil War. After graduating from Rush Medical College, Chicago, in 1869, he worked for several years as an assistant surgeon in the army, and joined the Marine Hospital Service in 1876.[1] There he climbed from the bottom of its ladder to the top rung in

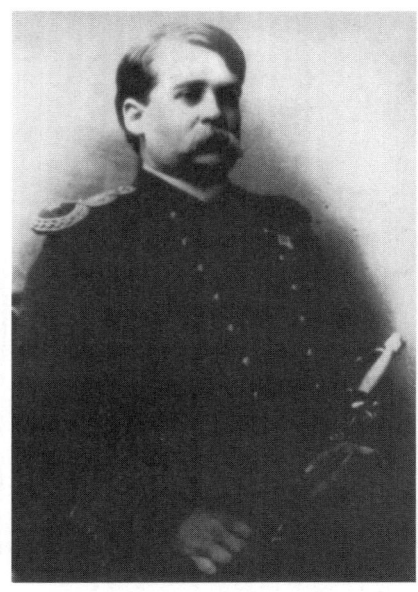

ABOVE
John Brown Hamilton, M.D., 1847–98. Courtesy of the National Library of Medicine.

just three years. As surgeon general of the MHS, he proved remarkably able—implementing the first national quarantine laws; winning from Congress the right to quarantine foreign ships entering American ports if contagious diseases were found on board; bringing in a system to prevent the transmission of those diseases from state to state; and insisting that merchant seamen be examined and passed as physically fit before enlisting.[2] When he accepted the chair of surgery at Georgetown in early November 1883, he was thirty-five years old and riding high in the headlines for his success in containing an outbreak of the dreaded yellow fever in Brownsville, Texas.

Hamilton's appointment, nearly six months after Ashford's death, did not please everyone. That same day, a student asked for his fees back, telling the dean he no longer desired to continue his course now that James Shields Beale, the former anatomy professor who had stepped in to teach surgery for the first two months of the session, had been "superseded by another professor."[3] But higher authority, in the person of the Reverend James A. Doonan, S.J., Healy's successor as president of the university, wrote to "heartily congratulate" the dean on acquiring Hamilton for the faculty.[4]

Everyone who knew Hamilton, even those who disliked him, had to admire his energy. In the words of his friend Llewellyn Eliot, he was "a man with unlimited capacity for work."[5] In his eight years as professor of surgery, Hamilton delivered his evening lectures at the medical school, took part in faculty meetings, ran a full surgical service at Providence Hospital, and regarded all this as partial employment. During the same period he continued to head the Marine Hospital Service, directed quarantine operations in the field, gathered data on unseaworthy vessels and infectious diseases, wrote reports and attended hearings, and constantly lobbied Congress to raise the authority of the MHS and give it equal standing with the Army and Navy Medical Corps.[6] He enjoyed both the work and the status, making it clear to his medical students that he liked to be addressed as "General Hamilton."[7]

In 1887, he also served as secretary general of the Ninth International Medical Congress. Held in Washington, it attracted physicians from twenty countries and was formally opened by the president of the United States, Grover Cleveland. Hamilton was responsible for producing the transactions of the Medical Congress: the texts of hundreds of papers read by delegates—some in their original German and French—and the comments offered in discussion. The compilation ran to five thick volumes, each containing more than seven hundred pages. Characteristically, Hamilton completed this mammoth task in ten months.[8] Three years later, he led the American delegation to the Tenth International Medical Congress in Berlin, a gathering distinguished by the presence of Joseph Lister and Robert Koch and by the delegates' unqualified endorsement, at long last, of antiseptic practices.[9] During his years at Georgetown, Hamilton also served as president of the first Pan-American Medical Congress, was twice elected vice president of the D.C. Medical Society, attended professional meetings at home and abroad, and still found the energy to turn out medical papers and books.

If Hamilton took any time off work at all, he seems to have spent it in plotting. His archenemies were the members of the recently established National Board of Health which, because it too had powers to enforce the quarantine laws, he saw as a rival to his own Marine Hospital Service.[10] Early in 1884, the board sought to discredit Hamilton's handling of the 1882 Brownsville yellow fever outbreak. Despite the newspaper headlines— "Public Health: Grave Charges of Inefficiency Against Surgeon General Hamilton"[11]—the board's case rested mainly on a complaint from a ferry boat owner, whose business had been halted by Hamilton's instructions to keep all travellers out of the Brownsville area, a safeguard which required securing a quarantine line over three hundred miles long. On February 14, 1884, Hamilton appeared before a congressional committee of inquiry in full fettle. He insisted on recalling every detail of the Brownsville operation, citing every communication he had received that endorsed its success, and dissecting and rejecting each of his accusers' points with surgical precision—so exhaustively that the weary committee members were obliged to extend the hearing into another day.[12] Hamilton routed his opponents on that occasion, and soon afterwards persuaded Congress to end the board's jurisdiction over quarantine, thereby destroying it.[13] His plotting, like his presentation at the hearing, typified the man: thorough, determined, and self-confident to the point of arrogance.

The same characteristics marked Hamilton's approach to surgery. His most famous operation was performed on Saturday, July 11, 1885.[14] That afternoon a nineteen-year-old waiter, carelessly handling a .32 caliber pistol, had shot himself in the abdomen, causing extensive internal injuries. The young man was brought to Hamilton at Providence Hospital. Until that day, only three successful operations for gunshot wounds of the abdomen had ever been recorded—two in the United States and one in Berne, Switzerland—and the textbooks still advised against surgical interference.[15] But Hamilton did not hesitate. "It is only by the reports of cases where an actual test is made upon the human subject that the truth will ultimately prevail," he declared in his account of the case.

Joseph Taber Johnson, then president of the Georgetown medical faculty, called it "one of the most skilful operations I have ever witnessed."[16] He described how Hamilton "cut open this man's abdomen, found and ligated the bleeding vessels, and safely stitched together not less than 13 intestinal wounds, any one of which would surely have caused death."[17]

The bullet had entered an inch to the right and above the navel; passing downward and inward under the rectus muscle, it had then entered the abdominal cavity. In Hamilton's precise words:

An incision was made in the linea alba about 6 inches long, the peritoneum raised and incised. A spurting artery was seen in the mesentery and the abdominal cavity was full of blood. The artery was immediately tied with a fine catgut ligature, the intestines drawn out loop by loop and the wounds stitched with Lembert's suture as fast as they could be reached. Eleven wounds requiring suture were found in the small intestine and two in the ascending colon. The wounds varied from a mere nick in the wall of the intestine to those where the ball had passed directly through it and all were everted, the mucus surface pouting.[18]

The patient made a complete recovery and in due course left the hospital ("without a word of thanks," Johnson commented), oblivious to how his life had been saved by Hamilton's boldness. More than two years later, the leading American authority on gunshot wounds of the abdomen, Charles T. Parkes of Chicago, spoke on the subject at the Ninth International Medical Congress. By then, thirty-six attempts had been recorded—nine had been successful—but Parkes still declined to commit himself on whether surgical interference was preferable to "conservative management."[19] The international debate on whether to perform surgery in such cases continued well beyond World War I.[20] But it is clear that as early as 1885, John Brown Hamilton—who concluded his own account by quoting surgeons from 1676 onwards who believed, like himself, that surgery should be attempted for abdominal injury—entertained no doubts whatsoever.

Barely nine years had elapsed between Johnson Eliot's most admired operative failure and Hamilton's triumphant success. But during that time, surgeons in Washington, as elsewhere, had finally begun to use antiseptics in the operating room. The revolution that would transform surgical practice was under way. Surgeons began at last to accept that the most powerful threat to their professional success, the factor that frequently determined their patients' recovery or death, was something they could not see.

Enlightenment had been a painfully slow process. Observations and experiments indicating the probable existence of invisible organisms as the cause of infection, their transmission by air or direct contact, and even their destruction by extreme heat or cold, had been recorded intermittently since the Italian physician Fracastoro had accurately described all these components of germ theory in a remarkable treatise published in 1546.[21] But such insights were ignored by the medical community even when the occasional perceptive practitioner produced results that supported the premise.

The greatest of these was Ignazc Semmelweis, a young Hungarian obstetrician practicing in Vienna. In March 1847, he noticed that a colleague who had died after pricking his finger during an autopsy exhibited symptoms identical to those of women who died from puerperal fever, and by painstaking investigation he correctly deduced how the infection was spread: "The carrier," he wrote, "is the examining finger, the operating hand, instruments, bed linen, atmospheric air, sponges . . . anything contaminated with decomposed animal organic material that comes in contact with the vaginal tract of the parturient." Moreover, Semmelweis immediately instituted a protocol for the rigorous scrubbing of hands, instruments, linens, and dressings, first with soap and water and then again with dilute chlorine, before every delivery. The result was that maternal mortality from puerperal fever dropped from 12 to 1 percent at the Vienna general hospital. "The significance of this experience for obstetrics and surgical wards is immeasurable," its director wrote, "and deserves the earnest attention of all men of science and recognition by the highest governmental authority." But for decades it received neither. Twenty years were to elapse before other Austrian and German obstetricians began to emulate Semmelweis's aseptic methods; thirty years before they were first used in surgery; nearly fifty years before they became standard practice. Semmelweis himself, more scorned than admired, was dismissed from his position in Vienna and returned to Budapest. There he continued to protect women from puerperal fever, until he died—ironically, from a septic cut on the hand—in 1865, the year that Joseph Lister began his researches on antiseptics for wound management.[22]

Semmelweis's discoveries, it is now recognized, were of more profound significance to surgery than those of Lister. Semmelweis realized that infection was transmitted mainly by contact, particularly by the physician's hands; for several years Lister, by contrast, believed that contamination came largely from airborne organisms and avoided scrubbing his hands. Lister's antiseptic sprays and solutions destroyed or retarded bacterial growth already present; Semmelweis's aseptic methods prevented bacteria from even entering the body. Semmelweis's prophylactic approach eventually became standard surgical practice; as soon as the sterilization of instruments and dressings had superseded disinfectants, Lister's antiseptics were relegated to first aid.[23]

But Lister had timing, publicity, and science on his side. His outstanding contributions were to demonstrate empirically that wound infections were caused by bacteria; to apply that knowledge to operating rooms and hospital wards; and to proselytize antiseptic practices throughout Europe and in the United States. His work, based initially on Pasteur's early research on putre-faction, published in 1864, was steadily vindicated in the laboratory: by Pasteur's landmark paper in 1878 on germ theory and its application to medi-cine and surgery; and by Koch's etiological proof, published the same year, that wound infections were caused by pus-producing organisms.[24]

By that time, the aseptic approach had also been vindicated by the German gynecologist Alfred Hegar, who was the first to use Semmelweis's techniques in surgery. In 1876–77, Hegar performed fifteen consecutive successful ovariotomies, an operation which normally carried a 60 percent mortality rate. Hegar not only insisted on scrupulous chlorination of hands, forearms, instruments, sponges, and sutures; he even forbade students from attending the operation unless they could prove they had not been with an infectious patient, at a postmortem, or in an anatomy room for at least five days beforehand.[25] Yet these practices, commonsensical to modern minds, were adopted much more slowly than Lister's.

In 1885, when John Hamilton performed his abdominal surgery for gunshot wound, even Listerian practices were still not entirely accepted. Two years earlier, a debate on antiseptics at the first meeting of the American Surgical Association revealed lingering skepticism—enough for a Philadelphia surgeon who wrote a review of operative practice in 1885 to declare that antiseptic surgery was "still *sub judice.*"[26] Hamilton did not share that view. He used antiseptics, including carbolized ligatures, iodized dressings, and a solution of bichloride of mercury (a corrosive agent which damaged tissue but was commonly used until after World War I[27]) to sponge the abdominal cavity. This places him among the enlightened—ahead, for example, of the great German surgeon Ernst von Bergmann, who did not capitulate until 1890 when Lister visited his clinic in Berlin.[28] In other practices, though, Hamilton remained very much of his time, on the cusp between old-fashioned and modern surgery. He did not scrub, nor cover his street clothes, for his famed abdominal operation; and when the patient complained postoperatively of pain in the scrotum (later diagnosed as being due to a rectal hematoma), he had six leeches applied.[29]

It is significant, however, that less than two years later, in August 1887, Hamilton established the first laboratory devoted to bacteriological research in the United States: the federally funded National Laboratory of Hygiene

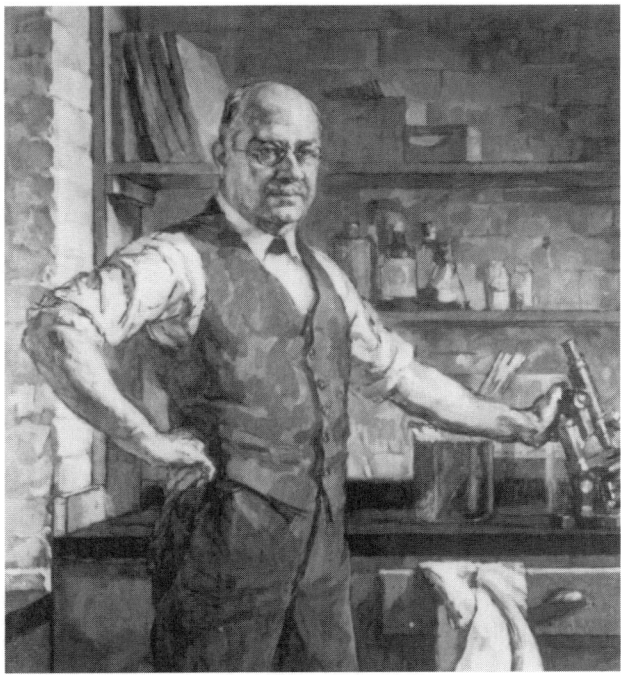

Joseph Kinyoun in his laboratory, from a
portrait painted by Lenhard Walmsley.
Courtesy of the National Library of Medicine.

at the Marine Hospital on Staten Island, in New York City's harbor. Undoubtedly, his motivation was in part political. The National Board of Health, stripped of its quarantine powers and moribund, was proposing to reinvent itself as a federal agency by conducting "continuous scientific investigations" into matters of public health. Hamilton moved fast to thwart this. When the House of Representatives Commerce Committee held hearings on the proposals in 1888, Hamilton dropped his well-timed bombshell: the Marine Hospital Service *already* had a laboratory performing such investigations, he announced.[30] Yet Hamilton was truly a progressive, utterly convinced of the importance of science to the future of medicine. "The business of the sanitarian today demands more than to wage a war of extermination against the unfortunate microbe," he said that same year. Young physicians should consider themselves lucky, he added, "in being sent out in an age when medical institutions seek to make experimental research the cornerstone of the medical superstructure."[31]

It was, in fact, a young physician who made Hamilton's preemptive venture into research such a resounding success. Joseph James Kinyoun had joined the MHS in 1886 with superlative qualifications: he had studied bacteriology with Robert Koch in Berlin and with Elie Metchnikoff at the Pasteur Institute in Paris. Hamilton, recognizing talent, appointed Kinyoun to direct the new laboratory—just one room—and had it equipped with apparatus similar to that used by Koch, including the latest Zeiss microscopic and microphotographic lenses. In his first year as director, Kinyoun tested the waters of New York harbor—and made the first bacteriological identification of cholera in the western hemisphere.[32]

In 1890, the laboratory moved from Staten Island to Washington. This was a windfall for Georgetown, because Hamilton made sure that Kinyoun, while continuing to direct it, also joined the faculty to teach bacteriology.[33] His expertise immensely improved the students' grasp of this new branch of basic science. When in 1894 he became the first in the U.S. to test and produce diphtheria antitoxin—only months after witnessing Emile Roux's first production of the vaccine in Paris—some of Kinyoun's investigations were in fact performed in Georgetown's own modest laboratory, which he had equipped at his own expense.[34] Though achieving no great discoveries himself, his major contributions to public health made him one of the leading figures of nineteenth century American science. The National Laboratory that Hamilton and Kinyoun established became, in the early twentieth century, the government's principal research and regulatory agency. Today, it is recognized as the pioneering forerunner of the National Institutes of Health.[35]

As discoveries proliferated, "progress" became the buzzword of those late years of the nineteenth century. From the bacteria revealed by the microscope to inventions like the telephone and electric light, science and technology promised to make life safer and easier for many; and for the industrialists who used that new knowledge to exploit the resources of an untapped continent in the service of mass production, the discoveries

brought unimaginable wealth. That wealth bred philanthropy, as the
"robber barons" began to divert some of their gains to charitable
endeavors—a development that did not go unnoticed at Georgetown.

Speaking to the medical alumni at their annual dinner in June 1886,
John Hamilton declared:

> The medical school looked over to New York and saw the great laboratory
> founded by the Pittsburgh iron merchant Andrew Carnegie; the
> $500,000 college building given by Vanderbilt; the $200,000 building
> now nearing completion in Cleveland, and we felt that unless help came
> from some quarter we could no longer with credit to the University main-
> tain a separate department. The ill-provided building on E Street, occupied
> for so many years, was inadequate for the purposes of medical teaching;
> this age of learning had left our school behind in the march of progress.[36]

Once again, a new building had become necessary; and this time the
faculty had built its own at a cost of $50,000. The professors formed a
corporation and borrowed most of the money, but they also persuaded the
easygoing university president, James Doonan, to pay the interest on the
loan and also to invest $18,600 of university money in the construction.[37]
It was the first funding the medical school had received from the university;
and it marked the end of nearly forty years of independence. But the
geographical separation remained. The new school—a three-story red brick
structure—was erected in downtown Washington at 920 H Street; it
opened for the new session in October 1886. It was, Hamilton said, "a
modest building compared with some of the mammoth structures lately
erected for similar purposes; but . . . ample for the accommodation of the
class." Which was no more than the simple truth. In 1886–87 the school
was still suffering the costs of insisting on a three-year course and had only
thirty-seven students.[38]

Two years later, however, enrollment had more than doubled to eighty-
four students. Perhaps it was this surge that provoked the controversy of
November 1888 with the school's next-door neighbor, Saint Joseph's
Orphan Asylum. The orphanage's board of managers brought a lawsuit
against the school, complaining about the "smell of corpses" and alleging
that their children could look through the windows into the anatomy

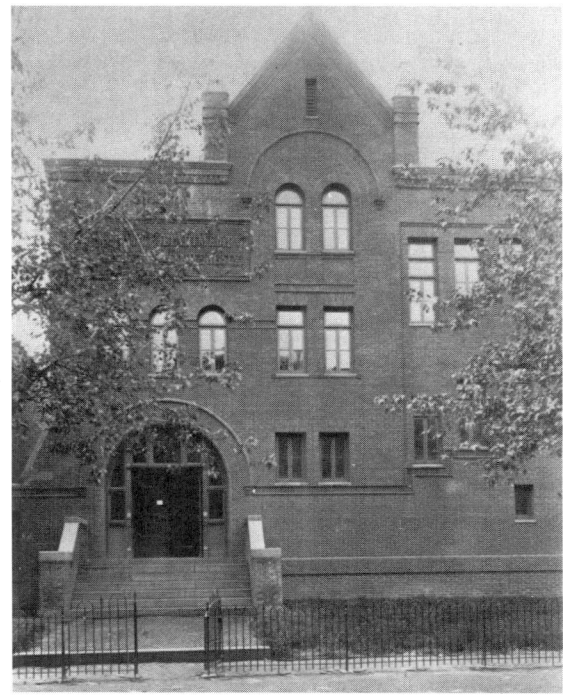

Georgetown Medical School occupied this building at 920 H Street, its first custom-built premises, from 1886 to 1930. Courtesy of Georgetown University Archives.

room and see cadavers laid out for dissection. The orphanage president declared that the medical school would "have to move somewhere else, for it is an outrage that the lives of the children and the health of the whole neighborhood should be so imperilled." The school's lawyers replied that blinds prevented anyone seeing directly into the dissecting room; but noted that "the occupants of the college had seen women on chairs and some people with opera glasses trying to look into the dissecting room." When a woman claimed she had seen "a human heart, dripping with blood, standing outside in a bucket," Professor Kleinschmidt protested that "it was merely the heart of an ox intended for purposes of anatomical demonstration." The press reported the story with glee, most luridly in the *New York Times*, which declared that the dissecting room "threatens the health of people throughout the District of Columbia"—adding, with Gothic relish, that "the bloodstained porch and backyard of the college . . . told a story too revolting for description." In the end, the medical faculty agreed to fix the ventilating shaft in the dissection room, which was found to be blocked. Smell and scandal abated together.[39]

By the prevailing standards of American medical schools at this time, Georgetown students were getting an education better than average. The course was still a year longer than the vast majority of schools offered; and the curriculum widened considerably in the 1880s to embrace a new and growing trend in medical practice: specialization. This had long been a controversial issue. "The chief objection brought against specialties," an AMA report of 1869 noted, "is that they operate unfairly toward the general practitioner, in implying he is incompetent to properly treat certain classes of diseases and narrowing the field of practice."[40] But the obverse also held true: physicians with the ability to specialize still hesitated to branch out, lest in giving up general practice they lost the bulk of their livelihood. Charles Liebermann was a classic example. Celebrated as an ophthalmologist from the time he arrived in Washington in 1840, and never without a heavy case load, Liebermann always remained a general practitioner.[41] But times were changing. As early as 1867, Johnson Eliot had pointed to the prejudice against specialization in America, contrasting this with Europe where, as he said, many specialists in diseases of the eye and ear, dermatology, and orthopedics were already established. Eliot did not share the prejudice. "Some of you gentlemen may discover . . . that you possess talent for some particular branch of medicine or surgery," he told the that year's graduating class. "If so, encourage it, develop it and adopt it!"[42]

The national debate ended in 1869 when the American Medical Association finally recognized specialization as an ethical practice. At the same time, bending to substantial opposition in its ranks, it forbade specialists from advertising.[43] No doubt this rule did inhibit many at first, but by 1894 there were nine ophthalmologists and ten laryngologists engaged outside of general practice in Washington.[44] It was no accident that the first specialties were surgical. Practiced by relatively few physicians, they posed less of a threat to the general practitioner than, for example, obstetrics or the diseases of children. (In 1889, there were no more than forty pediatricians in the whole country, and nearly all of them also treated adults.) In any case, surgery had reached the point where specialization was the next logical development. Refinements in technique and the invention of instruments permitting more accurate diagnosis meant that more time had to be devoted to study and to familiarization by practice.[45] Through the late 1870s and early 1880s, Georgetown, like other medical schools, offered lectures on the surgical specialties through optional classes, usually in the summer months.[46] But by 1887 these had all been incorporated into the regular course and their lecturers were promoted to full professors.

Ethelbert Carroll Morgan became the first professor of laryngology. The son of James E. Morgan, a former Georgetown professor, he had studied his specialty in Vienna, Paris, and London and in 1888 was elected president of the American Laryngological Association.[47] Joseph Taber Johnson, who had served for years as Georgetown's professor of obstetrics, was finally also named professor of gynecology in 1884. As Washington's leading and busiest gynecologist, Johnson provided service at two city hospitals and, from 1887 onwards, at his own private fifteen-bed sanatorium, which he built next to his home on K Street specifically for gynecological and abdominal surgery patients. President of the Medical Society of D.C. in 1887, Johnson was also a founder of the American Gynecology Society. In 1889 he was among the first Northerners invited to join the prestigious Southern Surgical and Gynecological Association (later simply the Southern Surgical) one year after its foundation; ten years later he was elected its twelfth president.[48]

The most eminent of Georgetown's surgical specialists was Swann Moses Burnett, a leading figure of nineteenth century American ophthalmology. A native of Tennessee and a graduate of Bellevue Medical College in New York, Burnett had arrived in Washington in 1876 and soon established himself as one of the first eye specialists in the city. He began lecturing Georgetown students in ophthalmology and otology in 1878, and the following year he also began a private postgraduate course in the subjects.[49] His teaching and clinical practice resulted in a number of textbooks, of which the most famous, *A Theoretical and Practical Treatise on Astigmatism,* was published in 1887, the same year he was appointed a full professor at Georgetown. It was one of the earliest works on astigmatism in the world.[50] Altogether, Burnett made more than sixty contributions to the medical literature, including two papers he delivered in person to the 1890 International Medical Congress in Berlin.[51] One of his oddest cases, reported in an 1899 issue of the *Journal of the American Medical Association (JAMA)*, was an operation to find the cause of a persistent headache. Removing the patient's right eyeball, Burnett discovered a flattened lead minié ball in the bones of the temporal fossa, "so firmly bedded as to form a part of their structure." The bullet had been there for thirty-six years, ever since the patient, two weeks after joining the Confederate Army as a seventeen-year-old enlistee, had been shot in the head at Gettysburg.[52]

For all his surgical eminence, Swann Burnett was best known in nonmedical circles as the husband of Frances Hodgson Burnett, world-famous author of *The Secret Garden* and other children's classics. She modeled one of her characters (Richard Amory in *Through One Administration*) on Burnett, and another (*Little Lord Fauntleroy*) on their son Vivien. Burnett named a bacteriological and pathological research laboratory he founded in Washington after their other son, Lionel, who had died of consumption in Paris in 1890.[53] The Burnett's tiny row house on I Street was a salon for the literati—among them Oscar Wilde, visiting from London[54]—and a showplace for their serious art collection, including Japanese art which, it is said, they were the first to bring into the United States. But the marriage did not last; they separated in 1897 and later divorced. Burnett continued as professor of ophthalmology at Georgetown until his death in 1906.[55]

The prowess of these three specialists and of Hamilton himself gave Georgetown a deserved local reputation for surgical instruction. Hamilton was an outstanding and exacting teacher. "In surgery we meet three times a week and any student who for one moment has forgotten the rule of Guthrie would deem himself happier had he remained at home," one student noted.[56] Yet Hamilton, regardless of the other claims on his time, went out of his way to help his students.

Repeatedly, as they struggled with the dense textbooks of the time, they asked him to recommend some practical text on tumors written in English. "I was obliged to say," he later wrote, "that I knew of no single treatise which brought together the varieties of tumors set forth in our present nomenclature and gave the symptomology and treatment." Characteristically,

Hamilton decided to produce one himself. He hired a stenographer to record his lectures on tumors verbatim. "[As] the subject is always considered a bugbear by the student," he pointed out, "the lectures only aim to impart the current information in a form intended to fix it in the memory." The result was his best-known book, *Lectures on Tumors from a Clinical Standpoint*. A model of clarity, it distilled the topic into 143 pages of practical information. At twenty-five cents in paperback and fifty cents in hardback, it was an instant success, running to three editions between 1891 and 1898.[57]

The surgical demonstrations given by Hamilton in general surgery, Johnson in gynecology and Morgan in laryngology at Providence Hospital, and Burnett in ophthalmology at the Central Dispensary and Emergency Hospital, were popular. Though intended for Georgetown students, they attracted hordes from other schools who arrived early and took the best seats. The Georgetown students protested to the faculty that they were being "crowded out."[58]

Yet Georgetown still had a long way to go. One of the protesting students was Austin O'Malley, who in his second year at Georgetown, 1890–91, was president of the student body.[59] O'Malley spent the following academic year at the University of Berlin, still Europe's leading medical school. His experiences there, described in vivid letters to the new president of Georgetown University, Reverend Joseph Havens Richards, S.J., speedily convinced him that Georgetown was "way behind" in medical education. "You can see more surgery here in a week than you would see in Washington in six months," he wrote after attending von Bergmann's clinics. "The operations are actually grouped to follow the lectures and if a patient is brought in with a certain tumor on a part of his body, they will usually bring in two or three other patients with similarly appearing growths on just the same spot and operate to show the differential diagnoses. The students won't wait for such trifles as amputation." O'Malley also found that Georgetown's courses on histology, pathology, and bacteriology lagged far behind Berlin's: "Some bacteriology is absolutely necessary if we would keep up with the times in antiseptic and aseptic surgery."[60]

O'Malley had a point. Georgetown had only just purchased its first microscopes—fifteen of them, bought in Berlin by the professors who attended the International Medical Congress there in 1890.[61] Things improved after Joseph Kinyoun began to teach bacteriology. When he brought glass jars full of cholera bacilli to Washington to study in January 1892, the event was headlined in the local newspapers, and students crammed into the Georgetown lecture hall to hear him speak on the subject.[62]

But Hamilton's influence on the faculty was beginning to wane, for the other professors had tired of his conceited and bombastic ways. According to O'Malley, whose letters give fascinating insight into the personality clashes of this time, the faculty were antagonized by Hamilton's "wire-pulling" and his "boast that the [medical] college was managed by himself."[63] They were disgruntled that the university had, without consulting them, honored him with an LL.D. degree—the first awarded to a Georgetown medical professor.[64] And they were dismayed that he had passed over James Kerr, an outstanding surgeon who had arrived in Washington in 1888, and had instead appointed Walter Wyman to the Georgetown clinical staff. Wyman was Hamilton's second in command at the Marine Hospital Service, but he was regarded as a mediocre surgeon. There was "too much Marine Hospital Service influence and social pressure buzzing about the place," O'Malley wrote.

Resentment against Hamilton came to a head in 1891. One Sunday in mid-May, the Georgetown students showed up at Providence Hospital for one of the scheduled surgical demonstrations and were turned away at the door.[65] The reason was that Thomas Mallan, an 1880 Georgetown medical graduate who now headed the surgical clinic at Providence, had severed relations with Hamilton. Apparently, Hamilton had promised Mallan an academic position at Georgetown and then reneged. The alarm of the faculty at this turn of events can well be imagined; Providence Hospital provided an essential part of the school's clinical facilities. A deputation dispatched in haste to Providence found Mallan intractable: he told them, O'Malley quoted, "as politely as I could, Georgetown College may go plumb to hell and I'll do all in my power to help it along."[66]

At the next faculty meeting, held on May 31, 1891, it was announced that John Brown Hamilton was resigning the chair of surgery "to move to Chicago." It seems that Hamilton, perhaps galvanized by the increasing criticism from all sides, had already accepted a new appointment as professor of surgery at Rush Medical College, his alma mater.[67] Hamilton also resigned as surgeon general of the Marine Hospital Service, using his influence to ensure that his old friend Walter Wyman would succeed him. Within a year, however, Hamilton regretted the move to Chicago and decided he wanted to be surgeon general again—assuming, characteristically, that Wyman would obediently step down. When Wyman demurred, Hamilton took a fast train to Washington and stormed into his old office. There he found that its main decoration, a full-size portrait of himself, had been relegated to the water closet. Whereupon the current and former surgeons general forgot friendship and dignity and fell into a fist fight.[68]

Wyman held his job, and Hamilton returned to Chicago, where he continued to serve the MHS as surgeon in charge of its local hospital, in tandem with his chair of surgery at Rush. Never flagging in energy, always in need of money, he secured a third appointment in 1894 as editor of the *Journal of the American Medical Association*, and excelled himself by pushing its circulation in four years from four thousand to ten thousand. Ebullient as ever, Hamilton continued to perform surgery, teach, edit, and write at his usual furious pace; but despite the homilies he had published in a strange little book called *Lessons in Longevity* (1884), he died aged fifty-one on Christmas Eve 1898 of perforation of the intestines after contracting typhus.[69] His collection of books, said to be "the largest private surgical library west of the Alleghenies," eventually came back to Georgetown, donated by his son Ralph who graduated from the medical school in 1904 and later became its professor of pathology.[70]

James Kerr was appointed Georgetown's sixth professor of surgery on the day Hamilton resigned. Graceful manners were never Kerr's strongest characteristic—typically, he neglected to acknowledge the university president's letter offering him the position until prompted ten days later—but he was regarded by everyone as Washington's finest surgeon.[71]

Kerr's breadth of surgical experience derived from his vastly colorful life.[72] He was from the north of Ireland, born in December 1848 at Portstewart, a coastal village near Coleraine in County Antrim where his father, a wealthy landowner, bred horses as a hobby. Kerr received a bachelor's degree at the Royal University in Coleraine in 1868, and his medical degree from Queen's University in Belfast in 1870; he also earned a degree in surgery. In his last year at Queen's, he was exceptionally fortunate to serve as "dresser" to Professor William MacCormac. The experience was crucial to Kerr's subsequent success in surgery. MacCormac, the great Irish surgeon later made a baronet by Queen Victoria, was the first in Ireland to put Lister's ideas into practice. He was already using antiseptics. Kerr thus began his career applying carbolized dressings to wounds—twenty years earlier than some of the most eminent surgeons of his day. A year or so later, while practicing in England, Kerr took the opportunity to visit Edinburgh and see for himself how Lister's work was revolutionizing surgery.[73]

In 1873, Kerr joined the British army's expedition to the Gold Coast of Africa (now Ghana), a campaign led by Sir Garnet Wolseley, the brilliant military reformer lampooned by Gilbert and Sullivan as "the very model of a modern major general." The Gold Coast expedition passed into history as "the engineers' and doctors' war" because the army had to hack a road through seventy-three miles of jungle and build 237 bridges over swamps, all in tropical conditions that brought widespread fever.[74] Kerr served as surgeon on a troopship carrying the famous 42nd Highland regiment, the "Black Watch." On the voyage out, he displayed the bravura that would become a trademark. In a heated argument about the sharks following the ship, Kerr maintained that no shark would attack a man who had not been wounded—and to prove it he dived in.

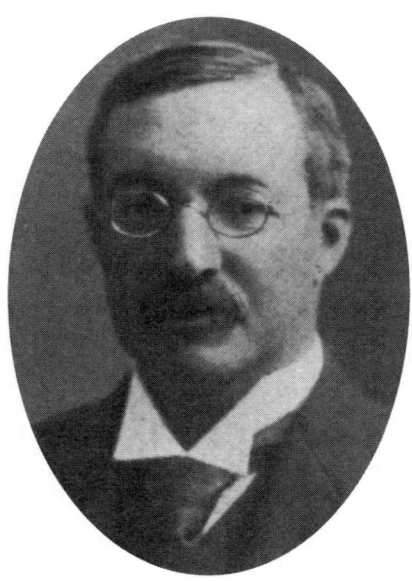

Returning to Europe unscathed, he got a job as surgeon on ships plying between England and Canada. Then, in 1875, Kerr settled in the wilds of Nova Scotia, as surgeon to a company mining iron ore. It was here that Kerr forged his skills, dealing with the multiple injuries incurred in accidents in the mines and the nearby blast furnaces that converted the ore into steel—all the while keeping precise case records and using the early antiseptic techniques he had learned from MacCormac. In the summer of 1876, he married Laurie Bell, whom he had met on one of his trans-Atlantic crossings. Laurie was the cousin of

James Kerr, M.D., 1848–1911. Courtesy of the Medical Society of the District of Columbia.

Alexander Graham Bell, and it was in Bell's house at Brantford, Ontario, that the wedding took place, just four months after the inventor had transmitted the first message ever sent by telephone—the wedding guests, indeed, were treated to a demonstration of this extraordinary new device.[75] Kerr's best man, also destined for fame, was a young Canadian professor of medicine named William Osler.

The young couple spent their honeymoon visiting the Centennial Exposition in Philadelphia, the nation's showiest celebration of its one hundredth birthday. For Kerr, however, the main attraction there was the International Congress of Medicine, the first ever held in America, where he heard Joseph Lister himself speak on antiseptic surgery. After six years practicing the great man's methods with good results, Kerr could not help noticing that most doctors in the audience were far less enthusiastic. Lister, confronting his detractors head on, began his presentation by answering the objections often raised against the use of antiseptic dressings. "The first objection," he said, "is that it is 'too much trouble.' I grant that it is somewhat troublesome, and yet I believe that . . . it is worth some trouble to be able to seal up an amputation, an exsection, or a large wound, with the absolute certainty that no evil effects will follow." He spoke persuasively for two and a half hours, demonstrated his dressings and antiseptic spray, and took questions for another hour. But comments from the floor revealed an ingrained skepticism. One surgeon spoke in favor of adding earth to wounds to dry them. Another, one of Canada's leading surgeons, said he found it "impossible to entertain the doctrine of germ putrefaction."[76] None of their opinions shook James Kerr's belief in Lister.

In 1880, after a spell in Montreal where Kerr's friend William Osler was teaching at McGill medical school, the couple settled in Winnipeg. It was a shrewd move. Winnipeg was a tiny frontier town, but the following year the Canadian Pacific Railway (CPR) finally reached it. In the ensuing economic boom, Kerr prospered. He became the CPR company's chief surgeon, medical health officer of both Winnipeg and the province of Manitoba, and federal medical supervisor of the Indians. (He once removed a stone from the bladder of a tribal chief who had arrived at the hospital with a full guard of warriors.) In 1883, Kerr helped establish the Manitoba Medical College in Winnipeg, Canada's third medical school and the first in the west, and he served as its first professor of surgery and dean. He also designed the city's new general hospital.

In 1887, Kerr traveled from Winnipeg to Washington to attend the
Ninth International Medical Congress, for which John Hamilton acted as
secretary general. It is possible they met on that occasion.[77] By this time
Kerr's in-laws, the Bells, were living in Washington, and Alexander
Graham Bell persuaded him to move to the city with his wife and four
small children the following year.[78] One reason for Kerr's decision was his
hope that a warmer climate might ease the rheumatism and nephritis that
plagued him.

Kerr quickly established a solid reputation, a standing recognized by his
appointment in 1890 as chief of surgery at the Central Dispensary and
Emergency Hospital, by then the largest clinical facility in the city. When
he accepted the chair of surgery at Georgetown the following year, he also
became a senior surgeon at Providence and Garfield Hospitals.

Having been one of the first (some said *the* first)[79] to introduce antiseptics to Canada, Kerr was equally quick to seize on the principles of aseptic
surgery, which finally began to be practiced widely in the 1890s. Describing
a year of surgical cases at the Emergency Hospital, 1891–92, Kerr wrote:

> In the emergency room we are *antiseptic*, and in the operating room *aseptic*,
> as far as the interior of wounds is concerned ... We use heat for sterilizing
> everything that goes into or near the wound, except our hands and the
> skin of the patient, which are prepared by scrubbing alcoholic, carbolic,
> and sublimate dressing respectively. We add the precaution of a perman-
> ganate and oxalic acid bath to our own hands.

He advocated the use of iodoform gauze packing in the treatment of wounds
within the serous cavities; he could, he said, "instance case after case where I
am confident fatal results were averted by these means." The old scourges of
surgical wards—infections like erysipelas and pyaemia—were now, he
maintained, "practically banished from our hospital."[80]

The practice of prophylactic asepsis gave surgeons far more confidence
of success than they had ever had before; patients too began, very gradually,
to change their attitudes, perceiving an operation as perhaps a chance for cure
rather than a likely passport to the morgue. As operative mortality lessened,
accountability rose. Hospitals which in the past had refused to divulge
mortality statistics on the grounds of "inexpediency" began now to publish

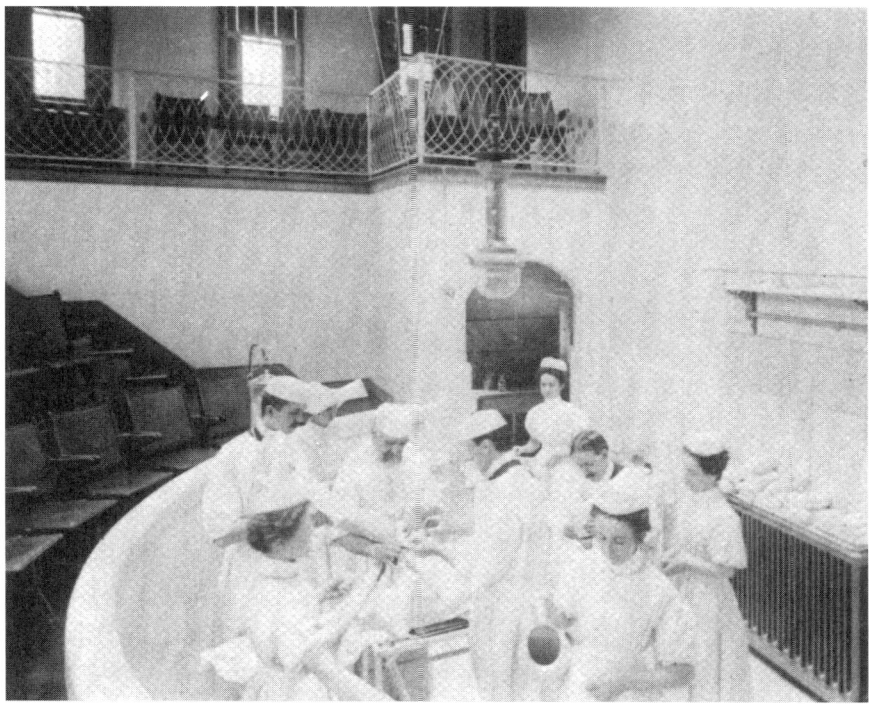

James Kerr, shown here operating in the amphitheater of Providence Hospital in 1895, was an early proponent of aseptic surgery and reputedly the first surgeon *in Washington to wear scrubs. However, note the absence of surgical gloves and masks. Courtesy of Providence Hospital.*

them. Surgeons who had explained away postoperative deaths by blaming everything except the act of surgery itself—or who had, more commonly, avoided any explanation at all—now began to report cases more accurately. Kerr's account of the record at Emergency Hospital, for example, ran: one death out of twenty-two amputations; one out of seventeen operations for concussion; one out of six penetrating wounds of the chest; none out of seven fractures of the cranial vault; none out of two gunshot wounds to the head—even though one of these patients, a "suicidal maniac," had put seven bullets into his own skull. Kerr was proud, too, to report that out of 885 wounds treated, only "half a dozen" had become infected. This success he attributed to "taking every available precaution that will avert sepsis," adding: "Until we are able to deny the assertion that antiseptic surgery is not always 'cock-sure' surgery, we cannot, except under peculiarly favorable conditions, afford to dispense with any detail that ensures additional success."[81]

For Kerr, that "detail" demanded that he and every member of his operating team wore white caps and gowns; almost certainly he was the first Washington surgeon to don scrubs. It required, too, a new kind of operating room: one that could be kept scrupulously clean. In 1891, a specially designed surgical amphitheater was built at Providence Hospital to meet those standards. The architect had been instructed "to spare neither effort nor expense to make this room conform to all requirements for perfect aseptic surgery." Housed in a two-story octagonal brick building, standing apart from the main hospital, the amphitheater had a floor and walls of marble—"woodwork having been avoided as far as practicable"—and, opening off it, a patients' room and a well-plumbed washroom, also finished in marble. The small operating area, illuminated on three sides by windows and from above by a large skylight, was overlooked by a curve of platforms climbing steeply in tiers and equipped with folding chairs to seat 150 students.[82] An 1895 photograph shows Kerr operating in this amphitheater, and all Washington surgeons were inordinately proud of it. Georgetown University's president, Richards, called it "one of the greatest events in the history of medical science in the District of Columbia."[83]

James Kerr, according to a 1961 history of Providence Hospital, was "a very skilful surgeon, a strict disciplinarian in the operating room, and at times authoritarian and autocratic. Some of the older physicians now living remember him well. One of them stated that Dr. Kerr always started things humming when he entered the doors of old Providence. He also said that Dr. Kerr always made an operation a great event, and that everybody in the hospital knew when he was operating as one of his favorite pastimes was throwing instruments." This the authors attributed to pressure of work "with a touch of showmanship thrown in."[84] But in truth Kerr was notorious for his irascible nature, salty language, and unbridled bursts of temper, characteristics that were later to overshadow his brilliance as a surgeon and diminish his career.

☙

The opening of Johns Hopkins school of medicine in Baltimore in 1893 was a landmark event in American medicine. It at once became the "gold standard" of medical education against which all other U.S. schools were measured, and it thus triggered a movement for reform which, within twenty years, brought to an end the old proprietary practices of the nineteenth century. Modeled on the leading schools of Europe, Johns Hopkins controlled its own hospital for integrated clinical teaching and postgraduate training. It attracted professors of the highest caliber, with the goal from the start of establishing a full-time faculty. William Osler was its first professor of medicine. No doubt it was on Osler's recommendation that James Kerr was offered the chair of surgery.[85] When he turned it down—because, it was said, he considered the conditions "too restrictive"[86]—the chair went to William Halsted. Meanwhile, under the direction of William Welch, who had trained with Koch, the school established the nation's first systematic program of medical research.

Long before Johns Hopkins actually opened, its advent was watched with trepidation by the region's other medical schools, among them Georgetown. Austin O'Malley, in one of his forthright letters to Richards from Berlin in 1892, recognized its importance. "After a few years I think that American students will go to Johns Hopkins for laboratory work in connection with medicine [instead of to Europe]," he wrote. "Those people in Baltimore know what is needed and they have money enough to work towards the right end . . . [and Hopkins] gets professors that do not live in the last century."[87] An editorial in *The Medical News* at around the same time voiced a more common view: "There is certainly nothing more needed by American medicine and American civilization than uncommercialized medical teaching."[88]

Probably it was the coming of Johns Hopkins, and maybe O'Malley's comments, that persuaded Richards to allocate ten thousand dollars to the medical school in July 1893, for which its dean, George Lloyd Magruder, had been negotiating for some time. The money paid the costs of virtually doubling the size of the building on H Street, extending it by eighteen feet and adding a fourth story. The improvements included a new chemical laboratory, a new dissecting room on the top floor, a new bacteriological laboratory equipped "with all the latest appliances for scientific research, including high-power microscopes," and electric light. Richards clearly intended the funding as an investment in quality, since in return he asked the faculty to find ways of raising standards and improving the curriculum.[89]

The grant—which the medical faculty was expected to repay at a rate of fifteen hundred dollars a year, but never actually did—came only in the nick of time.[90] Four months later, in November 1893, Richards was ordered by the Jesuit superior in Rome to refrain from any effort to further develop Georgetown's medical and law schools. The superior had received a complaint from Pope Leo XIII himself that Georgetown was seeking to rival the new Catholic University of America which had just been established in Washington—to the chagrin of existing Catholic institutions like Notre Dame, Fordham, and, in particular, Georgetown. Catholic University, which initially offered only graduate studies, was the pope's pet project. He wanted no hint of competition.[91]

A few weeks later, the hierarchy delivered another blow. Monsignor Francesco Satolli, the first papal delegate to Washington, decreed that Catholic University should simply take over Georgetown's medical and law schools. Reluctantly, Richards went so far as to draw up terms: $150,000 each or $175,000 together.[92] But the deans of both schools threatened the resignation of their entire faculties if the deal went through. Magruder, not attempting to conceal his anger, put his case bluntly in a letter to Satolli:

> I am positively of the opinion that a purely sectarian medical school would not prosper in this country. Consequently I would not be willing to serve as a member of such a faculty. As there are but few Catholics in the medical faculty, the wishes of the Catholic University, or even his holiness Pope Leo XIII would not have the slightest influence upon them. . . . From my knowledge of the faculty, I am sure that even were extraordinary inducements offered they would almost to a man decline to join the Catholic University. . . . Any attempt to bring about this affiliation would, without benefitting the Catholic University, absolutely destroy the Medical Department of Georgetown.[93]

The idea of annexation was dropped; but for years afterwards, the professional schools had to tread lightly for fear of offending the pope; and while the politically dexterous Richards strongly supported their endeavors, he did so covertly.

Nevertheless, progress was made. In 1895—again in response to the impact of Johns Hopkins and in accordance with Richards's wishes—the Georgetown faculty extended the medical course from three to four years, insisted that applicants pass an entrance examination, and switched its teaching from evening to daytime hours. This last step was a drastic one, but Georgetown decided that "sundown medicine," the mainstay of many American medical schools for so long, had had its day.

For forty-four years, Georgetown students had begun lectures at about 5:00 P.M., usually after putting in a full working day elsewhere. One of the last students to take the old evening course was Bailey K. Ashford, son of Frances Ashford and the future expert in tropical diseases, who graduated in 1896. Years later he recalled the "sundown" system in disparaging terms:

> Dissecting rooms were icy cold, lecture halls dimly lit, distances [to clinical facilities] far without proper means of transportation and . . . lectures were held at night. The doctors were too busy practicing medicine to lecture in the daytime. Furthermore, government clerks with a prying appetite for medical wisdom found in this profession a feasible escape from bureaucratic slavery, and since they formed the majority of the student body at Georgetown and the Government took their daylight hours, the Medical School had to conform its schedule to their convenience.[94]

Despite his father's early death, Ashford had clearly not needed to support himself with a daytime job; and because his father had been a professor, his tuition fees were halved.[95] But George Kober, who had worked to put himself through the same schooling in the class of 1873, took a more charitable and perhaps more accurate view: "The students who attended the evening lectures in those days earned their own living, appreciated the cost and value of a professional education and hence were ambitious, earnest and devoted to their work." These men, young and not so young, he said, "knew nothing of and cared less for alluring amusements, and many times the wee hours of the morning found them working together in the anatomical laboratory."[96] Kober often in later years expressed his gratitude for this system, which alone had enabled him to qualify in medicine. For some, however, it proved too tough. One student, working in the U.S. Signal Office by day, dropped out of the course because of his deteriorating eyes: "I am unable to use them at all at night and as I am confined in my office till four each day, I have no time for study till after lectures at night."[97]

The faculty decided on the change in early 1895, to take effect the following October. "All future matriculates will be required to devote all their time to the study of medicine," a professor explained. "The hours of instruction have been extended in consequence of the increased demands of modern medical education."[98] The change was necessary, but it came at a cost: it denied men of lower income the opportunity of a medical education, at least at Georgetown; it cut enrollments and the school's income; and for a few years it imposed a fresh burden on the faculty. The school guaranteed it would "rigidly carry out its contract" with students already enrolled in the evening.[99] This meant that the professors had to fit lectures and clinical instruction for the new daytime students into their morning and afternoon schedules, already filled with the demands of professional practice, while continuing to instruct upperclassmen in the evening—without, needless to say, any extra pay.

The professor who had argued most vigorously for the change to daytime teaching was James Kerr. Like Liebermann, Antisell, and Kleinschmidt before him, Kerr was in favor of reforms that would bring Georgetown closer to the European standards he knew. He was also an ardent advocate of the importance of clinical instruction. Students, he believed, could not adequately study diseases or the techniques necessary to surgical education unless they were free to attend clinics in the hospitals and dispensaries by day. Consequently, Kerr was elected chairman of the faculty's five-member "Committee on the Curriculum," appointed to design the new four-year course and the transition to daytime instruction.

At first, all went well. In an early discussion between the committee and the president of the university, Kerr spoke persuasively on the need for this change.[100] But thereafter he failed to attend committee meetings and, despite repeated urgings, neglected to give any recommendations on future arrangements for his own surgery course. He did show up at the final meeting, however. It ended in uproar. Losing his temper, Kerr dramatically called for a copy of the medical school catalogue and crossed out both his own name as professor of clinical surgery and all the clinics given by him and his assistants. "He informed the committee," his colleagues wrote in their subsequent report, "that it was his intention to post a notice stating that he would give *private* clinics, issuing tickets for them himself and making the matter his own personal affair, charging a fee for the same if he thought it proper."

Given Kerr's earlier insistence on the importance of clinical instruction and the need for daytime hours, the committee was baffled as to his reasoning. But for the faculty, it was the last straw. Their patience had long been stretched by Kerr's unpredictable and ill-tempered ways; this incident was only the latest in a series of incidents. Another had occurred when Kerr, surgeon in charge of the Emergency Hospital, had angrily rejected the Georgetown students' formal protest that the hospital's six clinical professors were each charging five dollars for tickets to their lectures, in sum more than most could afford on top of the overall tuition fee.[101] In yet another clash, Kerr had flunked an otherwise able degree candidate in surgery and denied his request to retake the examination. The faculty instructed that the student be re-examined by Kleinschmidt, who was impressed and passed him with a respectable score. Kerr, perhaps with some justification, was furious.[102]

By the spring of 1895, and despite Kerr's undoubted professional abilities, the faculty already had had enough of him. Behind the scenes, the university president was quietly trying to find a replacement. "There is one, and only one, really first class surgeon in Washington—Dr. James Kerr," Richards wrote in mid-May. "[But Kerr,] by his rough, arrogant and dictatorial ways, is said to have embittered greatly against him the remainder of our Faculty and the whole staff of the Emergency Hospital, as well as the profession generally." Richards, not a man of hasty judgment, gave this sweeping condemnation in a confidential letter beseeching a former Georgetown graduate to accept the chair of surgery. He was Ernest La Place, a distinguished surgeon and professor of surgery at the Medico-Chirurgical College in Philadelphia, and one of the few American physicians who had studied with Pasteur.[103] Richards offered La Place flattery ("I should be overjoyed to have your energy and genius engaged in the service of your Alma Mater, in whom you have already reflected credit . . ."), the promise of high reward ("You would command at once an extensive practice in consulting and operating. In a year you would be by far the greatest man in Washington . . ."), and even the inducement of an honorary LL.D to be conferred at the university's commencement in July.[104] Richards also sent Ryan Devereux, one of Kerr's assistants, on a personal mission of persuasion to Philadelphia.[105] La Place still declined the appointment. But Richards, clearly desperate to replace Kerr with a surgeon of at least equal stature, persisted. On May 31, he wrote asking La Place to reconsider and to accept the professorship of surgery at Georgetown not immediately but the following year (1896). "The chair in the school can, with great patience and care on the part of the Faculty, be held in status quo for that time . . . I know I urge a sacrifice upon you, as far as the present is concerned. But Georgetown University has been built upon self-sacrifice."[106]

Less than three weeks after this letter, however, the troubles with Kerr reached crisis point. At a special faculty meeting on June 18, 1895, the other members of the curriculum committee submitted not only their recommendations for the coming changes but also a lengthy report on Kerr's extraordinary announcement that he would in future offer only private clinics to students. They wrote:

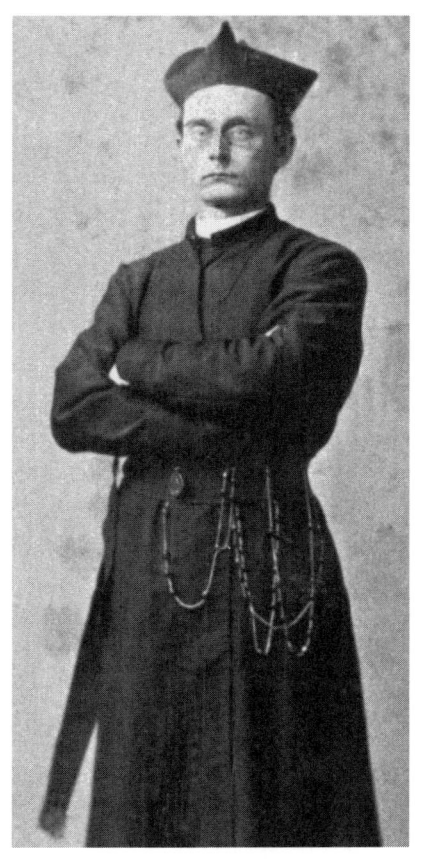

Reverend Joseph Havens Richards, S.J., president of Georgetown University, 1888–98. Courtesy of Georgetown University Archives.

We, as a majority of the committee, wish to earnestly protest against this course. Having received certain concessions from the University in consideration of improving the method of teaching, the individual members of the Faculty are severally and personally bound in duty and honor not to reduce the standard by depriving students of essential instruction . . . If [the professor of surgery] ceases to be an acknowledged clinical instructor and removes from the list four out of the five men that gave instruction last year without apparent intention of replacing them, it is evident that the School can no longer be certain that its students will be thoroughly instructed in clinical surgery.

They then came to what they saw as the crux of the matter, given the difficult transition to daytime teaching that lay ahead:

> It seems evident to us that the change in the curriculum . . . cannot be successful unless the individual members [of the faculty] meet it in a proper spirit. The change was inaugurated solely because it was felt that proper medical instruction cannot be given by evening lectures alone but that it must be supplemented by a considerable amount of clinical and laboratory work. To carry this out will require patience and personal sacrifices from each member of the faculty . . . more careful supervision of assistants and instructors, and more hours, all without any hope of immediate pecuniary reward. We believe that it is quite possible to do this, but the action of the professor of surgery does not seem actuated by this spirit and is therefore not approved by us.[107]

Kerr was present at this meeting. He was asked to explain his action, and he was entreated to "continue to conduct his chair as he had done during the past year." He refused to do either. Instead, he denounced the report as "a conspiracy to misrepresent and injure" him, became "very personal and abusive" of the committee members, and accused Dean Magruder of lying and betrayal. Finally, Joseph Taber Johnson made a motion that Kerr's "refusal to perform the duties of his chair as laid down in the prospectus be not allowed." Again, the professors appealed to Kerr to reconsider; again he insisted that his clinical teaching was "entirely a private matter." When the ballot was taken, everyone voted against him. Kerr at once stood up and announced he would resign the chair of surgery. Told he would have to do this in writing to the president of the university, Kerr promptly sat down again at the table and there and then penned a curt note to Richards: "Dear Sir, I regret to have to state that owing to the personal animosity evinced towards myself it is impossible for me to continue to hold my position as professor of surgery. I therefore beg to resign. Yours faithfully, James Kerr."[108]

Richards, pleading pressure of the university's commencement arrangements—but probably trying to buy time while he negotiated with La Place—did not reply until June 27, nine days later. He then urged Kerr to propose some way of settling his differences with the rest of the faculty: "I find that their dissatisfaction with the personal relations which have existed between them and yourself is even deeper than I had supposed; but if there be any means which you can suggest of reaching an amicable understanding with them, I shall of course be most happy to employ it." Kerr, not yielding an inch, replied the next day that he had no intention of withdrawing from the stand he had taken: "I write this as your letter seems to infer that *I* should do something to affect a reconciliation. I consider myself aggrieved." Richards gave up; two days later he accepted Kerr's resignation.[109]

The catalogue for the 1895–96 school year was printed with an ominous blank for the chair of surgery, with a footnote announcing that it would "be filled before the opening of the session." But no appointment was made. After months of making approaches to "several eminent surgeons outside the city," the faculty was forced to leave the chair vacant and construct the course around a hastily-recruited group of local surgeons.[110]

At the opening ceremony of the session on September 30, 1895, Dean Magruder tried to put the best gloss on the debacle. He announced:

> The chair of surgery has been divided. Deputy Surgeon General Forwood, United States Army, has consented to give a number of lectures upon such portions of military surgery as will prove of decided interest to the general surgeon. He will also treat of surgical pathology and the technique of operations. The faculty consider that they have been specially fortunate in securing the valuable assistance of a gentleman so distinguished in the branch upon which he will lecture.

It was significant that the guest speaker at this opening ceremony was the army's surgeon general himself, William Sternberg, no doubt invited to strengthen Forwood's standing.

"Another source of congratulation," Magruder continued gamely, "is that word has been received from Professor Ernest La Place, in response to an invitation, that he will lecture on brain surgery. The work that he has recently done in this department of surgery has added fresh laurels to his reputation which has already placed him in the foremost ranks of the surgeons of the day." (In the event, La Place delivered four lectures.[111]) Magruder added that Arthur A. Snyder, son of Georgetown's second professor of surgery, and John Woart Bayne, the attending surgeon and president of the board of Providence Hospital, would both lecture on theoretical and clinical surgery. Ryan Devereux, the only remaining Kerr appointee, would continue instruction on minor surgery, bandaging, and dressings.[112]

It was hardly a satisfactory arrangement. A week into the session Magruder dropped a note to Richards about the surgery course: "There is some muttering among the students. I am trying to keep it down." But two weeks later: "All seems to be quiet at the present. The lectures seem to be going smoothly now . . . I do not hear any grumbling. Do you hear anything?"[113] The main problem, though, was that James Kerr still controlled surgery at Emergency Hospital. With fifteen thousand patients and five hundred surgical operations a year, it offered medical students more opportunities to study disease and injuries at first hand than any other hospital in the city.[114] But Kerr refused to let the Georgetown students attend surgical clinics there.[115]

It was for this reason that in early March 1896, Richards and the medical professors first began discussing the possibility of building their own hospital. Richards offered a plot of land which the university had recently acquired on the corner of Thirty-fifth and N Streets in Georgetown, and fund-raising quickly began.[116] In the effort to engage public interest, much was made of the lack of a hospital in the Georgetown area. In one circular sent out asking for funds, Richards went so far as to say that "instances are not infrequent where patients, for want of prompt aid, have died in transit to the Emergency, Providence, or Garfield Hospital."[117] There may have been some truth in this statement, but it was equally true that there were then fourteen hospitals in Washington—a ratio to population equalled by no other American city.[118] The real motive behind the plan, as the faculty minutes and frequent worried communications between Richards and Magruder make plain, was the urgent need to have a hospital under the absolute control of the medical faculty— not only to eliminate the problems such as they now confronted with Kerr, but because the absence of clinical facilities of their own was hindering their search for a new professor of surgery.[119] In a real sense, therefore, James Kerr left the medical school a lasting legacy: he was the spur for the foundation of Georgetown University Hospital.

It took another two years beyond Kerr's resignation from Georgetown for the staff of Emergency Hospital to succeed in ousting him too.[120] Kerr afterwards served briefly on the faculty of Columbian medical school, then practiced privately until his retirement in poor health in 1907. He moved to his country estate in Warrenton, Virginia, where ninety-seven rolling acres surrounded a colonnaded antebellum mansion he called "Antrim" in nostalgic memory of Northern Ireland. He spent his last years there breeding racehorses, as his father had before him, and died there in February 1911.[121] His son, Harry Hyland Kerr, became a distinguished Washington neurosurgeon, serving as president of the Southern Surgical Association in 1941.[122]

Meanwhile, the Georgetown search for a new professor of surgery also dragged on for two years. Magruder mentioned many possible names in his regular notes to Richards, but nothing came of them. Eminent surgeons were invited to give visiting lectures at the school, both to enrich the course and to be courted for recruitment. Among them was Professor Friedrich Fehleisan, formerly of Berlin but now living in San Francisco, who was famous as the discoverer of the micrococcus that caused the infectious "hospital disease," erysipelas. He barely spoke English, and he demanded a guaranteed twenty-five hundred dollars from the school in his first year in Washington—a transfer fee the faculty seriously considered paying until Fehleisan, alarmed at the prospect of taking a local medical examination, as required by the District of Columbia, abruptly returned home. "So now we have to start all over again," Magruder said wearily.[123]

Not until March 1897 did the faculty at last find the professor they were looking for.[124] He was a man who, in contrast to the truncated terms of Hamilton and Kerr, was to occupy the chair of surgery for a record thirty-six years: George Tully Vaughan.

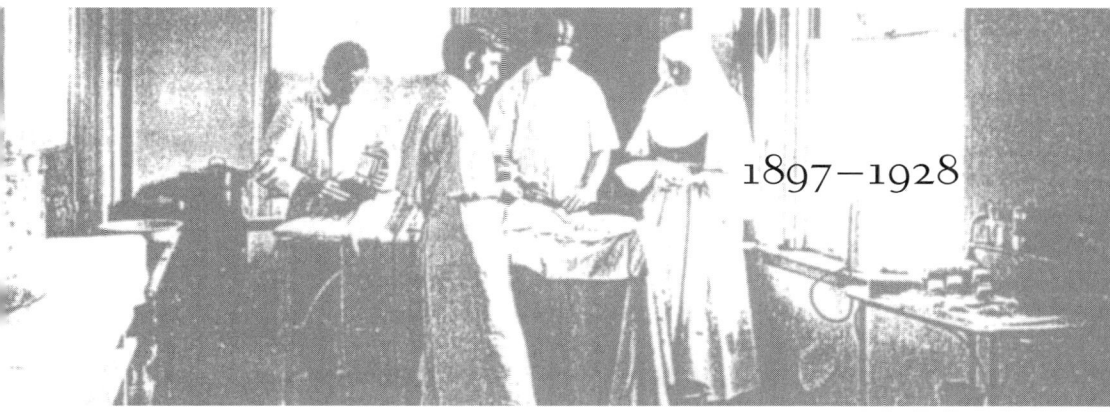

1897–1928

CHAPTER FIVE

STRUGGLES TO SURVIVE

*Georgetown University Hospital, Early Heart Surgery,
and the Impact of the Flexner Report*

GEORGE TULLY VAUGHAN'S active years as a surgeon spanned nearly two-thirds of a century, from his graduation in medicine in 1880 to the last operation he performed in 1943 at age eighty-four. His career began in the earliest days of aseptic practice, when abdominal surgery was still rarely attempted, before the term *appendicitis* was even coined, and before any surgeon had dared apply a knife to a living human heart. It ended on the eve of the modern era, just before the dawn of the age of antibiotics, organ transplants, and open-heart surgery.

Like John Hamilton, Vaughan was a product of the Marine Hospital Service. He had served his time at MHS hospitals in Massachusetts, Illinois, and Indiana, and in 1892 was transferred to Washington where he became assistant to Walter Wyman, Hamilton's successor as surgeon general.[1] In his later years, Vaughan said he owed most of his success to Wyman[2], and it was probably Wyman who recommended Vaughan to the Georgetown medical faculty in their desperate search for a professor of surgery.

From the caliber of the surgeons Georgetown had already approached—not just La Place and Fehleisan, but also J. M. T. Finney of Johns Hopkins, later to become the first president of the American College of Surgeons[3]—it is clear that they were looking for a man of outstanding academic qualifications. Vaughan had them: after medical degrees from the University of Virginia (1879) and Bellevue Medical College, New York (1880), he had taken postgraduate courses at the New York Polyclinic Hospital, at Jefferson Medical College, and at the University of Berlin. He had visited other great European centers— Vienna, Leipzig, Dresden, Padua, Berne, Paris, and London—to study the methods of celebrated surgeons. By 1897 he had published a dozen papers in scientific journals.[4] He was also known as a skillful operator who had already performed exacting procedures on the liver, the skull, and the aorta.[5] Even so, the bruised

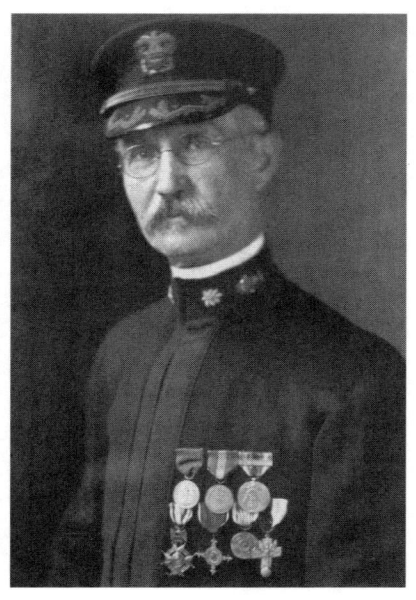

George Tully Vaughan, M.D., 1859–1948. Courtesy of Georgetown University Archives.

Georgetown medical faculty acted cautiously. They asked Vaughan to give a few lectures. Only then, satisfied with his teaching potential, did they invite him to take the chair of surgery.[6]

George Tully Vaughan was at this time thirty-seven years old, married, and the father of two children. A tall, spare, erect figure, with wire-rimmed eye-glasses and the obligatory moustache of his generation, he was "a very impressive, austere, southern-plantation gentleman, and a tremendous surgeon," in the words of one of his later students, Robert J. Coffey.[7] Decisive in the operating room, he was equally forthright in expressing his trenchantly conservative opinions in lectures, addresses, and letters to the newspapers. In the 1920s and 1930s, for example, he publicly advocated capital punishment for burglary and assault, the return of the whipping post for convicted criminals, and the "abolition" of defense lawyers.[8] He seldom missed an opportunity to declare his opposition to all constitutional amendments "from the thirteenth to the nineteenth inclusive," which included the abolition of slavery, the introduction of income tax, and votes for women.[9] Raised in the tradition of Southern courtliness, Vaughan truly could not imagine why any woman would want equal rights. "Has she really bene-fitted by these privileges or has she not rather been dragged down from the pedestal she used to occupy to a lower place on a level with the male who may no longer regard her as the superior being of former days?" he demanded with rhetorical flourish before what appears, at least to modern eyes, a singularly inappropriate audience: the graduating class of Georgetown's training school for nurses.[10]

Vaughan came of an old Virginia family. Originally from Wales, his forebears had settled at Jamestown in the early seventeenth century and later fought in the American Revolution. His father, Washington Lafayette Vaughan, had been a medical student at Jefferson Medical College in Philadelphia when George was born on June 27, 1859, on the family estate at Arrington, south of Charlottesville. The following October, the aboli-tionist John Brown led his raid on Harper's Ferry; by December, Vaughan later recounted, "feeling between North and South [had become] so intense and disagreeable that the southern students, including Dr. Hunter McGuire, my father and many others, withdrew . . . and were graduated from the Richmond Medical College in Virginia."[11] McGuire went on to become Stonewall Jackson's personal surgeon and amputated the general's arm in a vain attempt to save his life after he had been shot by his own side at Chancellorsville.[12]

Vaughan's earliest memories were of the Civil War, and perhaps it was for this reason that all his life he retained a fascination for military activities. A member of numerous military organizations and president of the Association of Military Surgeons, he was said to be the only medical officer to have held commissions in all three government services of his day: the Marine Hospital Service (which became the U.S. Public Health Service in 1912), the U.S. Army, and the U.S. Navy.[13] He liked to be photographed in military uniform, and this image was no mere pose. Whenever the United States became embroiled in a war—the Spanish-American War, the Mexican Civil War, and World War I—Vaughan volunteered his services at once.

The brief war with Spain (April to December 1898), in which the Spanish were driven out of Cuba and the United States acquired the Philippines, Guam, and Puerto Rico, broke out just before the end of

Vaughan's first year on the Georgetown medical faculty. Joining the army medical corps in June 1898, he served eight weeks of the summer vacation as a brigade surgeon with the VII Army Corps, commanding a tent hospital in Camp Cuba Libre at Jacksonville, Florida, and dealing mostly with cases of typhoid fever.[14] It was there, one day in August, that he opened a newspaper sent from Washington and read an item of great personal interest to him: "A notice," he later recalled, "that the Georgetown University Hospital would be opened on a certain day for the reception and treatment of patients, and giving a list of the physicians and surgeons and assistants connected with the hospital." Among them, he was pleased to see his own name as chief of surgery.[15]

꿍

The opening of Georgetown University Hospital was a landmark in the history of the medical school: the realization, at last, of an ambition that had taken nearly half a century to achieve. The first small brick building—four stories high, sixty feet wide, and fifty feet deep—stood at the corner of N and Thirty-fifth Streets, two blocks from the university. Construction was completed by mid-July of 1898. As soon as the workmen moved out, the nuns who were to run the hospital arrived. There were just three of them, all from the Congregation of the Sisters of Saint Francis in Pennsylvania: Sister Superior Pauline, Sister Edward, and Sister Adelfina. On their first visit to the hospital they discovered the basement flooded after a severe storm. For two weeks, they slept each night at the nearby Visitation Convent and by day cleared out builders' debris. Then the sisters moved into the hospital, sleeping on mattresses on the floor, toiling long hours to prepare the rooms, and going out to beg for furniture and donations.

After weeks of hard labor in hot weather, Sister Pauline and her assistants were at last ready for the grand opening. They sent out personal invitations and newspaper notices of the kind Vaughan read in his Florida tent hospital. Then, on the appointed date, August 15, 1898, they eagerly waited for visitors to drop by. But the sisters had forgotten—or perhaps did not know—that everyone who could get out of Washington in August did so, not only for their comfort but for their health. No one showed up. It was, as one chronicler wrote, "a tragically imperfect day" for the nursing nuns.[16]

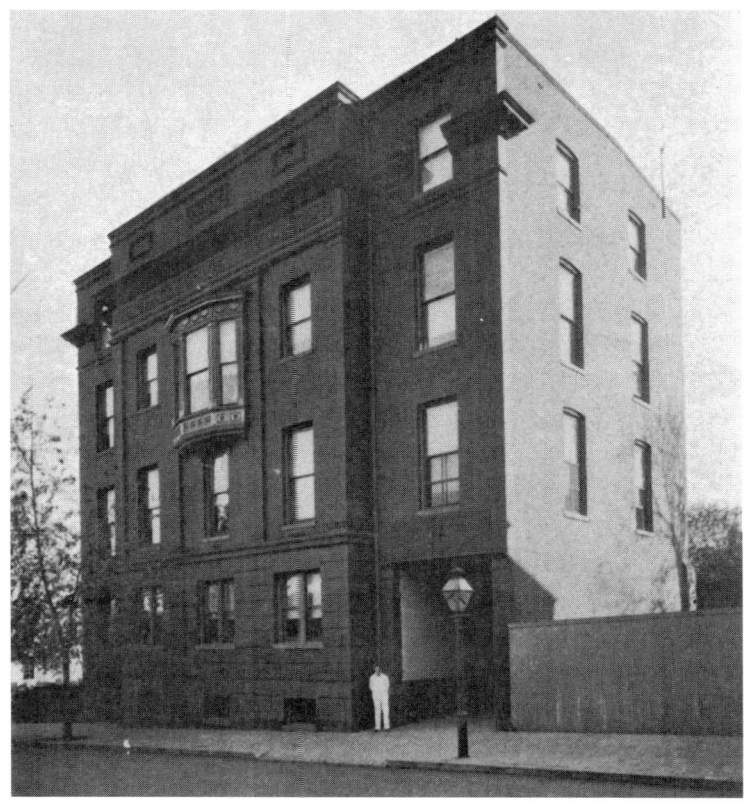

The original building of Georgetown
University Hospital, shown here soon after
it opened in 1898, stood at the corner of
N and Thirty-fifth Street, Georgetown.

The archway on the right was the entrance
for the hospital's horse-drawn ambulance.
Courtesy of Georgetown University
Archives.

Nevertheless, three patients were admitted that first week. The first,
who arrived unconscious, never revived; and the second, a severe case of
typhoid fever, also died after a few days. "When the undertakers' wagons
reached the hospital," Sister Pauline later recalled, "the children met around
the hospital door and said: 'Look at the slaughterhouse—killed two patients
the first week.'" But their third patient survived, and so did others. Before
long, a swelling tide of the sick and needy flowed to the hospital, sometimes
by horse-drawn ambulance, to occupy the twenty-four beds, undergo

surgery in the small first-floor operating room, and receive free treatment and medications at the outpatient dispensary. Soon the hospital was over-crowded and the sisters overworked. Until 1900, when an elevator was installed, they even had to carry incapacitated patients up and down stairs.[17] The hospital's first intern, William Clarence Gwynn, chosen by competi-tive examination from the 1898 class of Georgetown graduates, did duty as "porter, orderly, anesthetist, and assistant physician and surgeon as occasion demanded."[18] Years later he became one of the school's clinical professors of surgery.

In its opening year, the hospital dispensed more than two thousand prescriptions and treated 1,397 people, of whom only 93 were fee-paying patients.[19] The hospital was supposed to be self-supporting, for political as well as financial reasons. President Richards was still under tremendous pressure from Rome not to compete with Catholic University. In 1896, on reporting the need for a university hospital, he had been warned by the Jesuit general's office that establishing it might precipitate an order to close Georgetown University itself, if it were thought (presumably by the pope) "to stand in the way of a favorite plan." Richards persisted, but he was allowed to proceed only on the strict understanding that the University "would not incur any present nor future indebtedness for construction or maintenance." At least one communication from Rome, though, hints at a more collusive arrangement: "Can you leave the whole matter in the hands of the medical faculty? . . . Can the movement be carried through without your giving, or seeming to give, financial aid?"[20]

Richards played the game. The hospital accounts record constant fundraising efforts by the sisters, the medical professors, and even Richards himself. In fact, the university president privately described himself as "ex-officio beggar-in-chief" for the hospital.[21] But the accounts do not add up. They never fully explain how the subsequent expansion of the hospital, from one modest building housing 24 beds in 1898, to a 266-bed facility occupying much of a city block by 1913, was paid for.[22] In public, heartfelt thanks were given to generous donors like the banker Elisha Francis Riggs and his wife, who contributed the first $1,000 to the Hospital Fund and later endowed a whole wing.[23] Much was made of Sister Pauline's abilities to work financial miracles—a legend so strong that in 1951 the hospital's Ladies Board, in notes on its history, remarked that

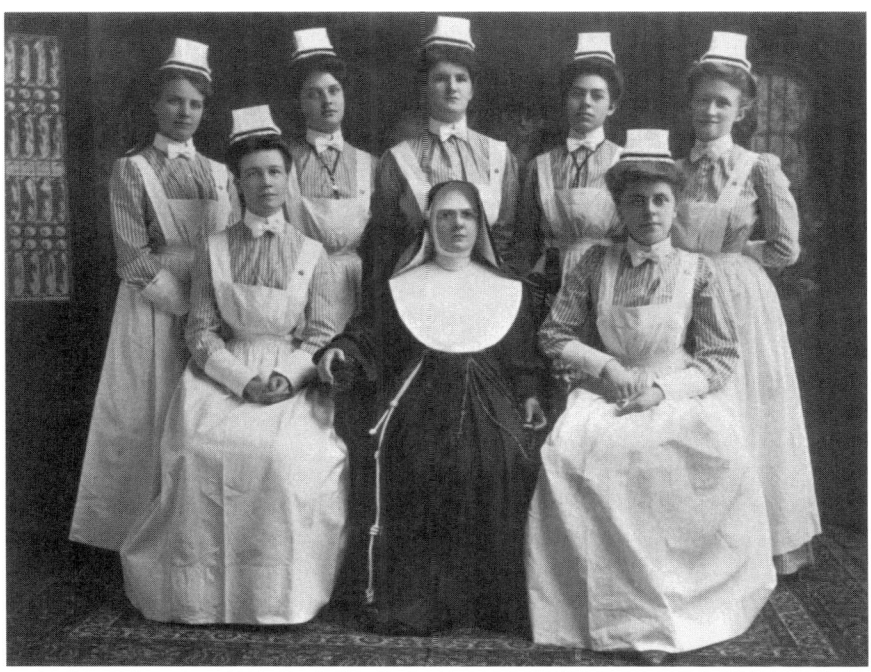

*Sister Pauline, first director of Georgetown
University Hospital, is shown here with
early graduates of Georgetown's Training
School for Nurses, circa 1903.
Courtesy of Georgetown University
Archives.*

after raising the first $40 to open the hospital, Sister Pauline "never had to
ask the College for further assistance."[24] That may have been true of day-
to-day operating costs, but not of the plant. Sister Pauline herself wrote that
"the debt on the hospital at the beginning was $7,500."[25] By 1912, the
dean registered the combined value of medical school and hospital as
$375,000, at a time when the school itself was valued at no more than
$50,000.[26] And two years later he noted: "It is not generally known that
the University is responsible for an indebtedness of over $200,000
contracted for the development and expansion of the school and the
hospital."[27] The hospital indeed received many gifts, in cash and in kind,
and it did rely heavily on the toil and endless penny-pinching of the
unpaid sisters; but it is clear that the hospital's principal and secret benefactor was the university itself.

Inevitably, this was an obligation that brought the medical school more closely than ever under the control of the university. Soon after the Reverend John Whitney, S.J. had succeeded Richards as president in late 1898, the medical faculty drafted new bylaws and, as a formality, sent them to him. Whitney promptly rejected them. He insisted that the president of the university was ex-officio the president of the medical faculty, and that the medical professor "now styled president be styled vice president." This protocol had actually been in effect for a few years back in the 1860s, but was long forgotten. Whitney now made sure it was revived and enshrined in the constitution of the medical school, and thereafter he presided whenever possible over faculty meetings.[28]

Whitney and his successors also assumed a pivotal role in the relationship between the medical school and the hospital. Sister Pauline administered the hospital and answered directly to the university president. The medical faculty's interests were represented by the Hospital Management Committee, which at its formation in May 1898 comprised Joseph Taber Johnson, Carl Kleinschmidt, George Magruder, George Kober, and George Tully Vaughan. Each clinical professor served in turn as executive director on a three-month rotation.[29] When friction between Sister Pauline and the committee occurred, as it inevitably did, each dispute had to be referred to the university president for decision.

The delicate task of smoothing difficulties and maintaining cordial relations in this tripartite balance of power devolved largely on the medical school's dean. George Lloyd Magruder, who had held the office with great ability since 1888, retired in 1901, though he continued to raise funds indefatigably for the hospital.[30] The faculty then unanimously elected George Kober as his successor. Kober, professor of "hygiene and state medicine" (now called public health), was at age fifty-one by no means the most senior member of the faculty. But he was an unmarried man of independent means who had no need to practice private medicine and therefore had the time—and certainly the inclination—to devote his considerable energies to the medical school. As events proved, the faculty could not have chosen a better man.

George Martin Kober personified the American Dream. He was the archetypal poor but clever immigrant who through hard work and frugality won both professional success and material wealth in the New World. Born in Alsfeld, Germany, in 1850, Kober crossed the Atlantic alone at age sixteen to live with his married sister in New York. The following year, 1867, he enlisted in the U.S. Army as a hospital orderly, working in an insanitary frame-built hospital on the edge of a marsh at Carlisle barracks, Pennsylvania. Typically, Kober spent his off-duty hours studying medical texts. When he was assigned to work in the library of the army's surgeon general in Washington in 1871, he found that Georgetown medical school was invitingly located just four doors down from his office in the old Ford's Theater on E Street. He promptly enrolled in its night classes.[31]

By day, Kober worked as sole clerk to the celebrated John Shaw Billings, cataloguing and indexing the library's huge collection. The other army clerks called him "Index." In later years, he treasured a poem written by a friend in honor of his twenty-fourth birthday, which began prophetically: "Index you are rightly named. Let thy future name be famed . . ." In his three years at the library, Kober considered himself "very fortunate" to be given the task of reading and indexing every communication sent to the surgeon general's office from army medical officers in the field from 1812 to 1874—an experience which left him with an enduring respect for military surgeons.[32] Each weekday night, regularly from 5:00 to 10:00 P.M. and often until midnight, Kober listened to lectures and practiced dissection at the medical school; on Saturday afternoons and Sunday mornings he attended clinics to watch operations. He was always grateful for this two-year education, and the only criticism he ever allowed himself was to concede that "the laboratory equipment was extremely meager." "No laboratory

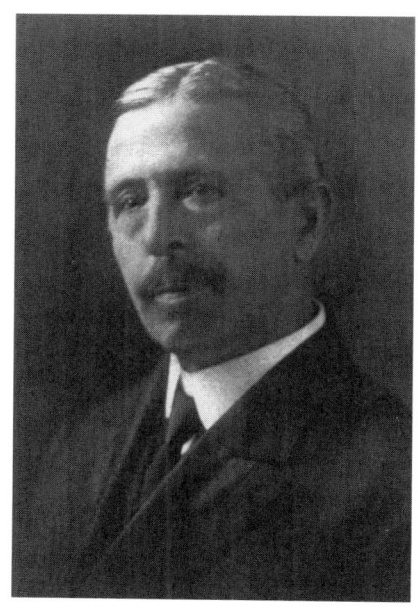

George Kober, M.D., 1850–1931. Dean of Georgetown University Medical School, 1901-28. Courtesy of Georgetown University Archives.

work in chemistry was done at the college," he added, "but a number of men fitted up a home laboratory for urinalysis which at that time was in its infancy."[33] In fact, it was Kober himself who set up that laboratory; his subsequent thesis on urinology, submitted for his degree in 1873 and published two years later, was one of the earliest American papers on the subject.[34]

After graduation, unable to afford to set up in private practice and prudently resolved not to try until he was financially secure, Kober joined the army medical corps. His first posting was to the bleak fortress on Alcatraz Island in San Francisco Bay, which was then a military prison. He served a few weeks there as station surgeon; and thereafter for twelve years he served continuously and with distinction on the frontier and in the Indian Wars.[35] It was a tough life, particularly for so gentle and bookish a man, but Kober's intellectual curiosity triumphed over physical hardship. During these years, in fact, he developed an interest in the sanitary issues that would become his lifework. His papers of the period leave a striking record of how, throughout his service, Kober—amid the everyday injuries and diseases of military life—relentlessly found the time to deepen his medical education. He frequently wrote to Billings in Washington, asking him to purchase and send the latest medical papers and books.[36] He even ordered 250 histological specimens prepared in the laboratory of the pioneering microbiologist Carl Ludwig in Germany.[37] In his military duties, too, Kober strove to excel. He worked primarily as a surgeon, and in 1876, with Billings' encouragement, he published a case of gunshot wound to the knee on which he had successfully operated and treated with injections of iodine. He was later recognized as the first to use iodine in this way, earlier even than Lister.[38]

Apart from money spent on study materials, Kober saved his modest army salary and invested it shrewdly in California's booming new economy. By 1889, he was worth around seventy-five thousand dollars and, at last, financially secure. He returned that year to Washington to attend Georgetown University's centennial celebrations. The second phase of his extraordinary career was about to begin. "I made up my mind that day," Kober later wrote, "to do as much as was within my power to promote the interests of public health and of my Alma Mater."[39] At Georgetown that fall, he created and occupied the first chair of hygiene and state medicine in the nation.[40] From then onwards, Kober devoted himself to the medical school and to researches into public health. He was a pioneer. He was one of the first to demonstrate the range of epidemics caused by unpasteurized milk.[41] In 1892, through diligent observation and "reasoning by way of exclusion," as he put it, he was the first to point to the role of flies in the transmission of typhoid fever.[42] There were many such contributions, for which he was awarded many honors.

By the time of his election as dean, Kober had already published more than seventy-five scientific papers[43] and was recognized as the leader in his field; but now he had also developed a consuming interest in medical education. That was the principal reason why his appointment proved, in time, such an inspired choice. Through the turbulent years that lay ahead, it was George Kober who was to hold the medical school together and, more than any other individual, ensure its survival.

The development that most excited surgeons in the closing years of the nineteenth century was the discovery of the Roentgen Ray. Only a few months after Wilhelm Konrad Roentgen first published his work on the X-ray machine in Germany in December 1895, surgeons in the United States were using it in diagnosis. Few understood how it worked—referring to it as "this mysterious force"—but they were quick to recognize the value of an apparatus that could see through skin and tissue to detect within the body the precise location of bone fractures and foreign objects. In Washington, Georgetown's Joseph Kinyoun started the first experiments to test the X-ray machine in April 1896. Its earliest recorded use for surgery in the city was at Providence Hospital in the summer or early fall of 1896; an unidentified surgeon used it to locate an elusive bullet in an old gunshot wound to the thigh.[44]

George Tully Vaughan first examined an X-ray machine in Philadelphia in February 1897 and brought it back to Emergency Hospital. He was enthralled by its possibilities, but presciently cautious of its use. "I soon gave up my part in its management as I was sure there were many things about it not then understood and I did not care to take the risk," he wrote later. "One of my friends who took charge of the work soon after, and has continued in it as a specialist, has lost one hand and several fingers on the other hand."[45] Others lost eyebrows and eyelashes. But from then onwards Vaughan, like other surgeons, relied increasingly on X rays for diagnosis. In 1899, he published a series of cases in which "skiagrams" (literally, "shadow pictures") had been decisive in locating bone fractures, tumors, several bullets, a broken needle in the knee, and a tin whistle in the esophagus.[46] Vaughan found the new rays particularly useful in cases where a bullet or other foreign object had fragmented within the tissues, something hard to detect with a probe. But he warned that "excessive or improper exposure to the rays . . . may cause a burn in which the tissues are destroyed, slough, and leave an ulcer which requires an unusually long time to heal." To avoid this he recommended that "the part exposed should always be protected by a light covering."[47]

Around this time, Vaughan brought another development to Georgetown: hypodermic injections of dilute cocaine as a local anesthetic. Carl Koller, the Austrian ophthalmologist, had discovered the anesthetic properties of cocaine in 1884. But it was Karl Schleich of Berlin who first used it in dilute concentrations by injection for many minor surgical procedures and even a few major operations (mastectomy and some abdominal surgery). Schleich's report of 521 cases caused uproar at the German Surgical Congress in 1892—not on account of the method, but because he injudiciously declared that surgeons who continued to use chloroform inhalation for minor procedures were guilty of malpractice.[48] In January 1895, George Tully Vaughan visited Berlin and watched Schleich operate. He returned home convinced that the mixed results Schleich's methods had brought in the United States were due to many surgeons' failure to follow Schleich's instructions strictly enough. He described in a subsequent paper the precise cocaine solution, the exact dose, and careful details of the procedure for injection—all of which had brought him, he said, "satisfactory results."[49]

Another development around the turn of the century was the use of sterile rubber gloves in surgery. These were introduced at Johns Hopkins, being reputedly first worn in 1889 by William Halsted's nurse because her skin could not tolerate disinfectants. Hopkins' surgeons did not use them with intent to protect the patient from infection until 1893, and not routinely until 1897. Even after that, many surgeons elsewhere rejected their use on the grounds of loss of sensitivity; and the debate on whether

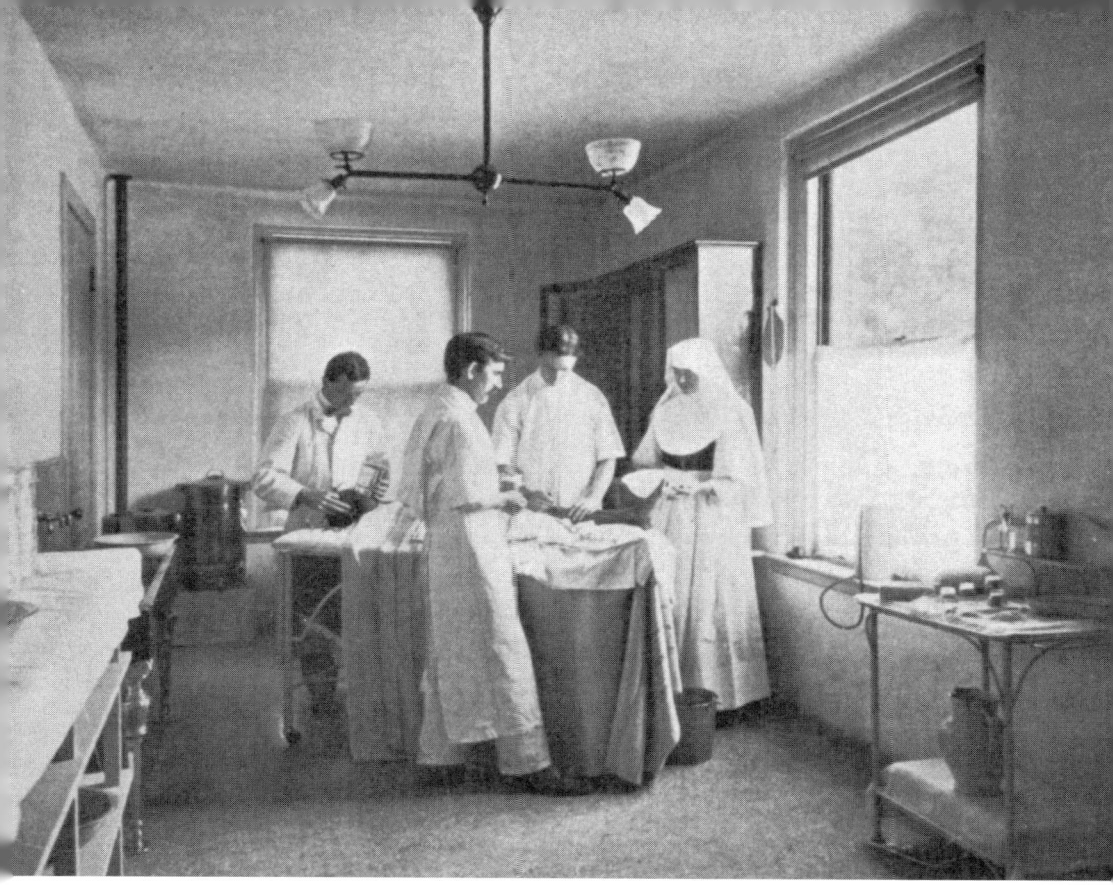

This photo, circa 1903, of the emergency operating room in use at Georgetown University
Hospital shows gaslights directed everywhere
except on the patient and still no surgical
gloves. Courtesy of Georgetown University
Archives.

they were truly necessary continued in some places up to World War I.[50]

At Georgetown, the first recorded mention of rubber gloves came in May of 1906 when Henry D. Fry, the professor of obstetrics, presented to the faculty a list of criticisms of procedures at the university hospital and "made a strong plea for rubber gloves in the operating room." He and other abdominal surgeons, Fry said, "absolutely would not operate in a hospital without the use of rubber gloves." The faculty's hospital management committee, agreeing that the hospital "could not afford to be in any way behind the times in modern methods," recommended that gloves be provided.[51] As usual, the matter was referred to the university president, now the Reverend David Buel, S.J. who replied sharply: "More than one member of the committee, ranking as highly as any surgeon in this locality, has made it his practice to operate without gloves, without incurring any suspicion of being behind the times in modern methods, and other surgeons who desire to use gloves have, and do gladly, provide themselves with them." Buel pointed out that a single pair of sterile rubber gloves cost one dollar—a fifth of the five dollar operating room fee which the hospital charged paying patients. He further pointed out that the surgeons themselves were charged nothing for use of the operating room and its equipment, or for the services of nurses, assistants, and cleaners, yet they charged private patients up to five hundred dollars per operation. Despite all this, he said tartly, he had arranged for Sister Pauline to provide gloves in future operations—and, in a final thrust, offered to pay for them himself if necessary.[52]

Whatever the identity of that "high-ranking surgeon" who never used gloves, it was not George Tully Vaughan. Three years earlier he had published his highly-regarded textbook *Principles and Practice of Surgery*, in which he made clear that "rubber gloves can be sterilized, while with the naked hand there is always some doubt as to its sterility . . . It is a good rule for the surgeon to have his assistants [also] use gloves, as otherwise he cannot always be sure that their hands are suitably prepared." His book insisted that the whole surgical team be clothed in sterilized suits and caps "to avoid all chance of infecting the patient," and—at a time when the debate on surgical masks was only beginning—suggested that "if the operator has to talk during the operation it is well to have a piece of gauze or a mask of some kind over the mouth."[53]

Vaughan's book, in which he thanked Georgetown's medical students and interns for their help, demonstrated his quality as a surgeon and teacher. One review judged that it

> . . . gives to the profession a clear, well-balanced presentation of a science that is inclining toward excessive elaboration rather because of the disinclination of the surgeon to entirely let go of the old while reaching out for the new. By avoiding this error and by infusing his well-known judgment and scholarship into the work, Dr. Vaughan has produced a distinct advance in surgical literature.[54]

These were the days of the earliest ventures into heart surgery. Vaughan devoted just two of the 569 pages in his book to the subject,

describing the only three procedures then attempted: tapping the cavity of
the heart to draw off blood ("This is a dangerous operation and should not
be lightly undertaken"); suturing wounds in the pericardium; and suturing
penetrating wounds of the heart itself.[55] This last operation, then regarded
as the ultimate in heroic surgery, was a new development in which
Vaughan had a deep interest. In 1901, he was the second surgeon in the
United States to attempt suture of the heart; in 1908, he became the sixth
American to perform it successfully.

   In the early 1880s, even the great German surgeon Theodore Billroth
had echoed centuries of superstition when he remarked: "Let no man who
hopes to retain the respect of his medical brethren dare to operate on the
human heart."[56] But in March 1896, someone did. Guido Farina of Rome
closed a stab wound of the right ventricle with three silk sutures. The
patient died of pneumonia six days later, but he had lived long enough to
validate the feasibility of the operation itself. Six months later Ludwig
Rehn of Frankfurt became the first to suture the heart of a patient who
recovered.[57] By the end of 1900, twenty-five similar attempts had been
made worldwide, with seven recoveries. This relative success stimulated a
further nineteen attempts in 1901, of which four were successful.[58]

   Vaughan made his first attempt on the evening of October 2, 1901, at
Emergency Hospital, less than an hour after the twenty-five-year-old
patient had suffered a one-inch stab wound in the left ventricle. Vaughan
sutured the wound, and drained and closed the pericardium, but then the
patient's heart stopped and efforts at resuscitation failed. "Death was caused
by hemorrhage," Vaughan wrote. Afterwards, reviewing the twenty-four
cases of heart-wound suture that had been published worldwide up to that
time—the first such tabulation in medical literature—he concluded that
hemorrhage presented the most immediate danger, but that infection had
caused six out of the sixteen deaths, probably because "the urgency of the
symptoms and the necessity for prompt and rapid action prevent the observance of proper aseptic precautions."[59] Vaughan's operation had been
performed six months after the first attempt in the United States had been
made by a surgeon in St. Louis, Missouri.[60] It preceded the first successful
American attempt, that of Luther Hill of Alabama, by eleven months. In his
account of that event, Hill noted that in any case of suspected heart injury,
"it is the duty of the surgeon to determine the nature of the injury by an

exploratory operation, as recommended by Professor Vaughan."[61]

Vaughan's second heart operation was performed six years later, on Saturday, February 1, 1908, also at Emergency Hospital. The patient, Richard Denton, was a thirty-two-year-old barber in an advanced state of alcoholic intoxication who had been stabbed in the chest an hour earlier. The blade had passed through the left lung and pericardium and made a wound one-third of an inch long in the lower end of the left ventricle. Vaughan later described how, using ether as an anesthetic and working under strict asepsis, he incised a U-shaped flap in the chest and cut through the fourth, fifth, and sixth ribs and the pericardium to expose the heart. "The lips of the wound were caught with hemostatic forceps and held together while a continuous suture of fine silk—five sutures—was made. The stitch holes bled, so that a second row of silk sutures was inserted . . . Two points continued to bleed and were caught up with forceps and ligated with catgut. Hemostatis was then complete and the heart beat well and strong." Denton made a steady recovery over the following five weeks—except for spasms of delirium tremens which were treated with hourly shots of whiskey. On March 11, he was discharged from hospital; and that evening Vaughan took him to a meeting of the D.C. Medical Society to demonstrate the case, which had already become celebrated locally. Less than three weeks later, the patient was readmitted to hospital "on account of excessive drinking," but was later discharged "in excellent condition" and six months later was "apparently in perfect health."[62] The police waited to see whether Denton would recover, then charged his assailant with "murderous assault." Vaughan appeared as star witness for the prosecution at the trial. The judge listened to his evidence in fascination, and then congratulated him on his "wonderful feat of surgery."[63]

The Journal of the American Medical Association (JAMA) confirmed that before the Denton case, only nine such operations had been performed in the United States, with five recoveries.[64] Following his own success, Vaughan again tabulated and analyzed all cases of heart-wound suture attempted worldwide. He presented the results in his presidential address to the Association of Military Surgeons of the United States in Atlanta, Georgia, in October 1908, and published them in the JAMA the following February. There had been 150 reported cases by then, with ninety-eight deaths and fifty-two recoveries—a mortality rate of 65 percent. This,

Vaughan pointed out, was "practically the same" as it had been in 1901. He demonstrated, again, that the main causes of death were hemorrhage and infection of the pleura or pericardium, showing that "there is room for great improvement in preventing infection." Even so, he concluded: "If Billroth could appear today he would be astonished to learn that not only does the profession approve of such operations, but that the mortality is no greater than he experienced in his own early work in abdominal surgery. Heart surgery is truly modern surgery."[65]

Vaughan wrote these words more than forty years before the advent of "open-heart" surgery. He performed his successful suture without benefit of intratracheal anesthesia, blood transfusion, oxygenators, or antibiotics. Primitive as they may seem today, his contributions rank him as a clinical pioneer of cardiac surgery. They also indicate his open-mindedness to new ideas in surgery, if not in politics and society, and the ego-strength that enabled him to test innovative techniques when opportunity presented.

Nowhere is this combination of qualities better illustrated than in Vaughan's work on transplants. For some years, he had closely followed the earliest experimental work of Alexis Carrel and others on the transplantation of organs, limbs, and joints. Then Vaughan, as early as January 1909, carried out the first transplant ever attempted at Georgetown University Hospital.

George A. Kelly, a thirty-year-old clerk, was suffering from a suppurating tuberculous knee joint. It had reached the stage when either amputation at the thigh or excision of the knee were necessary. Vaughan told the patient that a third option would be to attempt to transplant a sound knee joint taken from a deceased donor. He explained that this was an experimental operation he had never done before; Kelly chose the transplant. Vaughan removed the lower end of the femur and upper end of the tibia and replaced them with the donor joint, which was cut to fit and fastened in place by wires; then he replaced the patella in front of it. "There was almost immediate improvement in the patient's condition," Vaughan recorded. The operation attracted widespread interest; two surgeons visiting Washington from France and Germany even came to examine Kelly's knee. Vaughan was pleased the graft had succeeded, but was disappointed in his earlier hope that the patient would be able to bend his knee; the new joint remained rigid. Moreover, suppuration continued, requiring daily dressing, and eighteen months after the operation Kelly died. On autopsy, Vaughan found that "the transplanted parts had been largely absorbed and their place taken by new bone which had grown into them; at least two thirds of the foreign bone had disappeared." He concluded: "While the operation in this case was a failure, chiefly on account of the unfavorable conditions which existed, enough was learned to strengthen my belief in the success of the operation in better selected cases."[66]

Vaughan claimed no original breakthroughs of his own, and his pioneering work almost always followed up on recent discoveries by others: the knee-joint operation was based on the work of the German surgeon Erich Lexer, who had reported it only months earlier. But there was one exception. In 1902, Vaughan invented a technique for arresting hemorrhage from bone by plugging it with soft tissues, a procedure so simple that he described it in just two sentences: "The method consists in cutting a fragment of soft tissue, muscle or fascia, from any convenient place in the field of operation and applying the fragment to the bleeding surface or edge of the exposed, broken, or cut bone by means of the fingers," he wrote. "The advantages are obvious—the material is always present, it does not require special preparation, it does not act as a foreign body, and, according to my experience, it is always efficient." This technique was published in many journals in the United States and abroad, and was included in a standard textbook of the time, Da Costa's *Modern Surgery*.[67]

Having changed to a four-year curriculum and daytime teaching at the end of the nineteenth century, Georgetown had entered the twentieth century confident that it had attained a reasonably high standard of medical education. George Kober's work for higher standards at the national level seemed certain to sustain that momentum. His prestige was such that in 1906 he was elected president of the Association of American Medical Colleges (AAMC).[68]

Two years earlier, Kober had heard that the state of Michigan was proposing to introduce a new standard curriculum by mandating its medical schools to offer a minimum forty-two hundred hours of instruction over a four-year course. This was nine hundred hours more than the AAMC then thought an adequate standard and up to thirty-two hundred hours more than the poorest American schools were actually offering. Kober was impressed. So, at the AAMA's annual meeting in Atlantic City, New Jersey, in April 1904, he suggested that the Association should study curriculum differences between schools and develop recommendations for a uniform standard of hours nationwide. The delegates responded by appointing a committee and electing Kober its chairman.[69]

At the next Georgetown faculty meeting in May, Kober and the other professors discussed the Michigan schedule, which also specified minimum hours of instruction in each branch: 562 hours for surgery, for example. They decided to adopt it at Georgetown, to start in the new session in September.[70]

Kober delivered his report to the AAMC at its next annual meeting in Chicago in April 1905. His committee had found that between schools the total number of teaching hours varied from 958 to 10,244, with equally wide variations in specific subjects. "In some schools," he wrote, "such important subjects as physical diagnosis, pharmacology, etiology and hygiene are not taught at all, while one school devoted 780 hours to orthopedic surgery." This, he said, showed a "lamentable lack of uniformity."[71] The standard he proposed—the same that Georgetown had already introduced—was immediately adopted by the AAMC. On Kober's return from Chicago, the faculty recorded its congratulations: his achievement "could not fail to reflect credit upon the school and the author of the report."[72] The following year Kober, now president of the AAMC, became the second member of the medical faculty, after Hamilton, to be honored with an honorary LL.D. degree from Georgetown University.[73]

The euphoric sensation of being at the forefront once again no doubt inspired the faculty, with Kober's encouragement, to introduce another important new standard that the AAMC had adopted at the same meeting: two years of college as a requirement for admission into the medical school.[74] This went into effect at Georgetown in September 1905. The inevitable result was an immediate drop in enrollment. Only 23 new students registered that September, compared with 43 the previous year, reducing the total enrollment from 123 to 90. The next year brought a further disastrous drop to a total of 73, of whom only 13 were freshmen.[75] Reporting this setback to the university president, David Buel, Kober pointed out that the medical schools of Harvard and Columbia Universities had experienced similar falls in enrollment: "Higher entrance requirements may therefore be regarded as the principal factor."[76] But if other schools could sustain such drastic losses, Georgetown could not. The faculty was forced to abandon the college requirement and return to its old standard of four years of high school. It also accepted some students who had failed at other medical schools.[77] Enrollments rose again.

Although by 1907 only eight American medical schools insisted on two years of college for admission,[78] this failure was an intense disappointment to Kober. He also worried that a "large percentage" of Georgetown graduates were failing state board examinations. This, he told the faculty in October 1906, "strongly points to the fact that our final examinations are not sufficiently rigid."[79] Georgetown examinations then consisted of five questions in each subject; each question carried 20 percent of the final score, with an overall 70 percent required in each subject to pass. The quality of both questions and grading may be deduced from the recollections of James A. Gannon, later to become a surgery professor at the school, who graduated in 1906:

> One of the five questions in our final examination in medicine, which included pediatrics, was this: "A six months old baby has to be weaned. How would you feed it?" . . . My memory was hazy concerning infant feeding, and I just did not know how to feed this baby, and left this question till last . . . [Finally] I was desperate, so I wrote that I would do what most other doctors did and consult a good book on infant feeding.

Gannon later discovered that the professor of medicine, Samuel S. Adams, had regarded this answer as "so damned natural" that he gave him the maximum 20 percent score."[80]

The AAMC had no power at this time to enforce any of its recommended standards; it could raise them only by persuading member colleges to take an exemplary lead. The only enforceable standards were set by the licensing boards of each state, but they still commonly granted licenses to poorly trained graduates of low-grade medical schools. In 1906, the AAMC and the Council for Medical Education (CME), which had been established by the American Medical Association in 1904, took concerted action. They began by inspecting all medical schools. Within two years, they assembled a wealth of data which revealed that standards of education at many schools were even worse than they had supposed, particularly in the poorer southern and western states. But how could these be improved if such schools, and many licensing boards, would not, or could not, accept AAMC or CME recommendations? They needed more power and more public backing. So, in December 1908, the CME's secretary, N. P. Colwell, took the data to Henry S. Pritchett, president of the prestigious Carnegie Foundation for the Advancement of Teaching, and asked him to sponsor an "independent" inquiry into medical education across the country.[81] This study, conducted over the following year, was to become famous as the Flexner Report of 1910.

Abraham Flexner was a schoolmaster, classicist, historian, and reformer. He had training in neither science nor medicine and knew little about medical education (a cause of criticism later on). He began his Carnegie investigation in Baltimore at Johns Hopkins medical school, where he formed most of his ideas and which he used as a benchmark for the evaluation system he developed. Then, most often accompanied by Colwell, he visited every other medical school on the North American continent: 148 in the United States and 7 in Canada. He concluded that there were too many schools, often of negligible value, turning out too many doctors, often badly trained. It would serve the country better, he urged, to have fewer schools of greater quality graduating more proficient doctors.[82] Among the schools he deemed dispensable, after inspecting them in March 1909, were George Washington (formerly Columbian) and Georgetown.

Both schools, he wrote in summary:

> lack adequate resources as well as assured prospects. They are surrounded by medical schools—those of Richmond, Baltimore, Philadelphia— whose competition they cannot meet. Finally, the District of Columbia has relatively more physicians than any other part of the country. Should the district require, as it ought, a higher basis, or even enforce an actual four-year high school standard, both would suffer seriously. Neither school is now equal to the task of training physicians of the modern type.

Flexner's specific criticisms of Georgetown, which he labeled "a university department in name only," were: that its entrance requirement was in practice less than a four-year high school course; of its seventy-four teachers, only one (Kober) worked for the school full-time; although it had its own hospital with one hundred beds available for clinical use, this was "several miles distant" from the school; and although it had a "good" dissecting room, and "fair" laboratories for pathology, chemistry, bacteriology, and histology, it had no pharmacological laboratory, no library accessible to students, and no museum. The school's main weakness was lack of funds, its only resources being students' fees. Flexner also criticized Georgetown as one of the schools that allowed professors a share of the profits while failing to invest in buildings and equipment: "The medical department of Georgetown University has been in operation almost 60 years; its annual income is now estimated at $11,000. Its plant can represent only a small fraction of its receipts during its lifetime."[83]

Damning as Flexner's appraisal seems, Georgetown was in fact no worse than most other schools he visited and much better than many. Among the horrors Flexner documented around the country were schools that possessed not a single skeleton or microscope nor any clinical facilities; filthy laboratories and intolerable odors from putrid cadavers; a dissecting room that also served as a chicken yard; a gynecology room with no window, water, or equipment; a "library" without a single volume; a school with an adjoining "teaching" hospital on whose door was inscribed "No students admitted"; a school which had on its staff two teachers who had failed their state board examinations after graduating from the same school two years earlier; and a school with twenty-six professors and nine students which was, Flexner wrote, "a disgrace to the state whose laws permit its existence."[84]

Georgetown was not alone in struggling on a low income: fifty-one American schools, or more than a third, had annual incomes below $10,000—the lowest being $1,060. Nor was it the only medical school connected to a university which gave it little or no financial support: twenty-one other schools were in the same position. "It is important that our universities realize that medical education is a serious and costly venture," Flexner commented, "and that they should reject or terminate all connection with a medical school unless prepared to foot its bills and to pitch its instruction on a university plane."[85] Flexner was himself a graduate of Johns

Hopkins University, and its medical school remained his ideal.[86] With an income of more than $80,000 a year, plus a hospital endowment of $3.6 million which paid salaries to its full-time and part-time teaching and clinical staff, and its emphasis on premedica_ degrees, graduate studies, and research, Johns Hopkins was "the first medical school in America of genuine university type" and had "finally cleared up the problems of standards and ideals." At the other end of the spectrum, Flexner said, the "frankly mercenary" schools with nominal or no entranɔe requirements "should be summarily suppressed."[87]

The Flexner Report, published in 1910, caused a sensation. Its author's blunt conclusions and scathing wɛy with words—plus the fact that he named names—ensured that it was widely quoted. Flexner achieved what the AAMC and CME had hoped: public demand for higher standards. Modern medical historians have found deficiencies in Flexner's approach: he emphasized basic science at the expense of clinical applications; he evaluated each medical school's physical plant in detail but ignored the teaching qualities of high-caliber faculty members; and in promoting Johns Hopkins as ideal he gave more weight to research than to the training of competent physicians.[88] But at the time, the effect of the report was to strengthen greatly the power of the AAMC and CME, which had, after all, been the purpose of the exercise. After Flexner, both organizations and many state licensing boards imposed increasingly tough conditions for accreditation. So many medical schools were unable or unwilling to comply that by 1925 their number had almost halved, dropping from 148 to 80.[89] It was close to miraculous that Georgetown survived.

The faculty was, of course, shocked by Flexner's assessment. Its first reaction was to send a letter drafted by Kober to the president of the Carnegie Foundation, politely asserting that Georgetown's designation as "a university department in name only" was "not wholly fair," and offering a number of explanations to qualify Flexner's bald statements.[90] The unpalatable fact, however, was that his judgment was broadly correct; and some of the faculty's self-justifications hovɛred at the margin of truthfulness. Defending the absence of a proper library, for example, Kober said that students used one of the best medical libraries in the world, the surgeon general's; but since that library closed every day at 4:30 P.M., it is doubtful whether more than a few students ever went there.[91] His explanation that Georgetown had clinical facilities at many hospitals other than its own did not rebut Flexner's basic criticism that the University Hospital was "miles distant" from the school. As James Gannon recalled of his student days: "Much time was wasted on trips to widely separated hospitals."[92]

But Kober, despite the protestations set forth in that letter, was himself in no doubt Georgetown had to change. At the same faculty meeting on March 10, 1910, when Flexner's criticisms were first discussed, Kober said he was in favor of selling the building on H Street and relocating the school close to the University Hospital. The trustees of Emergency Hospital were then looking for new premises, and Kober got permission from the new university president, Reverend Joseph Himmel, S.J., to sell the H Street property to them for forty thousand dollars. The faculty invested one hundred dollars in having conversion plans drawn up, "to make a good presentation." But Emergency Hospital did not want the building; nor did anyone else.[93]

The faculty made other attempts to overcome Georgetown's shortcomings. It set about establishing its own library and museum, and appointed four "quiz masters" in an effort to improve the students' retention of knowledge. At this stage, even Kober thought that all would be well provided the school could demonstrate that its graduates performed respectably in state board examinations.[94] To that end—urged on by Kober, Samuel Adams, and George Tully Vaughan against the misgivings of several other professors—the faculty voted in March 1911 to bring back the two-year college entrance requirement. Vaughan said he felt it necessary "in view of the fact that 28 medical schools are now enforcing the two years requirement."[95]

But three months later, another blow fell. The New York Board of Regents, the licensing authority for that state, announced that from October 1, 1912, it would accredit only medical schools which employed at least six full-time salaried instructors in the basic science branches. After several meetings to discuss the implications of this, the Georgetown professors concluded: "It appears that the Regents are determined to suppress all schools that do not possess an ample endowment for teaching, and it may be impracticable for us to meet their requirements."[96] The following December, the AMA's Council for Medical Education introduced the same condition into its new set of recommended standards, which meant that other states would surely follow New York's lead.[97] Flexner had provided the regulatory agencies with teeth; now they were beginning to bite.

With hindsight, it is clear that two main factors saved the medical school from closure at this gruelling time. The first was the force of George Kober's tenacity, ingenuity, and, not least, his personal generosity. The medical school needed a library: Kober donated his own considerable lifetime collection of books and journals The hospital needed a pharmacological laboratory and more free beds for clinical instruction: Kober, at his own expense, built and equipped a new wing at the hospital to meet both needs.[98] But even Kober could not pay the annual salaries of six men.

The solution, and the second saving factor, lay in a development that had occurred ten years earlier, though no one had grasped its significance at the time. In April 1901, the faculty had been approached by the Washington Dental College, which was in financial straits, suggesting a merger. The medical professors took the proposal none too seriously and rejected it. But the university's president at that time, John Whitney, was eager to establish a third professional school and he insisted that they reconsider—which the faculty duly did, but only on condition that the new dental department pay two-thirds of the cost of extending the medical school building to accommodate dental students and thereafter share all expenses.[99] Thus, in the 1909–10 school year, the medical school received not only $11,816 in tuition fees, but a further $2,473 from the dental school.[100] It was scarcely a princely sum, but it made all the difference when the faculty began to calculate whether they could afford to pay six salaries—for which they needed around $9,000 per year.

It took months of agonizing to resolve the problem. Finally the faculty decided they could meet the requirements (barely) by paying minimal salaries to instructors in the laboratory branches for a total outlay of seven thousand dollars a year—about half the school's income. This was made affordable in part by the unanimous decision of the professors who taught the clinical branches "to relinquish all claims to financial compensation" themselves.[101] (For several years each had received dividends ranging from one hundred to seven hundred dollars a year). But that still left a shortfall. So Kober found an ingenious way of cutting the cost of two of the required salaries. He volunteered to reduce his own salary, as professor of hygiene, to a minimal five hundred dollars.[102] And he secured permission from president Himmel to appoint a college Jesuit, Father Francis Tondorf, to teach physiology. Tondorf came free, since Jesuits were not allowed by the order to earn money.[103] Nevertheless, he was not the most obviously eligible choice. An able physicist and astronomer, Tondorf had established an earthquake laboratory at Georgetown in 1911 and later was to become world famous for his work in seismology.[104] What he lacked was any medical training. Kober, desperate, decided that a course in biology that Tondorf had taken at Johns Hopkins in 1898–99—actually only sixty-four hours of instruction, as part of a broader course in math and physics[105]—was sufficient qualification. By May 1912, Kober had hopes that this precarious arrangement would meet the New York standard. As treasurer as well as dean of the school, however, he looked to the next academic year with trepidation. New students would have to meet the two-year college requirement; and the school, already stretched by the new salaries, might well suffer another drop in enrollment and fees.

Then, in July, another devastating blow fell. Kober received a letter from Colwell, informing him that the Council for Medical Education could no longer give Georgetown an A rating under the accreditation system it had established in 1906.[106] For Kober, a national leader of reform in medical education, this was personally humiliating; for the school, it threatened disaster. In correspondence with Colwell through the summer, Kober argued that the CME should never have taken this step without giving Georgetown the chance to rectify shortcomings, and he pointed to the many improvements it had already made since the last CME inspection.[107] In lengthy replies, Colwell insisted these were not good enough. In essence, he said, "Your school should have an annual income aside from students' fees of something like $20,000 or $25,000; otherwise we do not see how you can possibly engage an ample number of full-time teachers, strictly enforce your preliminary requirements, and otherwise properly conduct a medical school."[108] Kober responded in tones bordering on despair:

> You will agree with me that it will be much easier to secure endowments in the face of such contemplated action than after the act is accomplished—and who, may I ask, with two years of collegiate work, will

enter a school rated in Class B? Such action will either destroy the school or compel regressive steps in the matter of entrance requirements. I have been one of the pioneers in the matter of high medical education and under most adverse circumstances have accomplished creditable progress. I maintain that a school with our entrance requirements, a university hospital of 250 beds, improved methods of teaching and equipment, and other advantages . . . should not be destroyed without previous notice and a fair opportunity to meet the requirements of the Council.[109]

But in late August, the CME published in the *Journal of the American Medical Association* its list of accredited schools in category A; and Georgetown was not among them. It had in fact been relegated to category B: "schools which under their present organization might be made acceptable by general improvements"; but as the CME published neither those listed in category B nor in category C, defined as "schools which need a complete organization to make them acceptable," Georgetown's demotion was exacerbated by its ambiguity.[110] The faculty's bitterness was only heightened by the fact that, for reasons Colwell refused to divulge, the other medical schools in D.C., George Washington and Howard, had been given an A rating.[111]

Kober continued his bombardment of Colwell by letter; and there is some evidence that the new university president, Reverend A. J. Donlon, S.J. threatened the council with legal action. Certainly Georgetown enlisted the support of William Woodward, a graduate of the medical school who was both a lawyer and influential as the Health Officer of the District of Columbia. He drafted a letter to the council which Donlon signed.[112] In November, the council finally agreed to inspect Georgetown again. It afterwards made detailed recommendations, and the faculty agreed to adopt them.[113] Another month of suspense passed, as the faculty awaited the outcome. Then, on December 28, 1912, Kober sent Donlon a telegram from Chicago, where he had met with the CME: "Result of meeting satisfactory. School will be reinstated in class A . . . Much credit due to Woodward."[114]

As Kober had anticipated, freshmen numbers did drop precipitously because of the two-year college requirement; in October 1913, only eleven enrolled.[115] But steps to address this shortfall were already in hand. Kober had persuaded the university to introduce a two-year premedical course, the idea being that after 1915, all its graduates would swell the numbers in the medical school.[116] Meanwhile, he and the faculty struggled on, putting into effect as many of the council's recommendations as they could afford— although some were not actually implemented until years later.

One recommendation which the faculty did act on immediately was to reorganize the school into eight departments. In November 1912, therefore, George Tully Vaughan became the first chairman of Georgetown's department of surgery.[117]

The department comprised twenty-seven professors and instructors and included the surgical specialties of the time: gynecology, ophthalmology, otolorhinolaryngology, genito-urinary surgery, orthopedic surgery, dermatology, and syphilology.[118] Isaac S. Stone, who had been a clinical professor at Georgetown since 1892, now headed gynecology after the retirement of his longtime friend Taber Johnson. Stone, highly regarded as an excellent surgeon, followed in Johnson's footsteps to become president of the Southern Surgical Association in 1918.[119] Walter Wells, also well-known in his speciality, was the newly-appointed chief of laryngology, rhinology, and otology (later known as ear, nose, and throat surgery). A Georgetown graduate of 1891, Wells had spent two years training in Vienna, where he found stoic locals willing to hire themselves out to help students master the technique of using laryngeal forceps. For forty cents an hour, he recalled "they would drop a little ball of lead fastened to the end of a string down into the larynx and allow you to fish around for it."[120] Ophthalmology was now headed by William Holland Wilmer, a brilliant eye surgeon who had succeeded to the chair after Swann Burnett's death in 1906 and was now establishing an international reputation.

These were all first-class surgeons with large private practices. Indeed, for all Georgetown's shortcomings, one of the ironies of those difficult post-Flexner years was that many of its teaching staff were nationally prominent and made valuable contributions to the profession. This was one important ingredient in medical education that Flexner had set aside in his evaluation, choosing instead to promote the ideal of a "full-time" faculty. Flexner, much under the influence of William Welch of Johns Hopkins, recommended that clinical professors should abandon private practice and give their whole time to teaching and research at the medical school and its attendant hospital. This concept, accepted today as the norm, was considered hopelessly impractical in 1910. Even Flexner acknowledged that it depended either on clinical professors voluntarily foregoing large incomes for inadequate salaries, or on schools amassing endowments large enough to pay competitive rates. Even at Johns Hopkins, Welch never wholly succeeded in forcing through the full-time plan. Its great chairman of surgery William Halsted, who commanded huge fees for operations, resolutely continued in private practice until his death in 1918. His successor J. M. T. Finney also refused to give up practice and served as interim chairman at Hopkins for three years until a full-timer could be found. No schools, not even Johns Hopkins and Harvard, established complete full-time faculties until after 1945. Meanwhile there was much resistance and many resignations, not only on grounds of money but because many professors found that the requirement for research and the restriction to practicing only in the university hospital combined to limit their clinical opportunities and consequently their own professional growth and teaching capability.[121]

At Georgetown, there is no evidence that anyone even considered putting the clinical faculty on a full-time basis in the years immediately following the Flexner report. There was simply not enough money—either from the school's own meager income, or from the university which, as a Jesuit institution, had no tradition of paying salaries even to its own faculty. On the contrary, the clinical professors continued to subsidize the school as they had through its history. Giving up their modest dividends to pay for six basic science salaries was merely a continuation of long-established reality; though in truth it was not much of a sacrifice. For all his teaching and administrative work, Vaughan, for example, had received a dividend of five hundred dollars a year, less than his fee for a single major operation.[122]

Yet Flexner and Welch were correct in perceiving that medical education now required far more of the professors' time than ever before. Less than thirty years earlier, two men had taught the entire range of theoretical and clinical surgery at Georgetown; now twenty-seven teachers were required. Subjects given brief mention a decade before now needed hours of instruction; new courses to cover new techniques were added regularly. Administration had also become more demanding. In addition to his extensive private practice and his prominent role in several professional societies, Vaughan, as chairman of the department, was supposed to supervise not only didactic and clinical instruction at the medical school and the university hospital, but also at surgical clinics in five other hospitals in the city.

Vaughan and his colleagues did try to improve clinical teaching and bolster the range and quality of care at the university hospital. But much of their time was spent away from the school and hospital, and the lack of any alternative supervision (again, a direct result of the school's inability to pay salaries for hospital appointments) caused countless problems. The faculty regularly complained of the hospital staff's failure to keep good records, or maintain sufficiently sterile conditions, or implement the agreed system for paying anesthetists (an issue over which Kober himself threatened to resign).[123] The sisters, in turn, complained of irresponsible interns neglecting their duties, or ignoring hospital rules, or refusing to treat college athletes "because [the interns] had not received the usual complimentary tickets to the games."[124]

In 1909, the faculty had discussed ways to go beyond clinical demonstrations given to entire classes in the amphitheater—a practice Flexner criticized, observing that "most of the students see only the patient's feet and the surgeon's head."[125] At leading medical schools, such clinical performances had given way to small-group instruction on charity patients who occupied free beds in the university hospitals and came in still greater numbers for free treatment at their outpatient dispensaries.[126] At Georgetown, a faculty investigation in 1909 concluded: "In its present disorganized condition, the utilization of the dispensary for teaching purposes is next to impossible." The investigation recommended setting up a "clerkship" system: groups of senior students rotating through the university hospital for one month each to gain "general training and experience." But this, as Vaughan and others pointed out, was "quite impracticable" without someone in authority at the hospital to supervise them.[127] Not until 1920 was a full-time medical director appointed.

In 1914, Kober had to report that "cases of infection had occurred after surgical operations which ought not to have occurred," and a committee headed by Vaughan and Stone was appointed to investigate and come up with a plan for a "uniform technique for the operating rooms."[128] In the event, Vaughan played little part in that inquiry.

By April 1914, the political upheavals in Mexico had reached crisis point, and an American naval expedition was dispatched to Vera Cruz. On April 21, Vaughan read the first newspaper reports of the battle that had begun there. The next day, he went to see Surgeon General William Braisted and volunteered his services to the Navy Medical Corps. Pausing only to pack his bags and send a hasty message to the Georgetown faculty, Vaughan set sail from Philadelphia the following morning on board the *Morro Castle*. He arrived in Vera Cruz six days later and was given command of the field hospital for the marine brigade, which he organized in a one-story, four-room schoolhouse on the edge of town. "One of the rooms," Vaughan recalled, "was divided into two by means of a tarpaulin across the middle which could be rolled up or let down as desired—the front being used for the surgeon's office and the rear for the operating and sterilizing room." Brigade surgeon D. N. Carpenter reported: "Considering the primitive facilities of the operating room, the results obtained were excellent. There were 66 major [and 41 minor] operations with no deaths, reflecting great credit on the skill of Dr. Vaughan who performed the majority of the operations." Vaughan stayed in Vera Cruz for ten weeks; his free time he spent sightseeing, bird-watching, and attending bullfights. When it became disappointingly clear that American forces would not, after all, march on Mexico City, he asked to be relieved from duty and returned home.[129]

In Vaughan's absence, Isaac Stone had served as acting chairman of the surgery department; it was he who devised the plan to improve conditions for surgery at the university hospital. He introduced, among other reforms, a standard operating room technique which was printed and distributed to all staff and to private physicians who treated patients at GUH; established rules for behavior during operations ("Students will not stamp their feet or applaud"); and appointed a committee of three faculty members to supervise the entry qualifications and curriculum at Georgetown's Training School for Nurses (which had been established in 1903) so as to upgrade nursing standards. He also insisted that the rule requiring interns to write careful case histories on all patients be strictly enforced. This was a problem so acute that Stone even offered a twenty-five dollar prize to the intern writing the "most intelligent and satisfactory case histories during the year of his residence." Most importantly, from an educational viewpoint, he recommended that interns be allowed to perform, under supervision, surgical operations for which they were judged fit and to administer anesthetics in ward cases. The faculty recorded its delight at the "splendid efforts" of Stone "to bring about much needed reforms."[130]

By the time Vaughan resumed his duties at Georgetown, World War I had erupted in Europe. Although the United States remained neutral for nearly three more years, a number of American physicians soon joined Red Cross units in the war zones. Among them was Ernest Pendleton Magruder, professor of clinical surgery and third-ranking member of Georgetown's surgery department. He went to Serbia in November 1914 as director of American Red Cross Unit Number Three at Gevgalija. At the beginning of April in 1915, he wrote home: "I am looking after nearly 3,000 cases—operative and typhus, and for once in my life I have surgery to the full, yet it is not bullets but disease which makes it most dangerous here, especially typhus . . . People are dying at an alarming rate, and Serbia is quite helpless to combat the scourge now spreading rapidly." Shortly after writing this, Magruder traveled to Belgrade to care for the director of the first American Red Cross unit who had fallen ill with typhus; on the way, he too caught the disease and died. He was forty-three years old. In a memorial address to the Medical Society of D.C., George Tully Vaughan noted that of the eighteen American surgeons and nurses sent to Serbia by the Red Cross, only three had escaped typhus. He also read out a cablegram of condolence from the general secretary of the Serbian Red Cross, who said: "We ourselves have lost 105 doctors."[131]

Another early volunteer was John Breckenridge Bayne, son of a former Georgetown professor of clinical surgery and a graduate of the medical school. He went to England in 1916 and joined a medical unit sent to Rumania. His subsequent war service read "like a fairy story," an article in the *Georgetown College Record* later recorded:

At Bucharest he refused to leave the city while it was being bombed, although he had an attendant and two patients killed beside him. While assisting the natives he contracted cholera and subsequently diphtheria. For the latter he was obliged to operate on his own throat. When Bucharest was captured by the Germans, he was sent to a prison camp where he suffered incredible hardships. Finally escaping, he returned to America. He spent a couple of months recuperating in this country and then was sent back to Rumania in advance of the Red Cross ship.

Bayne's heroism won him the Star of Rumania, the country's highest honor.[132]

By 1917, it was clear that the United States would soon formally enter the war. That January, the Commission for National Defense called on medical schools to prepare by providing instruction in military medicine and surgery. Georgetown, of course, had been offering such courses on and off since 1863. Pledging full cooperation, George Kober could not resist adding that Vaughan and the current professor of military surgery, Walter Webb, were already lecturing on the subject.[133] As soon as the United States declared war on Germany on April 6, the faculty made 150 beds at the university hospital available to the navy, but insisted that so far as possible medical students should complete their degrees and one-year hospital internships before enlisting.[134] Almost at once, though, professors and instructors began requesting leaves of absence "for the duration."

George Tully Vaughan was now fifty-eight years old, some thirteen years beyond the normal limit for military service, but once again he followed the drum. Reporting for active duty as a lieutenant commander in the navy medical corps in June 1917, he served most of the next nineteen months on the North Atlantic as senior surgeon aboard the huge troop transport USS *Leviathan*. She was originally the German luxury liner *Vaterland*, star of the Hamburg-America line, but she had been confiscated—along with 103 other German vessels caught in American ports—on the day the U.S. declared war. Then the largest ship afloat, and one of the fastest, she was ideal for conversion into one of the transports the U.S. desperately needed to ferry more than a million troops to Europe.[135] "The beautiful staterooms," Vaughan recalled, "were torn out and iron standees from two to three in tiers were placed in the various decks—enough to accommodate 10,000 men. The ballroom, 90 by 60 feet, was fitted up as the chief hospital ward with beds in tiers two deep, while the orchestra platform was changed into two rooms for surgical operations with a sterilizing room adjoining."

The *Leviathan*, because of her speed, sailed mostly alone, without convoy. She could make the round trip from Baltimore to Liverpool or Brest and back in an unprecedented twenty-six days. Vaughan made the crossing twenty times. A prize target for German U-boats, the ship was "attacked five times by submarines and ran aground once, at Liverpool, but got off at high tide," he recalled. Had they ever abandoned ship, Vaughan was expected to take forty-seven passengers in his lifeboat. Despite the conditions—brutal storms and numbing Atlantic weather—and the fact that Vaughan was three times the age of many of the soldiers and crewmen he was caring for, he appears to have relished the experience. He claimed to have had no difficulty performing operations even with the ship steaming at full speed. His worst crisis was an epidemic of influenza (the deadly "Asian flu" of 1918) during one crossing from which ninety-one patients died.[136] Among the two thousand men who served as her crew, the *Leviathan* inspired such affection that in 1923 they formed an association which held reunions for more than forty years. Their abiding disappointment was that one of her crew, a signalman in the war, never showed up: he was the movie star Humphrey Bogart.[137]

In Vaughan's absence, the Georgetown faculty, after an outside search, appointed James F. Mitchell as acting chairman of surgery. Mitchell, a graduate of Johns Hopkins, was a distinguished surgeon; at Hopkins he had taken the famous 1893 photograph of the first operation in which a surgeon used rubber gloves.[138] But within months, Mitchell too went on active duty. By September of 1918, six professors and several instructors were absent from the department of surgery on military service, prompting the university president, Reverend John B. Creeden, S.J. to protest to the surgeon general that "the continued withdrawal of teachers is likely to threaten the very existence of the school."[139] The surgeon general arranged for a naval surgeon, Howard F. Strine, to take over as acting chief of surgery. Strine brought a certain resourcefulness to the task of teaching with a depleted staff; in late 1918, only four years after Charlie Chaplin had begun appearing in movies, Strine "introduced the unique plan of teaching the techniques of the most important operations by means of moving pictures."[140] In January 1919, Vaughan mustered out of the navy with the rank of commander and resumed his chairmanship of the department.[141]

In a commencement address the following June, the professor of ophthalmology, William Wilmer, reflected on the impact of the World War on Georgetown. "Seven men of the medical school have been decorated by our own and Allied governments, while eight have made the supreme sacrifice," he said.[142] Wilmer himself had received high honors. He had served through the war as surgeon in chief of the Medical Research Laboratories at Issoudun, in France, where he directed researches vital to early military aviation. He trained the first flight surgeons, studied the effects of high altitude and low oxygen on pilots, improved their performance, and reduced accidents. He was promoted to brigadier general, mentioned in dispatches, and awarded the U.S. Distinguished Service Medal and the French Legion of Honor.[143] At that commencement in 1919, both Wilmer and Vaughan were honored by Georgetown University with LL.D. degrees "in recognition of their scientific and patriotic services."[144]

One year after ending his military service, Vaughan performed another operation which earned him a footnote in the history of cardiovascular surgery. He appeared for a while to be the first surgeon to successfully treat an aneurysm of the abdominal aorta by ligation. This operation had first been attempted by the great English surgeon Astley Cooper in 1817, and over the next 103 years there had been eighteen further attempts. All had failed: twelve patients died within hours; Halsted's two lived for forty-one and forty-seven days; only one survived for six months.

Vaughan's patient was a thirty-nine-year-old bricklayer who had developed an aneurysm on the left side of the aorta behind the pancreas. The operation was performed on January 23, 1920. Vaughan recorded that he ligated the aorta by means of Halsted's method of incomplete occlusion of the lumen, so that blood flow would not be entirely impeded, but using soft tape instead of metal bands:

> A piece of cotton tape one-half inch wide was carried around the vessel
> about two inches above the bifurcation and just below the origin of the
> inferior mesenteric artery. Two turns of one end of the tape made the

surgeon's or friction knot, which was drawn gradually tighter and tighter until pulsation was no longer perceptible in the iliacs and barely so in the aorta below the ligature, then the knot was completed, the ends of the tape cut off and the abdomen closed.

Vaughan delivered his paper describing this, and the nineteen previously recorded attempts, to a meeting of the American Surgical Association in May 1921.[145] The patient, he reported, had made a good recovery: five months after the operation, against Vaughan's advice, he had returned to the heavy labor of bricklaying for eight to ten hours a day: "When last heard from . . . one year and four months after operation, [he] was in good condition, but just recovering from a spree." But the patient died the following February 1922. On autopsy, Vaughan found that the aneurysm had not ruptured, but it had swollen to five times its original size, displaced a kidney, and obstructed the ureter.[146]

Vaughan's patient had survived far longer than the others—two years and one month—probably because he was relatively young and fit. But it is of interest that Vaughan already suspected ligation was not the answer to such cases. Nine years earlier he had speculated: "Whether the future will bring a successful and reliable method of treating aortic aneurysms in the shape of gradual occlusion by Halsted's bands or the resection of the aneurysm and the implantation of a section of sound aorta from cold storage or otherwise, or some other yet unknown method, time alone can tell."[147] These were prophetic words: surgeons did not find a definitive cure for aortic aneurysms until the early 1950s, when ligation was indeed superseded by the technique of cutting out the damaged portion of the vessel and replacing it with a preserved or artificial arterial graft—a technique, Vaughan would have been gratified to know, invented by Charles Hufnagel, one of his successors at Georgetown.

By the 1920s, Vaughan had become the leading general surgeon in Washington and was known nationally from his many papers in medical journals. In 1913, he had been one of fifty-seven surgeons from the United States and Canada invited to be founding members of the American College of Surgeons (ACS), another product of the post-Flexner mood for reform. The college's declared goal was to create a "distinct degree in surgery . . . as a necessary qualification for practicing surgery," to be conferred on medical graduates who had fulfilled a required "apprenticeship in surgical hospitals, operative laboratories and actual operative surgery."[148] This goal was never actually realized (although the ACS did later establish a rigorous qualification system of board and fellowship examinations); but soon after World War I, the ACS did begin inspecting and accrediting hospitals where surgery was taught.

The first inspections in 1919 and 1920 criticized Georgetown University Hospital for poorly kept patient records, particularly in the matter of diagnostic and progress notes, and for the fact that "no combined monthly staff meetings were held for the purpose of analyzing and discussing the clinical experience of the staff."[149] Much stronger criticism came in 1920 from the Georgetown Clinical Society, a select group of alumni who practiced in Washington. They were alarmed that fewer and fewer physicians were sending patients to Georgetown and, after investigation of the hospital's management, blamed both staff and faculty for "chaotic conditions." The society's investigating committee was specially critical of the operating room: "There have been entirely too many infections." The committee concluded that "the ultimate solution of the problem will be found in placing in charge a thoroughly trained, competent graduate nurse" responsible for reporting at once "the name of any operator or assistant who fails to comply in every detail with the prescribed technique."[150] In 1921, the ACS went so far as to drop GUH from its list of approved hospitals; the number of patients attending the dispensary immediately fell by eight thousand—a drop of 65 percent.[151] The hospital was reinstated the following year after monthly conferences were established; but by 1923, the hospital was still not meeting the ACS's minimum requirements: "Your records were said to be so incomplete and inadequate in many instances as to be of little practical value from a clinical point of view," its report charged.[152]

Record keeping had indeed been a problem for years, mainly because it was the responsibility of inadequately supervised interns. From the hospital's opening in 1898, all interns at GUH had been recent Georgetown graduates serving a one-year residence to gain hospital experience—a practice that in 1920 was not yet a national requirement and, by ensuring a supply of cheap menial labor, commonly benefited the hospital more than the intern. Complaints of interns failing, even refusing, to perform what was expected of them were frequent topics at faculty meetings. One erstwhile student, good enough to have graduated head of his class, was said to have exhibited "only the most languid interest in the hospital," obeyed instructions "only when he considered them reasonable," and had remarked that he had accepted the internship "to secure a year's rest before settling down to practice." Even this incorrigible was allowed to complete his year.[153]

In these days before properly organized residencies were established, graduates who wished to practice surgery gained experience in the most haphazard manner. The career of James Gannon is instructive. As an intern at the university hospital in 1906–7, he had assisted in surgical operations, and for the next seven years, performed whatever surgery came his way through private practice and by serving in the dispensaries of several city hospitals. Then, in 1914, he was appointed chief surgeon at the new Gallinger Hospital (later known as D.C. General). He recalled years later:

> Of course, when I took up this work my surgical experience was quite limited, and I taught myself the operations with which I was not familiar in the following manner: Dr. Vaughan and Dr. Webb were named on the staff as consulting surgeons, and I would ask them to do the operation and I would assist. The second time the same operation was to be performed, I again asked one of them to do the operation and I would assist again. I would then follow some corpse to the morgue of the hospital and perform the operation there myself. The third time a like case presented itself in the hospital, I performed the operation.[154]

At Georgetown, the first real step in improving supervision over interns came in 1919–20 when the faculty finally found the money to appoint a full-time salaried executive director of the hospital, Colonel William Arthur.[155] It also chose Father Tondorf, now head of the physiology department, as the school's first dean of students (a position later expanded under the title "regent"). Tondorf thus gained authority to deal with complaints both by and against students, including those in the college's premedical classes, in the medical school, and among the interns at the hospital.[156] It was not a popular appointment.

Unaware of the financial background, the students could never understand why Tondorf was teaching them physiology when he had no medical knowledge and, moreover, appeared to constantly disapprove of them. Some even speculated that his appointment was some form of Jesuitic penance.[157] His genius in seismology they all accepted. By the 1920s, Tondorf was pre-eminent; a seismic disturbance anywhere in the world brought international news agencies seeking his comments. His finest moment came in 1923 when he announced, from Georgetown, that a severe earthquake had hit Japan, hours before the news was known anywhere else.[158] Within the medical school, however, Tondorf was regarded as a loner, an eccentric, and "just plain strange." Also considered an implacable disciplinarian, he was "cordially disliked by many of the students, who feared that he would fail them and ruin their careers," in the words of one, William McEvitt. "If he addressed you as 'friend,' you were not in trouble; but to be referred to as 'doctor' amounted to a condemnation."[159]

Tondorf was reputed to haunt neighborhoods in the vicinity of the medical school, searching for students frequenting bars or even "houses of ill repute." Wallace Yater, who graduated in 1921 and later became chairman of medicine at Georgetown, recalled that he and some others were once caught by Tondorf drinking beer in a saloon, shortly after they had taken an examination in physiology. He called them back to the school for a "disciplinary" oral test which, he said, would affect their score in the written physiology exam. He then asked them to answer "yes" or "no" to a single philosophical question on two theories concerning the energy state of the universe: "Does either theory conflict with Aristotelian-Thomistic philosophy or with the Church's teaching on cosmology?"[160]

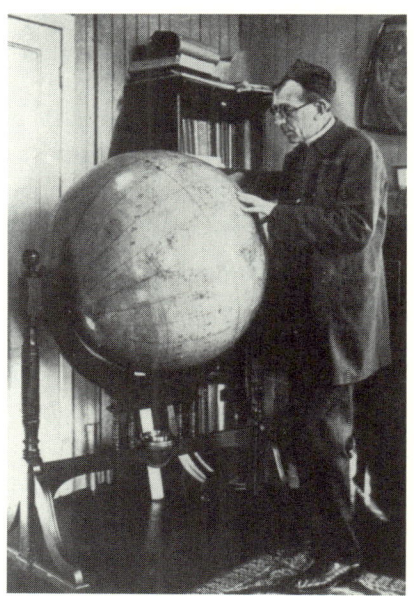

Tondorf, a famously hard worker, had no patience with even the most innocent forms of relaxation. One Sunday evening in January 1922,

Reverend Francis Tondorf, S.J., in his study. Courtesy of Georgetown University Archives.

during a storm that deposited twenty-eight inches of snow on Washington, several medical students were at the crowded Knickerbocker Theater watching a comic silent movie. Without warning, the roof caved in, killing 98 in the audience and injuring another 150. It was the city's worst disaster. "One moment we were all laughing as a clever caption was flashed on the screen. The next, all was horror," a survivor said. Five Georgetown students died, including two from the medical school, James F. Shea and William A. Walter. Four other Georgetown medical students were outside the theater and at once rushed into the wreckage and began heroic rescue work.[161] But during eulogies at the memorial service in Saint Patrick's Church, Father Tondorf chose to observe that had the dead students been at home studying, they would still be alive.[162] Students were outraged by this remark, believing it typical of the man's intolerance. Feelings against Tondorf— particularly among the interns—reached such a pitch that two years later Kober and university president Creeden reluctantly agreed "to bend to an almost universal opinion" and secretly arranged for Tondorf to resign his professorship and other duties at the medical school, ostensibly because of "pressure of work."[163]

Kober was greatly distressed by this. He admired and liked Father Tondorf and valued his services to the school, particularly in volunteering to teach physiology unpaid and so enabling the school to meet that require- ment for six full-time teachers back in 1912. Furthermore, in 1920, at a time when Georgetown had a poor reputation, Tondorf had brought credit to the school by taking the initiative on behalf of medical science in a national controversy over vivisection.

The growth of medical research in the first two decades of the century had spawned with it a vocal antivivisection movement which lobbied so successfully that by early 1920, the British government had appointed a Royal Commission to review the subject, while in the United States a bill was again passing through Congress to prohibit the use of dogs for experi- mentation in the District of Columbia. A strongly worded resolution of protest against the bill, drafted by Kober, was adopted by the 1920 national Congress on Medical Education.[164] But at Georgetown Tondorf called a faculty meeting and told them he thought "the time had arrived for a change from a defensive to an aggressive attitude on the part of the medical profes- sion." Georgetown, he said, should take the lead. James Gannon suggested a gladiatorial debate between Father Tondorf and "some chosen champion" from the Society for the Prevention of Cruelty to Animals.[165] Which, in fact, the redoubtable Tondorf did. But the faculty also sponsored nine public lectures on the importance of animal research in medicine and surgery. Simon Flexner (Abraham's brother), then director of the Rockefeller Institute for Medical Research in New York, gave the first lecture.[166] George Tully Vaughan gave another, in which he pointed out that research on dogs, monkeys, donkeys, and other animals was responsible for everything known about the brain and nervous system. Many formerly untreatable dysfunctions in the body, he said, could now be cured simply because the surgeon knew where to look for clots and tumors. He showed how research had led to successful operations on the abdomen, heart, and other organs, to transplants of tissue and bone, to vaccinations that prevented some diseases and treatments that cured or reduced the ravages of others—results that would have been impossible only fifty years before. In short, Vaughan said, animal experimentation had saved and extended the health and lives of countless human beings, whereas the "do-nothing method" propounded by the antivivisectionists had saved none. He castigated their "self-deceit," "distorting language," and "ridiculous logic."[167]

Father Tondorf edited these Georgetown lectures and had them bound into a one hundred-page booklet which he sent to medical institutions and newspapers nationwide. The demand was so great that he published a second edition in 1923. The campaign succeeded: Congress did not outlaw experimentation, and Georgetown received sheaves of congratulatory letters and telegrams for its well-publicized stand.[168]

The medical school needed that boost to morale. Its efforts to attract the endowment needed to raise the school's standing were still going nowhere. Hopes had been raised in mid-summer 1919 by a bill passing through Congress to give twenty-five thousand dollars apiece to Georgetown and George Washington medical schools, provided they raised matching funds.[169] The special predicament of both schools was captured by Surgeon General William Braisted in his letter of support to the House of Representatives:

In view of the fact that nearly all states in the Union make liberal provisions in many instances for their state universities and medical schools, and as it is well known that the tuition fees of students are wholly inadequate to cover the cost of education in modern medical and dental schools, in my judgment these two local universities, handicapped as they are for lack of adequate endowments, have rendered a great service in behalf of higher medical education and are deserving of recognition and financial aid.[170]

The bill passed the Senate, but failed in the House. Once again the two schools fell victim to their location: a stateless district, dependent on the whims of Congress.

Hopes rose again a few months later, when John D. Rockefeller announced he would give $100 million, at that time the largest philanthropic gift ever made, for the promotion of education, in particular to pay teachers more adequate salaries. Of this, $20 million was to be awarded to selected medical schools, with Abraham Flexner having principal say in the schools selected.[171] Kober at once went into high gear, enlisting the help of Georgetown's most illustrious and influential alumni.

One was Bailey K. Ashford, now an army medical officer in Puerto Rico. In 1899, he had discovered that the main cause of death on the island, endemic anemia, was caused by hookworm infestation. This breakthrough had prompted John D. Rockefeller to finance a health commission—forerunner of the Rockefeller Institute—to eradicate the disease worldwide. Ashford became internationally famous and in 1918 founded the School of Tropical Medicine in San Juan, a city so grateful that they named an avenue and a square in his honor.[172] Another distinguished alumnus recruited by Kober was Fielding Garrison, class of 1893, who had published in 1913 his 996-page *History of Medicine*. This classic work established Garrison's reputation as the leading American scholar of medical history.[173]

Ashford, who from his student days had regarded Kober as a near-substitute for his dead father, and who remained grateful that the school had trained him and his two brothers on half-tuition scholarships, traveled to New York in October to plead Georgetown's case in person. He wrote Kober: "I have tried to repay loyalty with loyalty. I did my very best."[174] For his part, Garrison responded: "I shall take great pleasure in writing to

Dr. Flexner, whom I know very well, and will ask Dr. Welch [of Johns Hopkins] and some other friends to intervene in the matter if possible."[175] Their efforts failed. Flexner wanted the funds used to establish full-time faculty; he bestowed money on scores of medical schools, including four hundred thousand dollars to Johns Hopkins.[176] Georgetown got nothing.

So, once again, the medical school turned to self-help. Starting with a legacy of more than fourteen thousand dollars bequeathed by Carroll E. Morgan, one of several of that family who had graduated from Georgetown or served on its faculty, the school established an endowment committee in 1920, headed by the associate professor of surgery James Gannon.[177] President Creeden and his deputy, W Coleman Nevils, also approached the archdiocese of Baltimore and other Catholic institutions for money "in order to place our medical school on a permanent basis," but that appeal too failed.[178] A general fundraising drive for the university did bring sixty thousand dollars to the medical school as its share. But otherwise, the endowment fund grew slowly from contributions by the medical professors themselves—mainly the faculty dividends they had given up—plus investment interest and a few modest bequests and donations.[179]

It was slow work and, ironically, the one large endowment offered to a Georgetown man at this time brought no assets to the school but, instead, another setback. William Wilmer's skill in ophthalmology was attracting patients from all over the world; and in 1922 he saved the sight of a wealthy society woman, Aida Root-Breckinridge. As she lay in her bed at Georgetown University Hospital with bandaged eyes, she had plenty of time to think. "I realized fully the many handicaps under which Dr. Wilmer was working in that small hospital from lack of equipment," she later recalled. There and then she conceived the idea of establishing, in his name, a world center for the research and treatment of eye disease. Wilmer, she said, "admitted that such an institute was very much needed but was horrified at the suggestion that the financial aid of his patients be requested. He not only refused to give out a list of his patients, but said he would block every attempt to compile a list." Mrs. Breckenridge was undeterred. Helped surreptitiously by, among others, Wilmer's family servant and his secretary, she compiled a list of more than seven hundred of his patients and from them collected some three hundred thousand dollars. Then she went to see Abraham Flexner at the Rockefeller Foundation. He

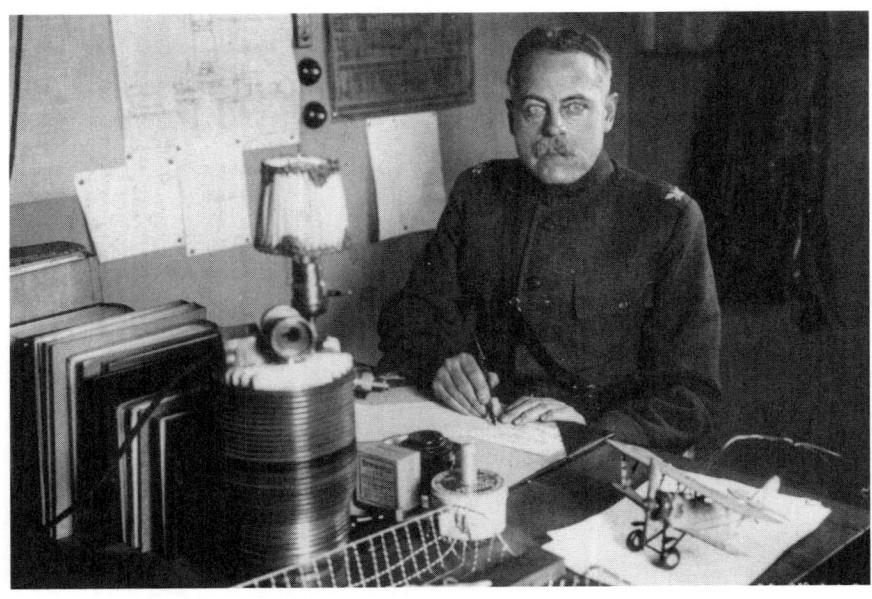

William Wilmer, M.D., 1863–1936,
photographed during active service in World
War I. Courtesy of the National Library of
Medicine.

considered the proposal a "very valuable idea," and offered to give $1.5 million
if a matching sum were raised, and provided that Wilmer himself would
consent to move to Baltimore so that his institute could be attached to Johns
Hopkins University.[180] Flexner too had his agenda.

Wilmer did not want to leave Washington. He had lived and practiced
there half his life. He had taught at Georgetown medical school for nearly
twenty years. And he came under great pressure to stay. A deputation from
the Medical Society of D.C. that included Kober and Adams called on him
in 1924 and "felt justified in stating," a minute noted, "that Dr. Wilmer
during the practice of his specialty for over 30 years in this city has acquired
a national and international reputation and hence the Wilmer Institute for
Ophthalmology should be located in the capital of the nation."[181] Kober,
who clearly saw the advantages to Georgetown if the institute were to be
established in Washington and its director continued as the school's

professor of ophthalmology, elaborated on this in private letters to Wilmer. But confronting the might of the Rockefeller Foundation, Kober recognized that his hope was a lost cause: "I feel that the offer is so tempting that you will hesitate to decline it," he sadly told Wilmer.[182] For a while, Wilmer did hesitate; but in March 1925 he resigned his chair at Georgetown and went to Johns Hopkins to become its first full-time chairman of ophthalmology and to direct the world-class institute which still bears his name.

Wilmer never lost his loyalty to Georgetown, though. When in 1934 he reached the age of seventy, he accepted the Johns Hopkins' rule of retirement at that age even though, exceptionally, he was offered a waiver. Instead, he returned to Washington. There, he was appointed to the Board of Regents of Georgetown University and continued to conduct research at a special laboratory made available to him at the medical school until his sudden death in March of 1936.[183] Out of an estate of nearly three hundred thousand dollars, he left one thousand dollars to Georgetown and five thousand dollars to the cause "dearest to his heart," Washington National Cathedral, where he is buried.[184]

Meanwhile, Georgetown's own efforts to raise funds from alumni and, occasionally, from wealthy patients were progressing but slowly. By 1926 the endowment fund had accumulated less than $155,000.[185] By then, in a twist of fortune, student enrollment was presenting a different problem: not scarcity, but excess. So many medical schools had closed in the wake of the Flexner report that Georgetown was now turning away dozens of applicants each year because the building on H Street was too small to accommodate them.[186] It became imperative to increase the endowment in order to construct a new school building.

In 1927, the professors made another appeal to the Rockefeller Foundation which, once again, was distributing grants to medical schools. This time Kober felt more confident. Over the past five years, he pointed out, every Georgetown graduate had passed his state board examinations, and the hospital had been extended to a capacity of 450 beds. The funds for that expansion, amounting to more than $1 million since the hospital's inception, he said, had come almost wholly from friends and alumni, so "we cannot hope for further aid from this source." Suspecting that the school's Catholic affiliation had gone against its previous application in 1919, Kober also emphasized a court ruling that Georgetown could not be considered a sectarian institution since it owed its existence to a congressional charter and admitted men of all denominations. Kober even felt it necessary to say that he himself was a Lutheran.[187]

This time another GU alumnus, the prominent New York attorney John G. Agar, served as the school's main advocate. But his meeting with Abraham Flexner did not go well. "I suggested that you were not looking for millions but for thousands only," Agar told Kober afterwards. "He replied that thousands would do you little good. You needed millions."[188] Once again, on the principle of "not spreading its funds over a large surface too thinly," the foundation gave further endowments to Johns Hopkins, Yale, Vanderbilt, and others—but nothing to Georgetown.[189]

So George Kober was again thwarted in his long-cherished hope of securing the future of the school so that he might retire in content. By the beginning of 1928, he was approaching seventy-eight years of age and he was tired. With the exception of Vaughan and John Hird, the long-time professor of chemistry, his generation of colleagues on the faculty had all died: Carl Kleinschmidt, Swann Burnett, George Lloyd Magruder, Joseph Taber Johnson, Frank Baker, H. D. Fry, and Samuel Adams. Only one of his fellow students from the class of 1873 was still living.[190] For nearly forty years, Kober had served the school. As well as paying for two additions to the hospital, he had invested seventeen thousand dollars of his own money in various endowments bearing his name.[191] They included scholarships, medals, and the prestigious Kober Lecture. (Established in 1923 as his gift to the school on the fiftieth anniversary of his graduation, the Kober Lecture ever since has been delivered on his birthday, March 28, by a distinguished member of the medical profession.) Even this tally probably underestimates Kober's true beneficence. According to a colleague, he presented the school's financial statement to the university president year after year with the comment, "Well, Father, I'm sorry the medical school didn't make any money this year but neither did it have a deficit"—never admitting that most of the time he had balanced the accounts out of his own pocket.[192]

Several times in his years as dean—a tenure now approaching three decades—Kober had resigned on a point of principle, then agreed to continue once the point was conceded. From time to time he had also announced his retirement to successive university presidents. He did so in 1917, pleading "advancing years"; Father Donlon talked him out of it.[193] He did so again in 1925, on reaching age seventy-five, and this time nominated Bailey Ashford as his successor. But Ashford, though flattered, declined the deanship; and Reverend Charles Lyons S.J., who had become president in 1924, would not accept Kober's resignation.[194] In June 1928, Kober refused to be nominated in the annual faculty elections; the faculty re-elected him anyway.[195] The problem was that no one could think of a worthy replacement. More practically, the faculty feared that nobody else would have enough stature to secure the endowment the school still desperately needed. As James Gannon commented at a fund-raising dinner: "Dr. Kober is the Atlas upon which the medical school has depended for many years. Take him away today and we close the school tomorrow unless this endowment can be had at once."[196]

But by July 1928, Kober had had enough. It was not just that his health was failing; he was angry. A few years earlier the university had introduced a new element into the administration of the medical school, appointing a Jesuit "regent" to oversee the school and to act as a conduit between its dean and the university president, who had formerly dealt directly with one another. Kober did not object to this arrangement in principle; he even saw advantages in it, particularly as the first regent was Father Tondorf, with whom he always worked amicably. But in 1926 another Jesuit, Walter Summers, took over as regent, and over the next two years relations deteriorated. Summers was a clever young man—later, he became head of the department of psychology at Fordham University and gained fame by inventing the first reliable lie-detector machine[197]—and he had go-ahead ideas. But from lack of experience he inevitably made blunders, which Kober, with twenty-seven years of intimate knowledge of medical school matters, found intolerable. Kober finally poured out his frustrations in a seven-page letter to President Lyons. He complained of interference and lack of consultation; it had become "more and more apparent to me that Father Summers considered himself authorized to do things which under our by-laws came within the duties of the Dean." His criticisms were "not personal," but "made in the interest of my successor . . . Wholehearted cooperation is essential for success and no school can function effectively if conflict in authority is tolerated."[198]

Lyons's reply spoke glowingly of Kober's value to the medical school, but did not address his concerns[199]—probably because he was himself in the process of handing over to his own successor. So Kober, on vacation at his country retreat in New Hampshire, prepared to do business with yet another Georgetown president (the ninth of his deanship), pondered the future of the medical school, and looked forward to realizing the goal he had sought so fiercely for eighteen years—the transfer of the school from downtown to the neighborhood of the university and the hospital.

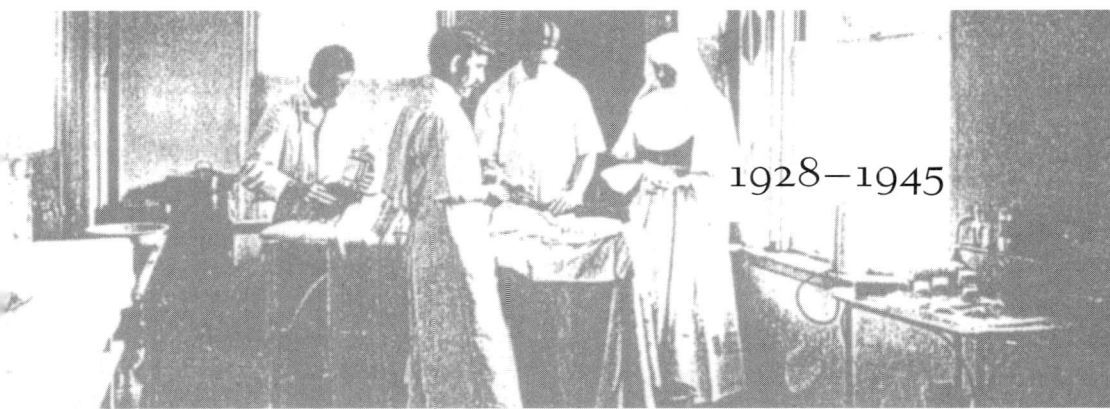

1928–1945

CHAPTER SIX

YEARS OF TURMOIL

GEORGE KOBER HAD pored over every detail of the new medical school building. He had the architect draw a rendering to show how it would look on the site: a ninety-feet-long redbrick building grandly surmounted by a cupola and cross. He determined how every square foot of its interior would be used. Above all, he took satisfaction in its location: the new school would be built only a block from the hospital—fronting onto Thirty-seventh Street, between O and N Streets—and would directly face Healey Hall, the central building of the university.[1] At last, Flexner's condemnation of Georgetown as "a university department in name only," and "miles distant" from its teaching hospital, would no longer sting.

But in August 1928, while Kober was still in New Hampshire on vacation, the Reverend W. Coleman Nevils, S.J. became the new president of the university, and he had different ideas. Almost his first decision was to insist that the new medical school be built on the other side of the university campus, facing Reservoir Road.[2] Eventually, Nevils thought, the hospital would move there too. He reasoned that a proper "medical center"—the unified teaching and clinical complex to which all medical schools now aspired—would need a large site to expand.

Years later, of course, his assessment proved to be wholly correct. At the time, however, the change of plan struck Kober aghast. He too envisioned a great medical center, but one which would grow outwards naturally from the hub of the existing hospital to occupy most of the six blocks bounded by Thirty-fifth, Thirty-seventh, Prospect, and P Streets. After thirty-two years begging for funds for the hospital, first to build and later to extend and equip it, and having invested so much himself, Kober was horrified by the suggestion that it should one day be abandoned. He called it a "violation of the interest of the benefactors"; and he recounted to Nevils how, in 1887, he had visited Saint Bartholomew's Hospital in London: "I saw bronze memorial tablets over beds endowed over 400 years before." Kober also had other, less sentimental, arguments. Reservoir Road, he pointed out, was in the middle of a "high-class residential section," too distant to be reached easily by the charity patients on whom clinical instruction depended; no tramcar lines ran there from the city, as they so conveniently did almost to the doors of the hospital on Thirty-fifth Street. But his chief objection was that to move the hospital would "involve an outlay of several millions of dollars." How and when could such a sum be raised?

To Kober, the whole point of the move from H Street was to bring medical school and hospital together—both to benefit clinical teaching and, finally, to meet the standards of the AMA and AAMC. For eighteen years, he had assured these authorities that Georgetown would comply as soon as possible; and they, believing in Kober's integrity, had accepted that he would keep his word. Now, he said, they were "greatly pleased" with the Thirty-seventh Street location. To switch the new school building at the last moment to another site a mile from the hospital would destroy all he had worked for since 1910. "To separate these two plants," he told Nevils, "would be fatal to the objects of a medical center."[3]

Nevils was unmoved. In September 1928, he accepted Kober's final resignation, made him "dean emeritus" and elevated him to the university's highest advisory body, the Board of Regents.[4] In November, Nevils received approval from Rome for the change of location.[5] In January 1929, he signed a building contract and instructed the architect to draw up new plans and specifications, sacrificing the twelve thousand dollars the medical faculty had already paid for the old ones.[6] Soon afterwards, site clearance began on Reservoir Road.

Meanwhile, the 1928–29 medical school year had begun as usual in the old building on H Street. Though none then knew it, four successive chairmen of the Georgetown surgery department were now working under its roof. George Tully Vaughan was still the current chairman. James A. Cahill, who would succeed him in 1933, was professor of clinical surgery. Fred R. Sanderson, who would succeed Cahill in 1942, was an associate professor of clinical surgery. And Robert J. Coffey, who would become chairman in 1947, was a newly enrolled student.

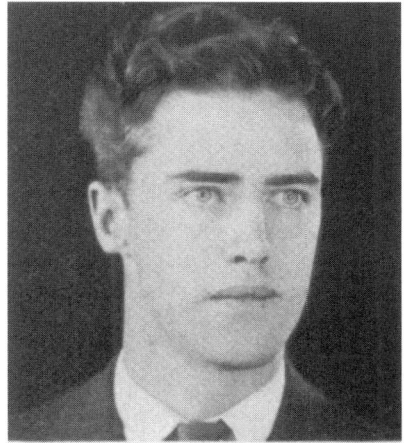

Coffey had arrived at Georgetown almost by accident. He was there, in a sense, because of Prohibition. The Eighteenth Amendment, ratified in 1919, had destroyed the livelihood of his father, Jeremiah Coffey, who until then had been a successful liquor wholesaler in Elmira, New York. For him, the ending was painfully abrupt: returning on the last haul, with a full consignment of liquor, as well as Robert's elder brother Jerome, then a young lad, on board, the Coffey truck was hijacked by armed men.[7] Forced out of the business he knew, Jeremiah switched to the grocery trade, but in this he was less successful and the family's income declined. So when, several years later, an affluent uncle offered to put Jerome through medical school, their mother decided to send his younger brother Robert along also, reasoning that the two could live almost as cheaply as one by sharing a room and textbooks.[8] The tuition fee

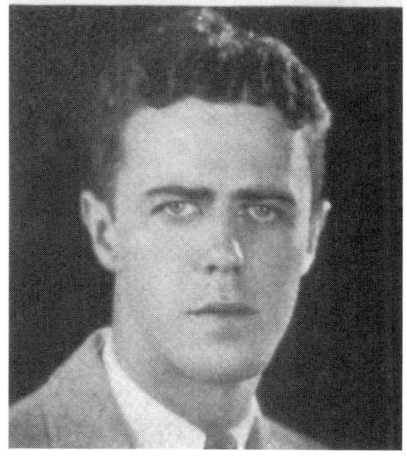

The Coffey brothers, Jerome (above) and Robert (below), in 1932, the year they graduated in medicine from Georgetown. Courtesy of the Georgetown University Yearbook (Domesday Book), 1932.

at Georgetown that year was three hundred dollars, plus a ten-dollar labora-tory fee and a further ten-dollar fee "for use of microscope."[9]

When he entered Georgetown in September 1928, Robert Coffey had completed his required two years at St. Bonaventure University, near Olean, New York, and was two months short of his twentieth birthday. More than sixty years later, he could still recall vividly his first impressions of the school on H Street. "It was a modest, slightly dilapidated, four-story red brick building that barely accommodated both the medical school and the dental school," he said. "Laboratory and lecture halls were quite limited, but the dental school got much the worse of the space allocation and equipment. Each time I passed by the dental clinic I used to shudder, because the students would be in there drilling teeth and operating the drill with a foot lever."

There were at least 155 medical students in that year's freshman class, chosen from a record 1,100 applicants.[10] In their first two years, the whole class was usually crammed in together for basic science lectures, most of which slavishly followed assigned texts. "We'd go into the physiology class on, say, Tuesday, and we knew that the subject to be discussed by the professor on that day would be covered by pages twelve to twenty-two in the book," Coffey recalled, adding dryly: "If you studied the text carefully, you were well prepared for the examinations." In those two pre-clinical years students never saw a patient or the inside of a hospital: "I didn't even know where the hospital was. It was strictly a didactic exercise." The funda-mentals of surgery were still taught by dissection. "They had a large pit with formaldehyde in it where cadavers were kept [before being] brought up to the anatomy lab. The odors were horrible. The lab was on the third floor, and I recall that one of the early high-rise apartments was being built alongside. When construction got up to the third floor, the workmen looked in and saw these cadavers; and they had a hard time keeping employees."

For a time, the Coffey brothers shared a room in the I ("Eye") Street apartment of Richard M. Rosenberg, a young instructor of physiology. Through him, they got to know some of the faculty members personally. This was unusual: students of that era were mainly taught by lower-level instructors, had little contact with their professors, and rarely even saw those who headed departments. When they did, all they saw as often as not were Olympian figures rushing into the lecture halls as though impatient at losing time from their private practice. One student recalled seeing the chairman of ophthalmology just once in four years, when he raced through his assigned lecture on diseases of the eye in twenty minutes, without removing hat or coat.[11]

Robert Coffey remembered some of his teachers with affection and respect—in particular George Tully Vaughan and Wallace Yater who became chairman of medicine in 1930. But with hindsight, he saw that others had been poor teachers, and at least one had indulged in questionable practices. Joseph Madigan, professor of anatomy, "insisted you buy his notes for about twenty or thirty dollars, which was a lot of money in those days. The notes were about that thick, but they weren't *Gray's Anatomy*. As I look back on it now, that was very unethical." Another of Madigan's practices was to invite marginal students to his home to take "special instruction." "But the special instruction was to go into a room, while the professor and his family had dinner, and read some notes he'd left." Such lapses, Coffey came to feel, were a response to the low salaries which the full-time teachers were paid—and it is true that Madigan, in contrast to his counterparts in the clinical branches whose private practices brought large incomes and luxurious homes, was paid three thousand dollars a year.[12] "This," Coffey said, "was probably a means of augmenting income." In fact, Madigan's practice of selling notes, home instruction, and even dissection instruments to students had already caused controversy within the faculty long before Coffey's time.

The subject had first been raised around 1924 by James Gannon, an associate professor of surgery, and in early 1928 he wrote a formal complaint to the executive faculty. The answer he received—in the form of a statement of unrecorded authorship to the faculty—so far from rebutting his charges, condoned them. Gannon's complaint that each freshman student the previous year had been charged thirty-five dollars for mimeographed notes was not profiteering, the statement said; instead, production of the notes had "meant a considerable loss to Dr. Madigan, both in time and money" and they had been used by students in other medical schools "to an extent which has necessitated copyright procedure on the part of Dr. Madigan." Selling dissection instruments? Madigan had purchased them as a job lot and sold them below retail price. Charging students for home instruction? This had been authorized by the university. Gannon's graver insinuation that Madigan was taking money from students in

return for passing them in anatomy was dismissed as calumny. This spir-
ited defense climaxed in a condemnation: "I shall recommend that Dr.
Gannon be publicly reprimanded. . . . This conduct is quite unbecoming a
professional man who is entrusted with the care of students."[13]

But Gannon's suspicions of Madigan turned out to be well-founded.
In July 1932, a recent graduate of the medical school (a classmate of
Coffey's) corroborated nearly ten years of rumor by offering evidence that
he had given $100 in cash to Madigan—less than the $250 Madigan had
demanded—in return for a passing grade in the anatomy examination, and
that he had acted as go-between to collect similar amounts from two
younger students. His statement was witnessed by several professors,
among them George Tully Vaughan.[14] Two days later, Madigan was told
his contract would not be renewed, and when he applied for a reference,
Nevils refused to give it.[15]

Coffey looked back on his student days with mixed feelings: "Our
education was not too well organized. A lot of what we did, we did on our
own. It was through our own curiosity, our own anxiety to learn, that
students carried out inquiries that weren't required on the course."[16] In
fact, the records show that Coffey's time at Georgetown were the worst
four years in the school's history. The Madigan scandal was only one
symptom of a malaise that debilitated the medical school at that time.

There were many other signs. The most obvious was that, beginning
in 1928, Georgetown's medical graduates began failing their state board
examinations in increasing numbers. In 1931, fourteen failed.[17] In 1932,
Georgetown's twenty-five failures (18.4 percent of that year's graduates)
were the worst in the nation.[18] After the pass-fail lists appeared in the
medical press, dozens of letters arrived from alumni. "There is something
wrong in Georgetown medical school," said one, "if our boys can't do
better than this."[19]

What *had* gone wrong? The basic reason, ironically, was the new
building on Reservoir Road. It was completed in January of 1930, and
teaching began there on February 3, when medical and dental students
returned for the second semester.[20] It was a splendid structure, far more

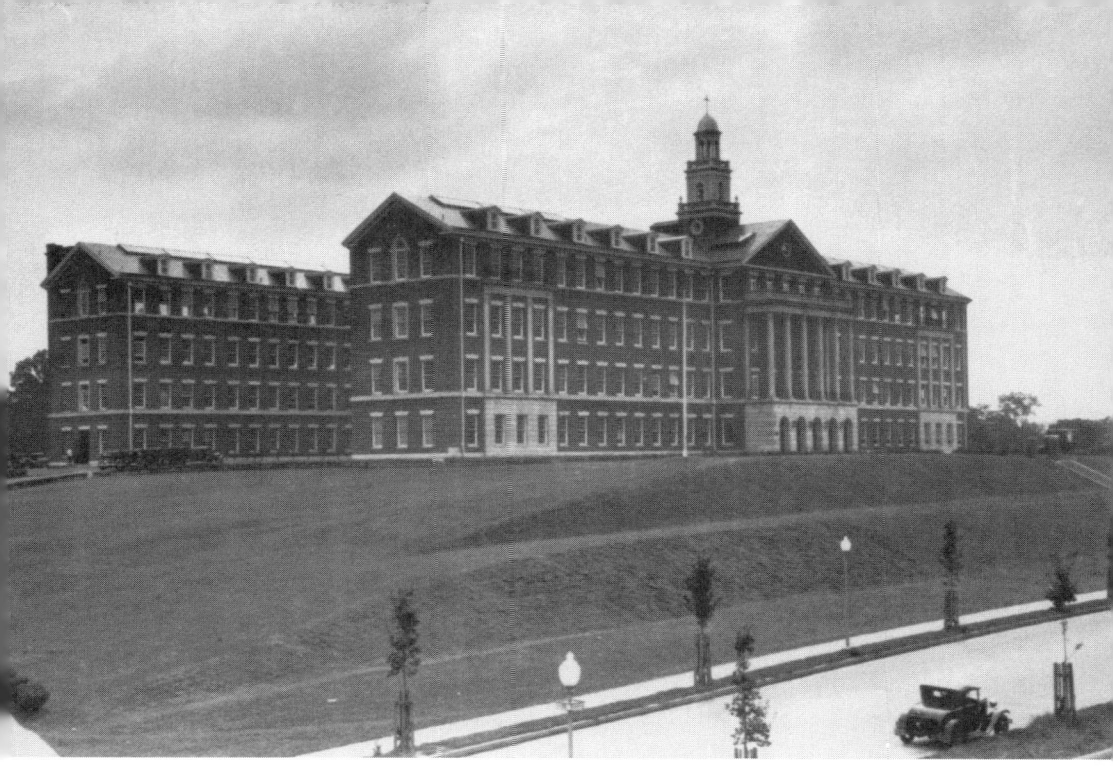

Georgetown School of Medicine's fourth and last building opened in 1930 on Reservoir Road in Georgetown, finally bringing the medical school and university together on campus after eighty years of separation. Courtesy of Georgetown University Archives.

attractive and well-appointed, or so it was said, than most medical schools of its day. Coffey remembered relishing its spaciousness and modern equipment, compared to H Street. "The whole milieu was an improvement," he recalled. "It was a nicer area, almost out in the country then. It was like a country club."[21] But all those years of fundraising had netted no more than $400,000, whereas the building had actually cost close to $1 million.[22] So, to begin paying off the debt, the school raised tuition to $450,[23] and increased the freshman class to a peak of 174 in 1931–32.[24] That year, the school had 593 medical students enrolled—843 including the dental students[25]—against an average enrollment in American medical schools of 284.[26] Georgetown did this in the face of warnings from the AMA and others that numbers were already too large for its staff and its laboratories.[27] The inevitable result was that many instructors had teaching loads two or three times higher than their counterparts at other schools, so students received even less personal attention than they had before.

The debt also meant that the school had neither money nor reputation to attract the best teachers. As its standing deteriorated through the 1930s, Georgetown increasingly recruited faculty from within its own ranks, appointing graduates of the school and relying on their loyalty to Alma Mater to work for low pay or—in the case of the part-time clinicians—for nothing. A few, like Yater, were excellent, highly qualified academics. The rest included basic scientists and clinicians who—well-regarded as they might have been in their fields—were indifferent and, in some cases, incompetent teachers.

These problems were compounded by the fact that, after Kober's departure, the administration of the school had fallen apart. After seven months of efforts by Nevils and by Kober himself to recruit a new dean from outside, the job went to John Ambrose Foote, valedictorian of the Georgetown class of 1906, who had been professor of pediatrics since 1921 and had become a distinguished practitioner in his field. But Foote, appointed dean in April 1929 and elected president of the Medical Society of D.C. the following month, was already in poor health.[28] So it was the new regent, Reverend John L. Gipprich, S.J., appointed the same year, who took over effective control of the medical school. Gipprich was a scientist: he had taken a postgraduate course in physics and mathematics at Johns Hopkins University and had taught physics at Georgetown University since 1915.[29] Perhaps that was why, at the medical school, he felt more comfortable with the basic science teachers than with the clinical professors. But Gipprich had no real grasp of the medical persona, and he was a manipulator, favoring those who agreed with him and labelling as troublemakers those who expressed different ideas. Within a year, the faculty was in a turmoil of dissension and intrigue.

Among those most critical of the way the school was going at this time was Wallace Mason Yater, the new chairman of the department of medicine. Yater was one of the few Georgetown graduates of his day to have trained at the Mayo Clinic, the prestigious clinical and research center established by William and Charles Mayo at Rochester, Minnesota. The clinic offered postgraduate medical training that was among the very best in the United States. A fellowship there was itself a high honor; Yater did so well in his three years that one of the Mayo directors described him as "far and away the keenest, brightest assistant" to work at the clinic "in all the years of its existence," and said that Yater "would have succeeded to a commanding position" had he stayed.[30] But in 1928, Walter Summers visited Yater at Rochester and offered him a position in Georgetown's department of medicine, with the understanding that he would become the first full-time chairman of the department as soon as its incumbent, William Barton, retired. Yater had been offered more money to remain at the Mayo Clinic, but he accepted the Georgetown post in the hope that he could reorganize the department on modern lines and help raise the school's performance to the standard set by Flexner.[31] The torch that Kober had for so long carried now passed, in effect, to him.

Yater became chief of the department of medicine sooner than he had expected, because Barton died—ironically, following an operation at the Mayo Clinic—in the spring of 1930.[32] Yater, thirty-five years old, became Georgetown's first full-time chairman of a clinical department, with a salary of five thousand dollars a year, an office and a secretary, the promise of research work, and the privilege of holding consultations with private

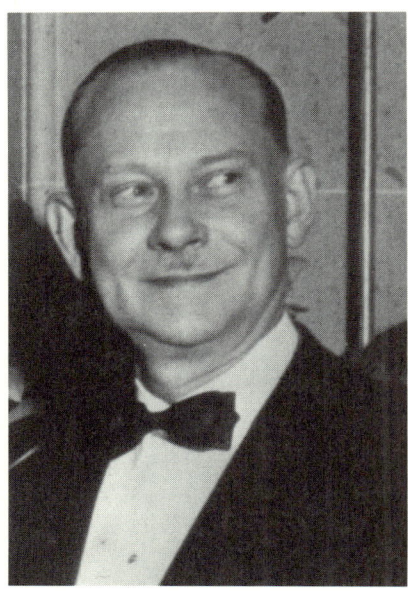

patients at the university hospital.[33] Almost everyone admired Yater's ability. His special talent was differential diagnosis—telling the difference between similar diseases. This, he drummed into his students, relied on knowledge gained from previous experience, extensive reading, and study of laboratory and autopsy findings, combined with keen observation and a meticulous examination of all the facts that a case could present. In 1927, before returning to Georgetown, he had already published his famous textbook *Symptom Diagnosis*, the first comprehensive work on the subject, which he had begun under the tutelage of William Barton in 1924 during a brief stint on the Georgetown

Wallace Yater, M.D., chairman of medicine, 1930–45. Courtesy of Georgetown University Archives.

faculty before moving to Rochester. The book ran to four editions and was translated into Russian, Polish, Chinese, and many other languages.[34]

Robert Coffey remembered the young Yater as "a god of the medical school—a brilliant, brilliant man who added tremendous life to the faculty at Georgetown." Coffey recalled:

> I got to know him in a very embarrassing way. In my senior year, I was working down at the old university hospital, and this woman came in who was extremely hyperthyroid. At that time Dr. Yater was doing some work on hyperthyroidism, and so he was called down to consult on this case. It was the first time I'd seen him. Everybody was just in awe of him, and unfortunately, he picked me out to present the case. Well, I'd never presented a case before and I stuttered through some history as best I could, then started on the physical findings. Dr. Yater said, "What is her heart rate?" Not knowing what it was, I said, "Ninety." Dr. Yater said, "What?" I very quickly changed that to a hundred and twenty. Dr. Yater said, "Coffey, you determine her heart rate yourself." I picked up her hand and started feeling her pulse. "No," he said, "I didn't ask for her pulse rate. I want her heart rate." At that point I realized I didn't have a stethoscope with me. I had to borrow one, and I think I put the earplugs in the wrong way, and started listening outside of both her dress and her overcoat. Dr. Yater corrected me on this, and I got the bell down against her skin, and listened for a bit. Then Dr. Yater said, "How are you going to count it?" At which point I realized I didn't have a watch. A friend handed me one of his very valued treasures—a gold watch that had belonged to his father and his grandfather. And as he handed it to me, I was so flustered I dropped the watch on the floor and broke it. That was my exposure to Dr. Yater.[35]

(Nevertheless, years later when Yater himself needed an operation for cancer of the colon, the surgeon he chose was Robert Coffey.)[36]

Though admired in general by his students and peers, Yater got off on the wrong foot with Father Gipprich. Soon after Yater's return to Georgetown, he and Barton sent the regent a letter listing improvements they felt the medical school should implement at once to meet modern standards. Gipprich merely returned the letter with four words scrawled in the margin:

"Yater is always criticizing."[37] Through the years that followed, Yater continued to speak his mind, and Gripprich continued to resent what he considered Yater's arrogance. Perhaps it was inevitable that Yater's ideas, based on his superior Mayo experience and not always diplomatically expressed, would fail to endear him to less well-trained colleagues. These tensions heightened after Yater, seeking to raise the level of research at the medical school, brought to Georgetown a brilliant young medical scientist from the Mayo Clinic named Jacob Markowitz. He had accepted the chair of physiology on the understanding that he could continue his researches in experimental surgery.

Jacob Markowitz arrived at Georgetown in the late summer of 1930, just before his twenty-ninth birthday. A Canadian, he had received both an M.D. and a Ph.D. from the University of Toronto; he had subsequently distinguished himself at the Mayo Clinic where he had gained a master's degree in experimental surgery.[38] By 1930, he was already known internationally from some thirty papers on researches into animal and human physiology which he had published in prominent journals. He was, in Yater's words, "one of the best animal surgeons in the world."[39]

Markowitz's appointment was an advance for Georgetown. He was its first medically trained professor of physiology in nearly twenty years. After Father Tondorf had been eased out in 1924, Father Summers had headed the department. Then, in September 1929, Tondorf had returned, but he died of a heart attack two months later; since then the chair had been vacant.[40] Yater had no doubts that Markowitz would drive the department to a level of excellence. "Jake, without doubt, had the best mind of all my contemporaries at Mayo's or anywhere else," he recalled years later. "He knew and could tell you all that was known in his own field, physiology, and in several other basic sciences: pharmacology, biochemistry, and anatomy. He was the best teacher I ever knew, and I learned a great deal from him."[41] Markowitz was, in addition, highly qualified to introduce experimental surgery to Georgetown.

Up to that time, the medical school had conducted little animal research. Markowitz was attracted to the challenge of building an experimental program from scratch; but after his experience of the Mayo Clinic's exemplary facilities, he must surely have viewed the task with misgivings. At Georgetown, he was given a small room in the attic of the school's north wing as his animal quarters. It lacked insulation, heating, or proper sanitation. No animals could be bred there, or even kept there properly for any length of time. So Markowitz had to buy animals individually.[42] He ran into trouble almost at once.

Markowitz was a humane man with much experience of working with animals, particularly dogs; he insisted they be treated with the same consideration as human patients undergoing surgery, with full anesthesia and sterile conditions.[43] He also knew, from hard experience, that his work provided a prime target for the antivivisection movement. Soon after arriving at Georgetown, Markowitz approached the D.C. Health Officer for help in procuring dogs from the city pound. Though animal rights supporters had regularly challenged the D.C. law, the city's medical schools were still legally permitted to buy dogs for research at two dollars each. In reality, the pound refused to provide them and the health officer declined to intervene, having himself, as he told Markowitz, almost lost his job under pressure from the antivivisectionists when he had supplied the government's own laboratories with dogs from the pound. Unwilling to face the headlines by taking this to court, Markowitz got permission from Dean Foote to advertise for dogs ("no puppies, no thoroughbreds") in out-of-town newspapers.

Inevitably, one of the replies was a "sting" from a leader of the Antivivisection League. "I was visited by a wrathful deputation," Markowitz wrote soon afterwards, "[who] promised to make a merry time for me. They were going to expose my monstrous cruelties of the past . . . and hound me out of town. These people are now in their element. They could do nothing about the Government laboratories using dogs. No other school in the District admitted using them. So they concentrated their efforts on my laboratory." Yet another bill to prohibit experimentation on dogs in D.C. was then under debate in Congress, and the antivivisection lobby used Markowitz's advertisement—together with quotes taken out of context from his published papers—to full effect. In January 1931, the lobby circulated notices offering a one hundred dollar reward to anyone who could prove that a stolen pet dog had been sold for research. "They wished to create the impression," Markowitz said, "that this was a common practice."[44] But three months later, a twenty-year-old Fairfax man, Stanley

Robinson, was convicted of stealing a pet collie which he had sold to Markowitz. Georgetown paid the dog's owner fifty dollars for compensation and stoically suffered the attendant publicity.[45]

Ironically, Robinson's trial took place only six days after Markowitz and Yater together unveiled an experiment that represented a landmark event in the history of surgical research. On March 28, 1931, doctors from across the nation, who were attending the American College of Physicians' annual meeting in Baltimore that week, spent the day in Washington visiting medical institutions. At Georgetown, they watched intently as the two men transplanted a dog's heart into the neck of another and showed that it continued to beat. It was the first time such a feat had been demonstrated; it was an important extension of Alexis Carrel's early work on transplants, and one of the pioneering bases for so many later successes in cardiovascular surgery and organ transplantation.

The immediate purpose of the experiment was to determine how thyroxine, a hormone secreted by the thyroid gland, affected the heart rate. The secondary purpose, Markowitz explained to the ACP delegates, was to demonstrate the current limitations of transplants. There had been much newspaper talk of "monkey gland" transplants—the controversial notion that monkeys could be donors for almost any spare parts surgery. Markowitz dismissed this as "sensational charlatanry," serving only to "discredit the field of organ transplantion in the eyes of the scientific world." He pointed out that transplantation worked only when an organ, such as a kidney, was transferred to a different site within the same animal. When transplanted to another animal it was treated as an invading organism and rejected. In this case, he said, the donor dog's heart would die within a few days—not because of any difference in blood groups, because dogs shared a single blood group. "This is one of the things we hope to find out— what it is that makes successful transplantation at present impossible."[46] The dog's heart transplant awed those who saw it and made newspaper headlines. Predictably, it fanned the fury of the antivivisectionists.

To Markowitz, such work was crucial not only to advance medical knowledge but also to train young surgeons. It was at this time that he began writing his famous *Textbook of Experimental Surgery*. Criticizing the lack of opportunities for graduate students to learn the actual practice of surgery, he argued that it served no purpose "to insist on post-graduate training in pathology, physiology, biochemistry, and then to let the student hold a retractor for his final year of the course, and perhaps open and close an abdominal incision or two. This is to insist on a proper training in everything but surgery itself."

Markowitz himself insisted that "only a small part of the art of surgery can be taught in the lecture room," and his book offered step-by-step tutorials in a wide range of operative procedures on dogs as an excellent means for graduate students to gain the "constant diligent practice" he considered essential to master surgical technique. "Surgery of the dog, in so far as it resembles human surgery, is in this instance of great value in training surgeons for the operating room. One who has seen able young men struggle through a cholecystectomy on a dog, can appreciate the full value of practice." Some clinical procedures, such as blood vessel anastomosis, "can be mastered only in the experimental laboratory," he said. For this, transplanting the heart of a small dog into the neck of a large one was a specially useful exercise, because the veins and arteries to be joined were unequal in size: "A surgeon who can successfully transplant the heart may be reasonably sure that he is adept in the technic of vascular anastomosis."[47]

With the demands of research, teaching, administration, writing, and ongoing skirmishes with the antivivisectionists, Markowitz carried a heavy workload during the 1930–31 school year. He was, nevertheless, drawn into the internal strife and personal animosities which were already sundering the medical faculty. There are always catalysts for discord. In this case, it was another new professor whom Father Gipprich had, without consulting the executive faculty, appointed in the summer of 1930 to head the department of histology and embryology. George A. Bennett was twenty-eight years old and, it turned out, had no medical degree and only minimal experience of teaching and research; yet Gipprich, again without consultation, authorized him to revise the first two years of the curriculum. This in itself created resentment in the faculty. Markowitz was incensed when Bennett tried to tell him how to conduct his laboratory.[48] Matters came to a head when Yater and Markowitz checked into Bennett's background. The upshot was that they issued a sworn statement accusing Bennett of being "an imposter": passing himself off as a doctor of medicine, and claiming credit for the authorship of two papers on the spleen which had actually been published by a Harvard professor who happened to have the same name.[49] Bennett maintained he had never claimed any degree other than an A.B., and "took it for granted" that no one would regard the reprints he had handed out as his own work.[50]

The issue split the executive faculty, with the battle lines drawn between, broadly, the basic science professors and the clinicians. Prentiss Willson, the highly respected chairman of obstetrics, who had taught at Georgetown for twenty-six years and was serving as acting dean because of John Foote's rapidly deteriorating health, sided with Yater and Markowitz. Appealing in March 1931 to President Nevils to intervene, he talked of "an atmosphere of personal bitterness and animosity in the Executive Faculty such as I have never known to exist before in the years of my association with the medical school." So naked had the animosity become, Willson confided, that the chairman of pathology had attempted to block the election of Wallace Yater to the American College of Physicians that month. This, Willson said, showed "total disregard" for the best interests of Georgetown since, "as no higher honor can come to an American physician," it might even help the school cling to its precarious A rating.[51] (Yater was, in fact, elected to the ACP at that time; in 1933 he was awarded the distinction of becoming its youngest ever district governor and later served as its secretary-general for fifteen years.)[52]

No action was taken on Bennett. Instead, in June 1931, Gipprich recommended that Markowitz be dismissed, on the grounds that "since his arrival at the school [he] has been continually giving trouble." Nevils complied.[53] Yater, shocked, protested that the dismissal of Markowitz, "the most outstanding member of our faculty," would mean virtually "the deathknell of scientific progress in our school." The reputation of any medical school, he argued, depended "largely upon the scientific attainments of its faculty even more than upon its teaching." He warned Nevils: "I am sure that if the matters which have been happening in our medical school were known, we should be the subject of a scandal which could never be lived down."[54] Markowitz, faced with academic disgrace, threatened legal action, and Nevils backed down.[55] Markowitz was reinstated, but the climate of hostility and intrigue continued. A year later, Gipprich succeeded in ousting both Markowitz and Prentiss Willson from the school.[56] Bennett remained.

So Georgetown lost, for the most capricious of reasons, one of the best medical scientists of his generation. Markowitz returned to his alma mater,

University of Toronto, where he continued research and completed his *Textbook of Experimental Surgery*. It became a classic and was used in medical schools throughout the English-speaking world for more than thirty years.

❧

Many of the faculty shared Yater's outrage at these events. In different times, perhaps, others might have voiced their opinions as strongly as he did. But this was the early 1930s, the era of the Great Depression. Every member of the faculty, from departmental head downwards, was now on a yearly contract, reviewed each June, and no one could afford to lose his job. In the letters which survive from this period, written by the professors to Nevils or Gipprich, those economic anxieties are a constant subtext: hinted in the extravagant thanks on having their positions confirmed; in the tentative way they tiptoed around issues the least bit controversial; and in the fulsome assurances of loyalty in which they wrapped the slightest criticism. Even Yater chose his words with care.

Nobody dared criticize Gipprich, at least not in writing. The most anyone ventured was to suggest that, because of Foote's absence through illness, he was "laboring under great disadvantages" in not receiving sound advice.[57] The more astute professors, however, realized that Gipprich's power derived from his friendship with the Father Provincial, Edward C. Phillips, who was head of the Jesuits' Maryland—New York province, and thus Nevils's immediate superior.[58] This sandwiched Nevils into a difficult position. He admired Yater, Willson, and Markowitz and regarded their fears for the medical school as well-founded. But he was also under orders. When rumors of the charges against Bennett and Madigan began to seep out—prompting the director of the Mayo Clinic, for example, to ask whether they were true[59]—Phillips brushed the charges aside as "by no means new," and instructed Nevils to reply that "the present complaints seem more in the nature of a blackmail affair than an honest endeavor to see actual or supposed defects corrected."[60]

Nevils, however, did take a decisive stand when it most mattered. In April 1931, John Foote died (followed closely by his predecessor, George Kober) and the medical school once again needed a new dean. An obvious candidate had now emerged. William Gerry Morgan, a prominent gastroenterologist

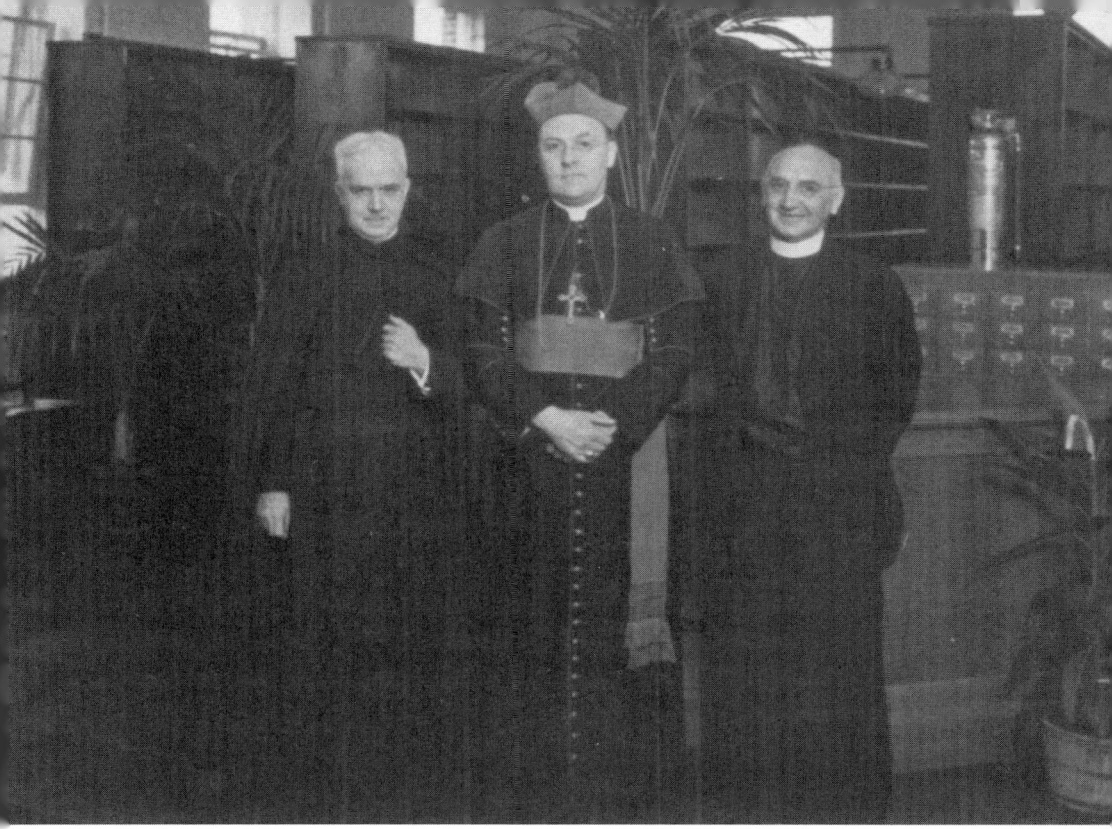

The new medical school was dedicated in February of 1930 by Most Reverend Michael J. Curley, archbishop of Baltimore, seen here in the library with (left) Reverend W. Coleman Nevils, S.J., president of Georgetown University, and (right) the medical school's regent, Reverend John Gipprich, S.J. Courtesy of Georgetown University Archives.

who had taught at Georgetown on and off since 1904, had earned the highest distinction of the profession in 1929 when he was elected president of the American Medical Association.[61] Here was a man who, like Kober, had earned national prestige and was utterly loyal to Georgetown's interests. The medical faculty, though divided on many other issues, were almost unanimous in wanting Morgan as dean. The problem was that Gipprich had one of his own protégés in mind. In this explosive situation, Nevils got word that the departmental chairmen and other senior professors had met in secret and decided to resign as a body if Gipprich's nominee were made dean. Using this intelligence to chasten Gipprich and persuade Phillips, Nevils acted swiftly to avert the crisis. To the astonished relief of the faculty, he publicly announced the appointment of Morgan, effective September 1931. From then on, Nevils confided in a letter written nearly twenty years later, "Dr. Morgan did a 100 percent job, under the most trying circumstances as Father Gipprich continued his underhand antics until finally [in 1934] I was able to persuade Father Phillips of the needed change."[62]

The only member of the executive faculty to remain aloof from this discord was George Tully Vaughan, mainly because from 1929 to 1931 he had suffered long spells of illness, endured two operations, and lost his beloved wife. In early November of 1929 (just three days after the great stock market crash), Nevils had hosted a grand ceremonial dinner in honor of Vaughan's seventieth birthday. George Kober was among the guests, and so was William Wilmer who—though he declined many invitations to Georgetown functions because of pressure of work in Baltimore—"laid everything aside" to attend this one.[63] Clearly it was expected that Vaughan, after thirty-two years as chairman of surgery, would now retire in favor of a younger man. But Vaughan showed no intention of stepping down.

Everyone revered him. "We are all devoted to Dr. Vaughan," Nevils wrote in several secret letters in a vain search for a sufficiently eminent successor.[64] Once recovered in health, moreover, Vaughan demonstrated he had lost none of his surgical skills, nor a particle of the clarity of mind which had for so long graced his lectures and writings. Ever the military man, he probably considered it his honorable duty to stay at his post, serving the school as long as he could. The drawback was that Vaughan was a product of the nineteenth century—already age forty when it turned into the twentieth—and of a generation of part-time professors for whom medical education was but an altruistic extension of a successful private practice. Times had changed; Vaughan had not.

By 1930, the surgery department, even though it had now lost gynecology to the department of obstetrics, had swelled to more than twice its original size.[65] For years, Vaughan had appointed clinical staff to teach varying hours in seven city hospitals, according to piecemeal arrangements worked out to suit their individual convenience. They were not paid, the prestige of a university appointment being considered sufficient recompense. Overall, it was a system that encouraged neither conscientiousness

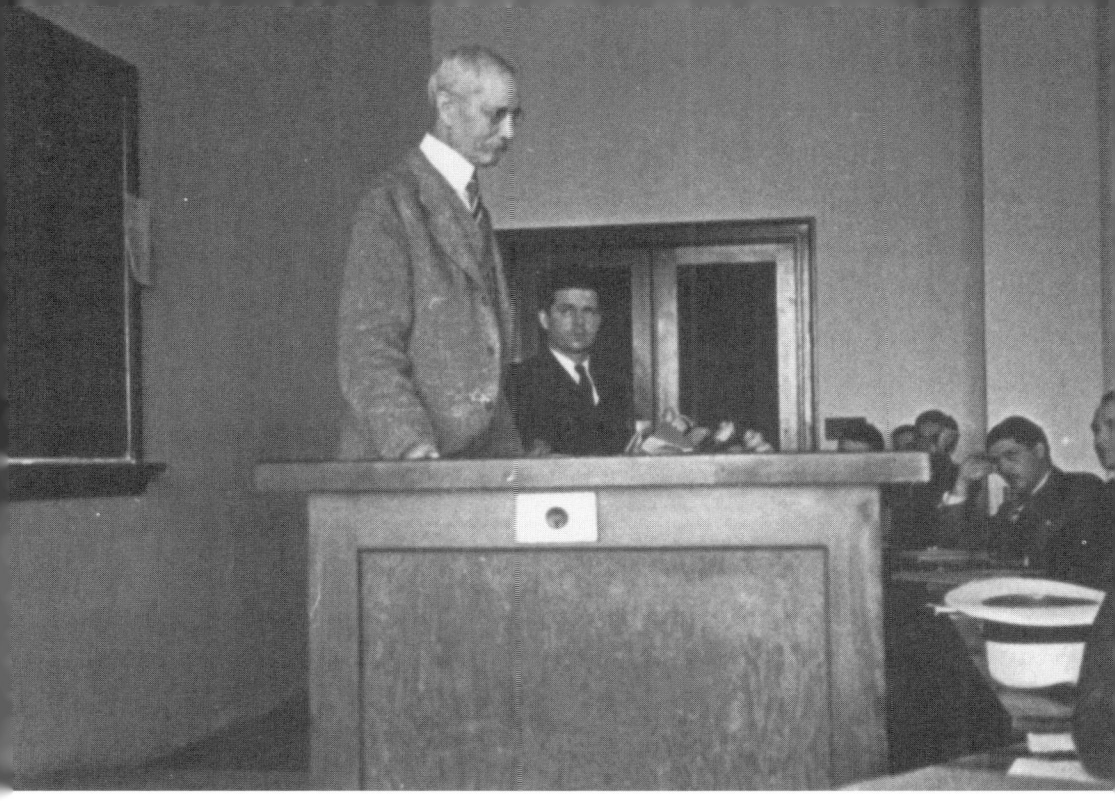

George Tully Vaughan teaching a class in the early 1930s. Courtesy of Georgetown University Archives.

nor efficiency, and as the demands on the department grew more complex, administration became increasingly disorganized. By 1931, it was clear that neither Vaughan nor anyone else knew exactly how many people worked for the surgery department, nor precisely what they did, nor when and where they were doing it. There was no detailed schedule and no complete list of personnel. The faculty list in each year's catalogue was never accurate: some newer teachers were left out, while the list retained names of others who had not taught for years. This was true of the other clinical departments as well, but over the next two years they established complete records, whereas Vaughan failed to produce any.[66]

Finally, and with due tact, the task was given to the professor of clinical surgery, James Cahill. His report, produced in February 1933, showed that seventy-eight people now worked for the department, spread between eight divisions which included roentgenology, anesthesia, and oral surgery. He recorded the exact number of hours each person contributed each semester to lectures at the school and to clinical instruction at various hospitals and dispensaries. This documented what everyone already knew: Vaughan, now approaching seventy-four years of age, still reserved for himself the lion's share of the work. In didactic lectures to the senior class alone, for example, he contributed ninety hours; whereas other senior professors put in between six and fifteen. Long-term surgeons on the faculty, already middle-aged themselves, were thus deprived of the opportunities and responsibility they considered their due.[67]

Back in 1930, John Foote had delicately suggested to Nevils that a rule be introduced requiring all faculty to retire at age sixty-five, to enable younger men with new ideas to develop the expansion of the school.[68] Nothing was done, because no one dared put the proposition to its immediate target, Vaughan. Three outside inspection committees visited Georgetown during 1932–33. Each urged reorganization of the surgery department under the chairmanship of a younger man. Vaughan, they added, should be made professor emeritus, "confining his activities to special lectures."[69] All other departments were being reorganized, and Dean Morgan was anxious for a start to be made on surgery. But still neither he nor even Gipprich felt able to confront Vaughan.[70] The old soldier had to be mustered out by the commander-in-chief.

In July 1933, Nevils finally agreed to make "the necessary arrangements." Drawing no doubt on all his acknowledged diplomatic skills, he had a long talk with Vaughan, secured his resignation, and then—evidently as part of a tough bargain—wrote him an extraordinary letter:

The President of Georgetown University with deepest regret accepts the resignation of Dr. George Tully Vaughan, and only does so because of pressure brought to bear from the outside that a younger man be placed as head of the department of surgery. In an interview with Dr. Vaughan the President said that in spite of the above pressure, Dr. Vaughan is still free to retain his position, and that his resignation has to be entirely voluntary.

Personally the President is convinced that no surgeon can render better service to the school than Dr. Vaughan, and he holds this in spite of full realisation of Dr. Vaughan's so-called advanced age. His accumulated wisdom is an asset no one else can at present bring to the medical school. In addition to this full conviction of Dr. Vaughan's fitness to retain his present position, and the desirability of his doing so, the President of Georgetown University feels nothing that the institution can do will compensate Dr. Vaughan for what he has been to the University.

Hence Dr. Vaughan's resignation has been accepted on the following conditions:

1. He is to be Head Professor Emeritus of the Department of Surgery, and he is subject only to the Regent and the Dean in the Medical School and Hospital.
2. He is to remain as a Member of the Executive Faculty that his invaluable experience may still be available to the Medical School which owes so much to him.
3. He is to be special lecturer on Surgery under direction of the Regent and Dean.
4. By special and entirely unsolicited act of the Board of Directors he is to retain the same salary as a life member of the Faculty. This act was passed several months ago even before Dr. Vaughan's resignation was contemplated." [71]

This letter—more in the nature of a contract than a termination—ended George Tully Vaughan's thirty-six-year tenure as chairman and chief of surgery, but not his career. The new "head professor emeritus," enjoying to the full the privileges he had exacted from Nevils, continued to attend meetings of the executive faculty, give lectures and clinics, and operate at the university hospital for a further ten years.

Nevils immediately appointed James Augustine Cahill as Vaughan's successor. He was the first Georgetown graduate to occupy the chair of surgery, and in the circumstances, the choice was wise. Nevils had looked for candidates elsewhere—hampered by the Provincial's specific instructions to select only a Catholic[72]—but no outsider could readily have fathomed Georgetown's peculiar problems and intricate politics; and if he had, he might not have stayed.

In contrast, Cahill's intimate knowledge of the medical school and its personalities dated back to 1911, his freshman year. Born and educated in

Washington, the son of a prominent local banker, Cahill had left his native city only twice: for a year's internship at a hospital in Ohio, and in World War I, when he served as an army medical corps captain at an evacuation hospital in France. On his return in November 1919, he set up in private practice as a general surgeon, and in 1921 joined the Georgetown faculty as an assistant to Vaughan. At the time of his appointment to the chair on July 17, 1933, he was forty years old.73

Cahill had neither the breadth of experience of Vaughan, nor the academic standing of Yater; he had published only fourteen medical papers, thirty-two fewer than Yater, a slightly younger man.74 But he was a fine surgeon, a fellow of the American College of Surgeons, and he also met the one condition that Father Phillips had insisted upon: he was a Catholic. Ideally, Nevils would have preferred a full-timer to develop the department of surgery as Yater was doing in medicine,75 but Georgetown's ability to pay no more than six thousand dollars a year was as unattractive to Cahill as it was to any other surgeon with a highly successful practice and, in his case, five children to support. Realistically, Nevils recognized, what mattered most in 1933 was loyalty to the school, understanding of its problems, and willingness to work altruistically on its behalf. Cahill had those qualities in abundance. In those trying times, his cheerful disposition counted for a great deal too.

Unhappiness within the faculty had not ceased with Markowitz's departure. His successor to the chair of physiology—Owen Gibbs, another brilliant young experimental scientist with a first-class reputation, who had invented one of the first mechanical hearts—lasted sixteen months before resigning in disgust.76 The prevailing climate was captured most succinctly by James Gannon. Having served as acting chairman of surgery during Vaughan's illnesses, Gannon had long considered himself Vaughan's heir apparent. When Cahill was appointed, he resigned, and, as one of the few faculty members who had never hesitated to express criticisms in the past, he took this last opportunity to tell Nevils exactly what he thought. He was resigning, Gannon wrote:

> because more students are enrolled in the school than can be properly taught . . . ; because the percentage of State Board failures is too high [and because] attempting to overcome the lack of endowment by accepting too

many students is a mistake . . . ; because the Regent has assumed the role of dictator . . . and exercises power which properly belongs to the faculty and the staff; because the interns at the hospital no longer earn their positions by competitive examinations, but are selected from the Regent's friends in the student body, and are appointed by him to the hospital; because the professor of obstetrics [Willson] was dismissed a year ago because he entertained views as to the conduct of the medical school which were at variance with those held by the Regent.[77]

Nevils privately agreed with this assessment, but it took another year before he was at last able to persuade Father Phillips to remove Gipprich.[78] In early August 1934, the faculty generously held a farewell dinner for Gipprich at the Congressional Country Club[79], but they were relieved to see him go. (He was assigned to parochial work in Maryland, returned to the university in 1946 as father confessor, and died in the hospital in 1950.)[80] The new regent, Reverend David McCauley, S.J., formerly a biology teacher at Fordham University, quickly won the faculty's confidence. He not only proved a capable and energetic administrator, but had the knack of getting along with people. He was able to relieve the personal tensions that had jangled nerves throughout Gipprich's reign. "I really enjoy, for the first time, my deanship duties," Morgan confided to Nevils a month after McCauley's arrival.[81]

If Gipprich had been the most tangible symbol of these troubled times at Georgetown, however, he was not the cause of its fundamental problems. For years, he and every other senior member of the faculty had known the degree to which Georgetown was falling behind the rising national standards set by the AMA and the AAMC. In 1931, someone (most probably Yater) had prepared a frank comparison of the school's record, point by point, with the AMA publication "Essentials of an Acceptable Medical College." On almost every point, Georgetown failed. The AMA's most crucial essential was bluntly spelled out: "Statistics show that modern medicine cannot be acceptably taught in a school which depends solely on the income from students' fees. No medical school should expect to secure approval, therefore, which does not have a generous annual income from state or private endowment in addition to students' fees." At Georgetown, the in-house comparison noted, there was "no endowment and no steps being taken or plans laid to obtain one."[82] Worse yet, by 1933 the accounts showed that although the school's "unusually high" enrollment had increased its income to around three hundred thousand dollars a year, only half of that went to instruction; the rest was used to pay off the debt on the building.[83]

Through the early 1930s, a number of licensing authorities inspected the medical school, and just as regularly their reports repeated the same criticisms: no endowment, too many students, too few full-time teachers, too little research, and a general want of organization in the school, its departments, and its clinical facilities. How then was Georgetown able to cling to the A rating it patently did not deserve? One explanation was that William Gerry Morgan and Wallace Yater, through their prestige and professional connections, were able to fend off the blow. Another was that, through these depression years, many marginal schools were given considerable leeway. Georgetown was not the only school to raise enrollment and accept less qualified students in order to survive.[84] In 1934, though, the AMA decided to enforce its standards more stringently.

That December, the AMA's secretary, William Cutter, took the unusual step of inviting the Father Provincial Edward Phillips to visit him. "As soon as we were seated in his room," Phillips wrote afterwards, "he rather surprised me by saying that he wished to see me to ask whether or not we considered there was any reason for continuing the medical school at Georgetown, and if not, he thought that this would be an opportune time to close it and withdraw from the field gracefully." Phillips, taken aback, assured Cutter that "the University should, and would, strive to make the school thoroughly efficient." But Georgetown had been making such promises since 1910, and Cutter pressed his advantage. He told Phillips that "every ordinary good school" needed, over and above tuition, resources of some five hundred dollars per student. He warned that Georgetown would be inspected again in February 1935; this time it would receive an appropriate rating.[85]

It is possible to discern the shadowy influence of William Gerry Morgan behind this conversation. The former president of the AMA, who knew Cutter well, recognized that nothing short of a proper endowment could save the medical school, and he believed that only a real commitment by the Jesuit hierarchy could raise one. But in 1935, the inevitable happened: Georgetown was inspected and duly placed on "confidential probation."[86] The AMA, sensitive to public opinion, no longer judged it expedient to publish comparisons of named medical schools, as the Flexner report had, or even to announce that a particular school had been found unacceptable. But the profession knew. Bowing to the inspectors' criticism of Georgetown's system of divided authority between dean and regent, Morgan immediately resigned. "There can be no question," he wrote, "but that the time has come when the office of Dean of Georgetown University Medical School requires the full time service of the incumbent."[87]

Soon afterwards, Coleman Nevils left Georgetown and the Reverend Arthur O'Leary, S.J. became president of the university. It was O'Leary's task to find a new dean, but Nevils so strongly agreed with Morgan that he intervened from a distance. The only way, he felt, that Georgetown could attract a first-rate medical professional to give up practice and devote his entire time to the school was by offering a realistic salary. Nevils found a way to do it. He talked to a friend, Ray Reiss, a Georgetown University alumnus who had become a wealthy furniture manufacturer in New York and a college benefactor. In consequence, Nevils confided years later, Reiss "offered to pay for five years $12,000 annually for a lay dean." It was a generous offer. Unfortunately, Nevils said, "Father O'Leary couldn't see it."[88]

O'Leary wanted the regent, David McCauley, to take over the dean's duties as well. The executive faculty—perhaps unaware of Reiss's offer; perhaps because they regarded McCauley as able; perhaps because they felt it offered the best hope of getting financial support from the university—unanimously agreed. All, even Yater, signed a letter requesting that McCauley be appointed regent-dean.[89] Thus, for the first time in its history, a Jesuit assumed sole control of the medical school.

Against this background, James Cahill's efforts to develop the surgery department were severely constrained. To function efficiently, it needed at least some full-time members. It had none, nor money to appoint any. An attempt to raise funds had been made in 1930, when the surgeons on the faculty voted to donate to a "surgical budget" 20 percent of their fees from operations on private patients they brought to the University Hospital. But it is unclear how much this voluntary levy raised or even how long it lasted. Only one donation is on record: fifty dollars from James Gannon.[90]

Cahill introduced monthly departmental staff meetings and kept close track of the work of both staff and students.[91] He initiated programs such as a cancer symposium led by Robert B. Greenough, then president of the American College of Surgeons and an authority on the surgery of cancer.[92] He helped organize a new clinic at the university hospital for the free diagnosis and treatment of all types of tumors; for the first time, this coordinated specialists from the departments of surgery, medicine, radiology, and pathology.[93] He helped arrange an annual five-day postgraduate training course for Georgetown medical alumni; it began in September 1936, and he directed the 1938 session. Cahill made local headlines on that occasion when, in front of an audience of visiting surgeons crowded into the amphitheater, he performed a successful splenectomy on a seventeen-year-old girl who had suffered since the age of six from a disease which caused excessive bleeding.[94]

In particular, Cahill introduced the first surgical residency programs at Georgetown, Gallinger, and Providence Hospitals; he won recognition for them from the American College of Surgeons and the American Board of Surgery, founded in 1937. Those early residents were in training for two years.[95]

In 1937, Cahill reported one of his most interesting cases at a meeting of the American College of Surgeons in Chicago. A twenty-five-year-old seamstress working in a Washington garment factory had had her entire scalp and right ear torn off when her hair caught in the flywheel of a machine. Over the next eight months, Cahill grafted an entire new scalp by using pedicle flaps of skin cut from her shoulder blades, and a new ear fashioned from the

James Cahill, M.D., chairman of surgery 1933–42, with early surgical residents at Providence Hospital, 1939. Courtesy of Providence Hospital.

skin of her neck and strengthened with cartilege taken from her seventh rib. The series of operations was remarkably successful—more so than most of the other ninety-six cases of complete scalping due to industrial accidents then reported in medical records—and the seamstress emerged from the treatment with only a thin scar visible on her forehead.[96]

Cahill had some excellent senior surgeons in the department in that period. Five of them had trained at the Mayo Clinic: Fred R. Sanderson, professor of clinical surgery; Fred C. Fishback, thoracic surgery; John H. Lyons, general surgery; Robert E. "Pete" Moran, the father of plastic surgery in Washington; and John Shugrue, the city's leading neuro-surgeon.[97] These and others gave strength to the department; but the fact remained that their services were for the most part voluntary and inevitably the department continued as one of the most disorganized in the school.

In September 1938, another Mayo graduate was appointed to the surgical staff: Robert J. Coffey returned to Georgetown as professor of experimental surgery. After graduating from the school in 1932, Coffey had gone back to his hometown of Elmira in upstate New York for a two-year internship at St. Joseph's, the local hospital. It was there that he first developed an interest in surgery. "I was interested in the completeness and finality of surgical care, as against medical care which very often is a matter of observing the patient over a period of years," he explained. "In surgery, you eliminate the disease—at least, that's the main objective." In 1934, with the encouragement of Wallace Yater, Coffey had applied for a surgical fellowship at the Mayo Clinic. He was turned down for surgery, but was offered a fellowship in medicine, which he accepted: "Anything to get to Mayo's." There, assigned to the service of J. Arnold Bargen, an authority on colon disease Coffey worked for his master's degree in medicine on polyps of the colon related to cancer. But he also developed an interest in the physiology of the pancreas. Since this work involved surgery, he was able to switch to the surgical fellowship he had first desired, and found it everything he had hoped: "The Mayo Clinic then was modern surgery at its zenith." The thesis he wrote for his Ph.D. in surgery, awarded in 1938 by the University of Minnesota, was the culmination of an experimental investigation of the role of the pancreas in the digestion and absorption of food.[98]

With these impressive qualifications—few surgeons then had Ph.Ds— Robert Coffey was invited back to Georgetown by Yater to be its first professor of experimental surgery. Jacob Markowitz had initiated a program eight years earlier, but the title was new and the work focused on instructing students in operative technique. Unlike Markowitz, Coffey now found at Georgetown all the facilities he needed for research and teaching. In fact, an animal house designed expressly for the accommodation and care of experimental animals had at last been constructed in the grounds of the medical school in 1938.

It was desperately needed. In the six years since Markowitz's departure, research had expanded in all departments. Some six thousand animals a year were being used, and their care was nothing short of a disgrace. "The present quarters in the old paint shop are so unsuitable that we have been forced to use evasions of all sorts in order to prevent the health authorities and the representatives of the SPCA from examining conditions in this place," a 1935 memorandum noted. "Moreover, the place is so small that we can keep only a few dogs in it at any one time. The other animals used must be kept in various parts of the medical school under conditions that are all but intolerable."[99]

Proper accommodation for research animals had been one of the AMA's specified "essentials for an acceptable medical college" since 1931. In the AMA's 1932 tour, the faculty was forced to ask the inspectors not to look at the animal quarters because "they would not give a just view of the school," but assurances were given that a suitable animal house would soon be constructed.[100] Detailed plans were immediately drawn up, and in every year that passed these were used to persuade a variety of professional inspectors, health authorities, and animal rights organizations of Georgetown's "serious intention" to erect the building.[101] Not until 1938, however, when the school needed to make visible effort to regain its approval rating, was it finally built. The school catalogue was then able to advertise "a new animal house where ample facilities are available for the care of animals and [where] special surgical work and instruction is given in this field by a most competent and well-trained instructor."[102]

That instructor was Coffey: his principal job was to give thirty-two hours of instruction in surgical technique to all senior students, who came to the animal house in small groups. "We split each group up into teams," he later recalled. "One would be the anesthiologist, one the surgeon, one the scrub nurse, etc. They would operate on the animals, of which we had a generous number at that time, and carried out various operative procedures. This was a very worthwhile course."[103]

For developing and directing this program, Coffey was paid nothing. At the same time, he was endeavoring to build a private surgical practice in Washington from scratch—no easy task in 1938. In that first year, virtually his only patient was a "beautiful collie dog" suffering from an obstruction in the throat. After the operation, Coffey steeled himself to ask the dog's grateful, and wealthy, owner for a fee of one hundred dollars (instead of a more appropriate twenty-five dollars), then kicked himself when she responded: "But I thought it would be at least a thousand." With no income from his professorship and heavy competition from every other established or struggling surgeon in town, Coffey's career might well have ended before it had begun. Fortunately, he had the support of a fond elderly relative, the widow of a multimillionaire who had been the mayor of Elmira and first president of the Bendix Corporation. Before Coffey left for Georgetown, she presented him with a new car (a sporty LaSalle), a charge account for clothes at a fashionable menswear store in New York, and a check for two thousand dollars. Her generosity carried the young surgeon through until, mainly by taking on dispensary work at Providence Hospital, he began to build a reputation and a practice. Life was good, and it became even better one Sunday early in January 1939 when, attending morning mass, he was introduced to a beautiful young woman named Mary Catherine. She was the daughter of Joseph J. Mundell, Georgetown's professor of obstetrics. Their meeting led to a date that same evening, their wedding the following September, five children, and fifty-five years of happy marriage.[104]

The medical school, meanwhile, had suffered yet another humiliation. In November 1938, the Association of American Medical Colleges confirmed the 1935 judgment of the AMA's Council on Medical Education and Hospitals when it, too, recommended that the school be placed on probation. The improvements Georgetown had made since 1935—the new animal house, a properly organized library, and a new enrollment policy that limited the freshman class to one hundred students—were simply not sufficient to meet the stringent standards which the educational authorities now demanded of all accredited medical schools.

The AAMC's report, based on an inspection made in April, 1938, insisted that enrollment was still "in excess of the facilities for thorough

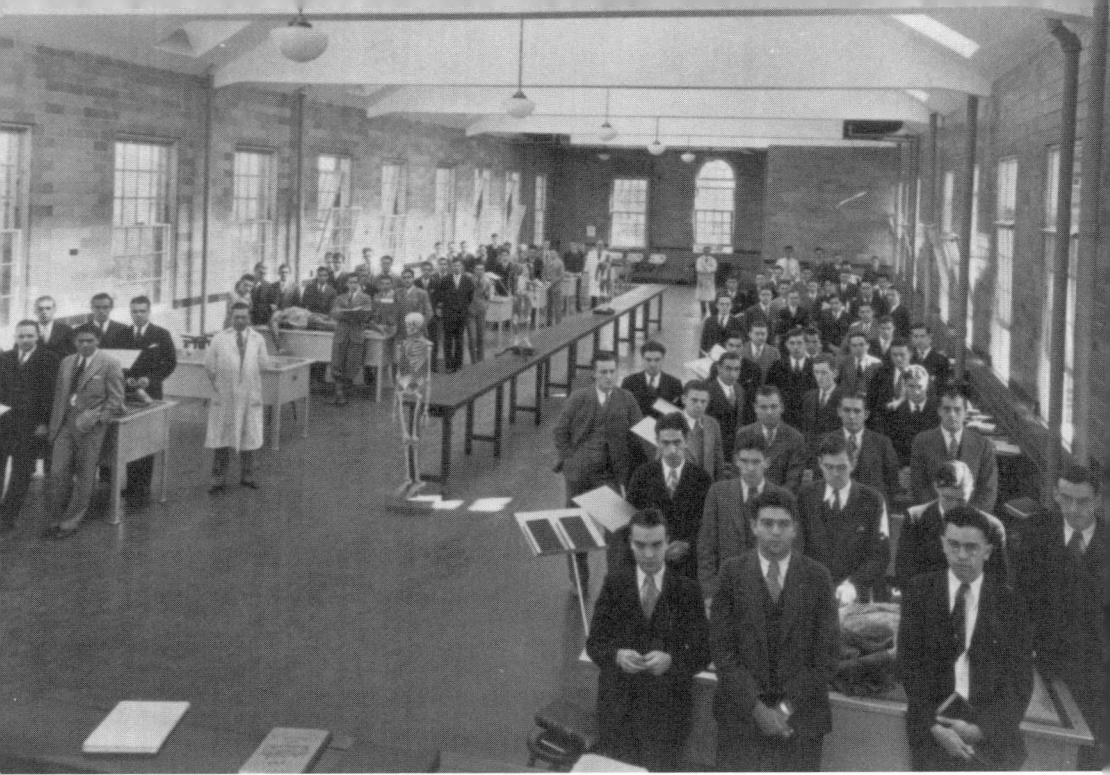

The size of the class, reduced to one hundred in 1935, but still criticized by the licensing authorities, can be seen in this photograph. The anatomy laboratory with cadavers on the tables, shown here in the late 1930s, was on the top floor of the new medical school, as it had been in its three previous buildings. Courtesy of Georgetown University Archives.

instruction; it probably should not exceed sixty in the class." Its main criticisms, however, were directed at the clinical program which, it said, was "neither effectively organized nor in agreement with the present conceptions of sound clinical instruction." The university hospital was still too small to provide more than a fraction of cases needed for instruction. Much of the clinical teaching with ward patients was done on the other side of the city at the 650-bed Gallinger Municipal Hospital which Georgetown shared with George Washington medical school. Georgetown students served clinical clerkships there on Tuesdays, Thursdays, and Saturdays; GW students on Mondays, Wednesdays, and Fridays. This system, the AAMC report said, "fails to give a desired continuity of thought, time, and effort." Far too much time was devoted to didactic lectures, even in the senior class, at the expense of patient contact; and far too much ward instruction was delegated to younger members of the faculty—"usually young men with only one previous year of hospital training."[105]

The medical school now had twenty-eight years' bitter experience of seeing its shortcomings thus catalogued, but the senior professors regarded this one as the last straw. A few days after receiving the AAMC report, they all—including the dean, McCauley—signed a strongly worded letter to the president and board of directors of the university. It was a demarche: "We, the Executive Faculty of the School of Medicine, are addressing you because we are greatly disturbed for the future of our school," it began. ". . . We are sure that without an endowment of at least three millions of dollars the school cannot only not progress but cannot even continue to exist." The letter then itemized, even more pointedly than the AMA or AAMC reports had done, the many problems caused by absence of financial support, particularly in the clinical departments:

> It is almost impossible to get the older and more experienced physicians to take an interest in the teaching of students in the dispensaries. It is almost entirely the younger men, who have lots of time and want more experience, who do this work. The students, of course, do not get the benefit, therefore, of the best teaching. . . . More and better supervision of the teaching of students in the wards is also quite essential, and here again, in order to get older men with experience to do the supervising, funds are necessary. In other words, there is no department of the medical school which can be run without ample funds.

Driving home their point, the professors wrote: "The time has come when the authorities of the university must make a major effort to procure an adequate endowment for the School of Medicine as soon as possible." They ended: "We address you thus sternly, reverend and dear Fathers, because we love our University and our School and because the situation is serious and one which we can no longer handle alone."[106] President O'Leary responded sympathetically. The board of directors had frequently discussed the medical school's plight, he said, but all the university's departments had suffered financially during the depression; there was simply no money for the school. O'Leary had one suggestion to offer: the board had decided that "one member of the university would be set aside for the purpose of securing funds for the medical department." The person selected for this task, however, was McCauley, already overburdened in his duties as regent and dean.[107]

So, once again, the executive faculty made the best of a critical situation and turned its attention to the immediate problem of averting the AAMC's threat of probation. The senior clinical professsors—Yater, Cahill, and Mundell—completely reorganized the curriculum of the junior and senior years, eliminating much didactic instruction and increasing hospital experience. The unsatisfactory scheduling arrangements at Gallinger Hospital were changed: the Georgetown and George Washington programs were divided into two separate services, each with its own wards, so that the clinical clerks now saw their assigned patients on an uninterrupted daily basis.[108] The faculty also demonstrated its commitment to higher standards when examination time came round: it failed 34 percent of the 1939 graduating class—a flunk rate never equalled before or since.[109] When the AAMC next examined Georgetown in November 1939, the inspectors reported they were "agreeably surprised to find so much had been accomplished since our last visit." AAMC secretary Fred Zapffe, in a personal note to O'Leary, added: "I feel that this closes the case of the Georgetown University School of Medicine."[110] But the probation imposed by the AMA remained, and so did the problem of the missing endowment. McCauley appointed a fund-raising committee, but there is no evidence that it accomplished anything.

Soon, however, the school was caught up in troubles wider than its own. War enveloped Europe and, with the bombing of the U.S. naval base at Pearl Harbor on December 7, 1941, spread into the second global conflict in less than thirty years. Men like James Cahill, who had served in the first, now saw the surgery and other departments once again deplete as younger colleagues applied for commissions or were drafted.

George Tully Vaughan, still spry at eighty-two and doubtless chagrined he could not volunteer again, watched events with interest. Soon after Pearl Harbor, he attended a Georgetown Clinical Society dinner in honor of John Moorhead, a New York surgeon who had been in Hawaii on a postgraduate lecture tour at the time of the Japanese attack. Vaughan, Cahill, and the others listened in fascination as Moorhead explained that he had been there to demonstrate a hand-held electromagnetic device of his own design which could be used "like a surgical divining rod" to detect the precise location of a bullet in

the body. Needless to say, Moorhead had been among the first medical volunteers to rush to the stricken American fleet. Dealing with wounds worse than
he had seen in France twenty-three years before, he said, he had put his
"bullet-finder" to the test by pinpointing fragments from bomb-blast.[111]

Many Georgetown medical men were commissioned into the U.S.
Navy. One was Gerald McAteer, chief resident in surgery at the outbreak
of war, who served as surgeon on the aircraft carrier USS *Hornet* at the
Battle of Midway in June 1942 and, four months later, at the Battle of Santa
Cruz Island, in which the ship was sunk. Though himself seriously
wounded, McAteer insisted that he be carried among the other wounded
and dying men to continue to give medical care. He was later awarded a
Silver Star for his gallantry.[112]

Robert Coffey was assigned to a coveted posting as the only general
surgeon on board the USS *Iowa*, leader of the Iowa class of battleships. "I
became what was known as a 'plank-owner' on that ship, because I joined it
in the New York shipyards when it was being built," he recalled. The *Iowa*
saw action in the North Atlantic and the Pacific, but its most historic role
was to transport President Roosevelt to the Teheran Conference in
November 1943, where he met with Churchill and Stalin to begin plans for
the Allied invasion of Europe.

On the way there, Coffey related, an incident occurred which came close
to changing world history. During naval exercises, one of the destroyers in
the convoy accidentally fired a live torpedo which passed within a hundred
yards of the *Iowa*, as the president and members of his cabinet watched from
its bridge. The offending destroyer was promptly returned to Norfolk to pick
up a new complement of officers. It was on this same trip that Coffey learned
what few Americans then knew, that Roosevelt was a paraplegic, permanently confined to a wheelchair, and he helped treat one of the more
embarrassing consequences of the president's condition. On the journey back
from Teheran, Roosevelt was stricken with a violent attack of diarrhea.
"Being a paraplegic and having little or no control over his sphincter muscles,
he developed a rectal prolapse," Coffey said. "His rectum actually turned
inside out, emerging by three or four inches." Called to the president's state-
room, Coffey fixed the problem. "I saw him at the White House several
times thereafter and apparently he had no further trouble."[113]

With so many of the faculty serving overseas, the professors who
remained at Georgetown carried heavy and stressful workloads. Like other

medical schools, Georgetown accepted more students for training. Moreover, under orders from the Wartime Commission for Education, it also accelerated its program, condensing the four-year curriculum into three years by virtually eliminating vacations: students worked three trimesters a year, separated by ten-day breaks.[114] As part of a national civil defense program, Georgetown was also one of five schools selected to train physicians in techniques to treat the effects of chemical warfare, for fear such weapons might be used against civilians.[115] The demands on the depleted teaching staff were thus immense.

"I was on the verge of a complete physical and mental breakdown," Wallace Yater recalled. "I had little or no rest or recreation during the war years; there just were not enough teachers to manage increased enrollments of students. The military took most of the best-qualified clinicians on my staff. I was left with only three or four assistants on whom I could rely for regular attendance at classroom lectures or on the wards in teaching hospitals."[116]

The same was true for James Cahill, and for him the strains proved too great. In October 1942, he fell ill at his home on Foxhall Road and a few days later died of a heart attack. He was a week shy of his fiftieth birthday. Six medical students bore his coffin into the funeral service at St. Matthew's Cathedral. Among the honorary pallbearers who followed it were his predecessor in the chair of surgery, George Tully Vaughan, and the man who was immediately appointed his successor, Fred Sanderson.[117]

Frederick Roman Sanderson, another native Washingtonian, had long been a colleague of Cahill's at Georgetown. They had entered the medical school together as freshmen in 1911 and graduated in 1915; in the university yearbook Sanderson was described as "the handsomest man of the class" and Cahill as "the most popular and universally beloved man among us."[118] Their paths had diverged only once, in World War I. Cahill traveled east to France with the American Expeditionary Force; Sanderson went west to Rochester, Minnesota, for a three-year fellowship in surgery at the Mayo Clinic, followed by two more years there as an assistant in surgery.[119]

This rigorous academic training earned Sanderson a faculty position at Georgetown, as an assistant professor of clinical surgery, immediately after he returned home in 1922. From then on, Sanderson and Cahill had a close professional relationship, though their chosen forms of relaxation were very different. Cahill, like many surgeons, enjoyed golf at the Chevy Chase Country Club. Sanderson's passion was riding to hounds; for several years he was master of the Potomac Hunt.[120] In February 1936, Sanderson saved Cahill's life by performing an emergency operation for a ruptured appendix. The problem, he discovered, was a gold tooth crown which Cahill had lost several months earlier, not realizing he had swallowed it.[121]

Sanderson was forty-nine years old when he became chairman of the department of surgery. He was by then prominent as one of Washington's leading general surgeons, a fellow of the American College of Surgeons, a member of Southern Surgical, and a co-founder and former president of the Eastern Surgical Society. He had gained further local distinction only months earlier by being elected president of the Medical Society of D.C.[122]

The medical school records which survive from the 1940s are so sketchy that it is impossible now to assess Sanderson's impact on the surgery department. He was the last of its part-time chairmen—running his large practice from an office on I Street and operating at Gallinger and Providence as well as Georgetown University Hospital—and his tenure took place in difficult times. He suffered the same wartime strains as Cahill and Yater, and for him the conflict also brought personal tragedy: his son, Fred Jr., was killed in action.[123] In the circumstances, maintaining the status quo was hard enough; development was out of the question.

World War II did bring minor gains to Georgetown. But for the most part, the stringencies of war hastened the medical school's decline. The AMA and AAMC had suspended inspections during the war, and only one yardstick of a medical school's standing now remained: each year's national and state board examination results. Disastrously, those of May 1943 showed Georgetown ranked second lowest in the country. Its failure rates of 11.4 percent in state boards and 7.1 percent in the national board compared miserably with the nationwide rates—2.4 percent and 2.2 percent respectively—and with those of its closest competitor, George Washington medical school: 1.9 percent and 1.4 percent.[124] These poor showings failed to improve over the next two years, unravelling still further the fraying nerves of an overworked faculty.

The crisis came in June of 1945. Again the spark was controversy over a faculty member: this time a man being considered for the chair of pathology despite objections from the chairmen of all the main clinical branches—Yater, Sanderson, Mundell, and Joseph Wall, head of pediatrics.[125] But the real issue was the perilous state of the medical school which, as Wall wrote in a blunt statement to the faculty, "has now reached a pinnacle of discredit."[126] Yater went further: he offered his resignation. And in a letter to Reverend Lawrence Gorman, S.J. who had succeeded O'Leary as university president in 1943, Yater listed the eleven reforms he thought were needed to put the school back on course. They included: an endowment of at least $2 million; realistic salaries to attract good teachers; personal interviews and a test of basic education ("grammar, spelling, and even handwriting") to admit better students; the culling of weak students in the first two years; more interdepartmental meetings to integrate the curriculum; and the need for "new blood" from outside to reinvigorate the faculty. More pointedly, Yater urged—as second only in importance to an endowment—that a medical man be brought back as dean. "It takes a physician, and a man of certain qualifications, to know and to handle the problems of running a medical school," he wrote, adding obliquely: "In the past there has been too much mysticism connected with the running of the school, and entire frankness should be fostered as to financial status and other things."[127]

Yater was talking in part of the general secretiveness into which the administration had withdrawn in Gipprich's time and to which McCauley was not immune. Specifically, however, Yater was referring to a discovery he had recently made which had shocked him: namely, that the university was not merely giving no financial help to the school, but was actually taking from it ten thousand dollars a year as a charge for McCauley's services. Yater tossed this fact, like a grenade, into a stormy meeting of the executive faculty. McCauley was incensed, but his subsequent account to President Gorman confirmed Yater's point: "There is dynamite in the fact that [Yater] knows it, and in the fear lest he or anyone else disclose it to our accrediting agencies. Where he got this information, nobody knows. The only people who knew it were Dr. Hird [faculty treasurer], his assistant and I, and all of us have been most cautious in regarding it as information of the most confidential sort."[128] The following year, McCauley told Gorman that the medical school could not afford the stipulated ten thousand dollars for his services, and asked for the charge to be cancelled "in the spirit of charity and generosity that has so enriched our Society." Gorman refused.[129]

Years later, Yater admitted that his letter to Gorman was intended not as resignation outright but more as an ultimatum. Exhausted as he was by June 1945, Yater still held hope that the university would accede to at least some of his suggestions. That possibility seemed strengthened when his friend Reverend Edward J. Walsh, vice president of the university and founder of its School of Foreign Service, approved the letter and insisted on accompanying Yater to a personal meeting with Gorman. After an hour's talk, Yater recalled, Gorman said: "Well, I'll think it over and perhaps, during the summer, we can do some of these things." Three months passed; Yater heard nothing. In September, he wrote Gorman again, inquiring if any of his recommendations were being contemplated.[130] Gorman's reply was prompt and curt: "I wish to state that I have decided to accept your resignation from the faculty of the medical school, effective October 27, 1945."[131] It was a dismissal, with one month's notice.

Yater remained bitter about this until the end of his life. What he never knew was that, shortly after his meeting with Walsh and Gorman, the university president had drafted a letter in which, in the friendliest terms, he assured Yater that steps were already being taken to address his concerns—in particular to find a full-time medical dean.

> On the necessity of such a professional man and competent administrator with standing in the field of medical education we are all agreed and to that point I am addressing all our energy. I am convinced that the appointment of such a Dean will go a long way towards solving many of the difficulties which you feel are operating to the disadvantage of the school. [I am] encouraged to hope that the improvements . . . which I am now undertaking may so change conditions that you will find it agreeable to continue at your post.[132]

That letter, written in Gorman's own hand and preserved in his papers, was never sent. It is impossible now to judge what happened in the summer of 1945 to change Gorman's mind. But there are clues. McCauley had responded to Yater's criticisms—particularly on the need for a medical dean—with hostility. "There is only one conclusion that can be drawn," he had told Gorman in July. "The continued association of Doctor Yater and myself with the School of Medicine and with the Hospital will be impossible. Our purposes and aims are so opposed that the effects of a prolonged association are bound to be harmful and even dangerous to both of these institutions."[133]

As soon as he heard what had happened to Yater, Joseph Wall also resigned. The efforts of Yater and others to improve the school "apparently have been ill-received by the authorities of the university when made solely in the spirit of good faith and constructive endeavor," he wrote Gorman in disgust.[134] The abrupt loss of two clinical chairmen within five days caused consternation among faculty and alumni. Yater was unquestionably Georgetown's best man; Wall was an eminent physician who had spent more than fifty years at the school as student and teacher and was now president of the American Academy of Pediatrics.[135] The Georgetown Alumni Association urged Gorman to bring back both men, sending him a petition signed by ninety-nine alumni, including seven current departmental chairmen, as well as Fred Sanderson and nineteen other members of the depleted department of surgery.[136] There is no evidence the university made any response.

So Yater severed all connection with Georgetown and went on to create a group practice in Washington, the Yater Clinic. Twenty years passed before the school offered conciliation, in 1965 at the behest of the then medical dean, John Rose, by conferring on Yater a long overdue honor, the title of Professor Emeritus of Medicine.[137] A further eleven years elapsed before the school awarded Yater an honorary degree, shortly before his death in 1976 at age eighty-five.[138]

Yet even as Yater left the school in 1945, events were in train which ultimately would bring about its transformation. The Lanham Act, approved by President Roosevelt in 1944, granted Georgetown $2,850,000 towards the building of a new hospital, on the understanding that an additional $750,000 would be raised by the university.[139] These were the first significant public funds the medical school had received in its entire history, now approaching a century. Within a few years, the medical center Kober had dreamed of would become reality, and most of Yater's hoped-for reforms would be realized too, as Georgetown entered a new era.

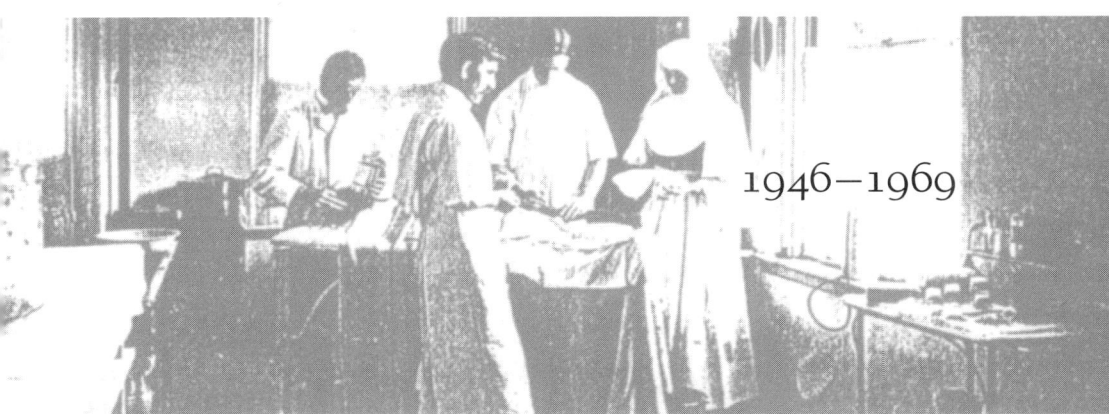

CHAPTER SEVEN

FOUNDATION OF THE MODERN DEPARTMENT OF SURGERY

THE NEW DEAN and regent of the medical school was not the physician that Wallace Yater had hoped, but another Jesuit. The Reverend Paul A. McNally, S.J. was an internationally renowned astronomer who had directed Georgetown's Astronomical Laboratory for eighteen years. He had also been a vice president of the university since 1942 and, since 1945, leader of the vigorous campaign which had raised $750,000 for the new hospital.[1] In both roles, he had demonstrated formidable abilities as an administrator. Nevertheless, his being made head of the medical school in September 1946 came as a shock even to McNally, and his reaction was equivocal: he asked to remain nominally director of the observatory "until he found out just what this medical appointment would mean."[2] In his new office, however, McNally quickly proved himself a man whose vision matched his energy. His actions enabled Georgetown at last to develop into a first-class medical school.

This was the turning point. For nearly one hundred years, Georgetown had struggled against tides of economic disadvantage and had come close to foundering several times. It had always possessed nearly all the necessary ingredients for success: being part of an old-established university; located in a growing city which happened to be the nation's capital; and blessed with a succession of professors passionately committed to high standards of medical education. Only money had been lacking. Over the next twenty years, however, from 1947 through the 1960s, this essential also became increasingly available as a prosperous nation, enamored of new visions of health and longevity, poured federal and private funds into medical research, training, hospitals, and medical schools. This was a new financial banquet—very different from the partisan philanthropic feasts of earlier years—and, finally, Georgetown had a seat at the table. The school benefitted too from a marked change in the attitude of the Jesuits towards it—a rapprochement brought about by the intelligence and utter obstinacy of one of their own, Paul McNally.

Like his predecessors, McNally knew nothing of medical education; the difference, however, was that he was willing to learn. The mentor he chose was a physician who had arrived fortuitously at Georgetown only three months earlier with just the knowledge and experience that McNally lacked. He was Harold Jeghers, Yater's successor to the chair of medicine. Already a renowned educator, Jeghers had been professor of medicine at Boston University School of Medicine and chief of its medical service at Boston City Hospital, where for years he had worked closely with colleagues from Harvard and Tufts. He thus arrived at Georgetown with a masterly grasp of the interaction between academics, clinical education, and research in the leading medical schools and teaching hospitals around Boston.[3]

At Jeghers's suggestion, Paul McNally's first act as dean was to head north to Massachusetts, to see for himself. Through one hectic week, Jeghers introduced McNally to professors and administrators at all the Boston area schools and teaching hospitals.[4] The visit had a profound influence on McNally. On his return to Georgetown he set in motion a series of administrative changes designed to raise standards and to weld the academic and clinical components of the medical, dental, and nursing schools, and the new hospital into an integrated modern "medical center"—an idea still regarded by many at Georgetown as utopian.

His most significant change was to replace the part-time chairmen of the clinical departments with salaried full-timers who would, in turn, gradually increase the number of other full-time faculty within their departments. In 1947, "full-time" did not mean what it does today, as defined under the faculty practice plans introduced in the 1960s and 1970s. The new contracts merely obliged full-time clinical professors to limit their private

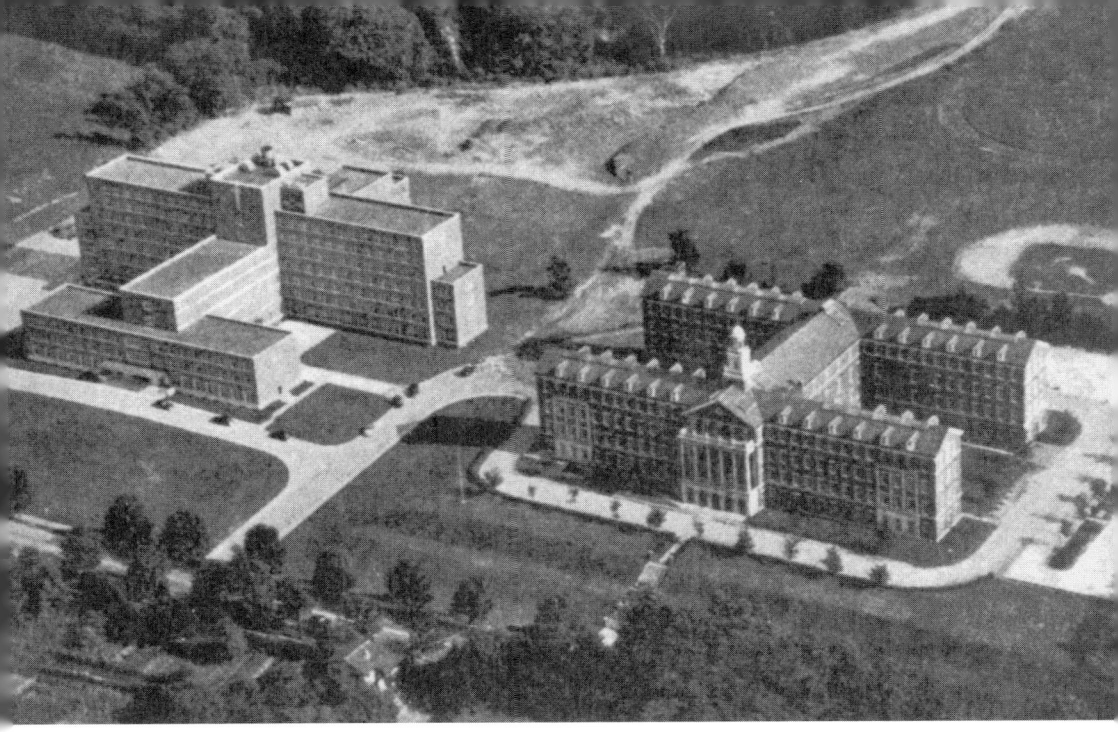

After nearly fifty years of being "miles distant" from each other, Georgetown University Hospital and School of Medicine finally came together with the opening of the new hospital in 1947. Today, the sprawl of the modern Medical Center surrounds both buildings. Courtesy of Georgetown University Archives.

practice to the university hospital, while allowing most of them to keep fees for service over a certain agreed level. This arrangement was known as geographic full-time, and it created a self-supporting salary structure which the Jesuits were willing to sanction because it cost the university virtually nothing: as soon as a full-timer became established, his "salary" was met from the private fees he generated at the hospital. Inevitably the introduction of this system—new to Georgetown though used in many other medical schools—was vigorously opposed. But McNally had the authority and he held firm.[5]

The timing helped. In 1946, many highly qualified men were returning from the war, eager to resume their interrupted careers. McNally, counselled by Jeghers, was determined to recruit the best: men of prestige whose academic backgrounds and professional connections would swiftly elevate Georgetown's standing. By July 1947, six new chairman (out of fifteen who then comprised the executive faculty) had been appointed on a full-time basis to head clinical departments. All six had impressive academic credentials.

Willi Baensch, the new chairman of radiology, had as a young man assisted Wilhelm Konrad Roentgen in Munich and for several years had been Marie Curie's assistant in Paris. Founder and director of the University of Leipzig radiology institute (1926–45), president of the Roentgen Congress in Europe (1934), and secretary-general of the International Congress of Radiology (1937), Baensch had long been distinguished in his field. Married to an American, he came to the United States after the war. McNally heard, by chance, that he was seeking a professorship and invited him to Georgetown.[6] Edward B. Tuohy, chairman of anesthesiology, was also internationally known in his field and had devised many new instruments and techniques. He came to Georgetown after twelve years at the Mayo Clinic, and in 1947 he was president of the American Society of Anesthesiologists.[7] Charles F. Geschickter, chairman of pathology, was a national authority on cancer. During the 1930s, after a tour of cancer centers in Europe, he had returned to direct the Garvan Cancer Research Laboratory at his alma mater, Johns Hopkins. Through the war years, he directed the pathology laboratories at the Naval Medical Center in Bethesda, Maryland, and for this won the Legion of Merit.[8] Murray Copeland, chairman of a new department of oncology and radiology, was also an authority on cancer and had worked closely with Geschickter ever since they had trained together at Johns Hopkins and the Mayo Clinic. They had collaborated before the war on several highly regarded textbooks on breast cancer; Copeland, too, had won the Legion of Merit for exceptional medical service in the Pacific.[9] Andrew Marchetti, chairman of obstetrics and gynecology, was another Johns Hopkins graduate. He had been a senior professor at Cornell School of Medicine where, among other notable achievements, he had helped develop the Pap smear to detect cervical cancer.[10] Even the new professor of surgery, Robert J. Coffey, the only Georgetown graduate of this group, had higher academic qualifications than most surgeons of his time; with an M.S. in medicine and a Ph.D. in surgery from the University of Minnesota, he had already contributed to experimental and clinical research in pancreatic disease, an especially difficult area of surgical intervention.

When he took over as chairman on July 1, 1947, Robert Coffey was thirty-eight years old and had been out of the navy for eighteen months.

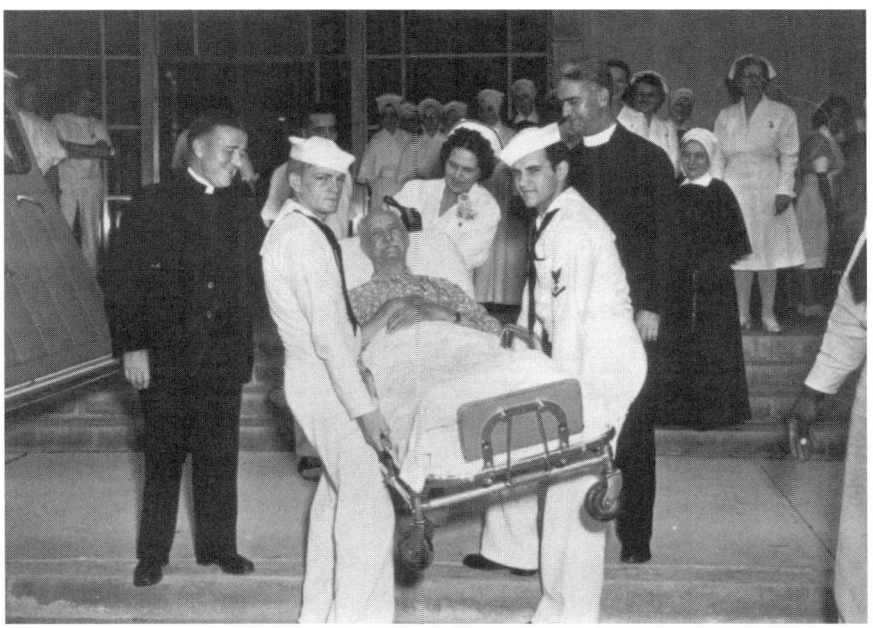

The eighty-eight-year-old George Tully
Vaughan was transferred from the old
Georgetown University Hospital to its new
building on Reservoir Road on the day it
opened, July 31, 1947. The new medical school
dean, Reverend Paul A. McNally, S.J.,
stands at the left, welcoming him. Courtesy of
Georgetown University Archives.

Back in private practice in Washington, he had been serving as consultant in surgery at the National Naval Medical Center in Bethesda, the Army Air Corps Hospital at Bolling Field, and the Veterans Administration Hospital at Mount Alto (where the Russian Embassy now stands). He had also been working with his old mentor Wallace Yater as general surgeon in Yater's new group-practice clinic, located at that time—before it moved into its present home in the sixty-one-room former Belgian Embassy building on Massachusetts Avenue—in a modest suite of offices on the corner of Eighteenth and K Street NW.[11]

Coffey accepted McNally's offer of the surgery chair at an annual salary of twenty-five thousand dollars. "Three or four months later," he recalled, "Father McNally came to me and said that finances were pretty strained and asked if I would accept a reduction to twenty thousand dollars a year. Which I did. There were advantages compared with private practice: you

had no rent to pay, no overhead, and you didn't need malpractice insurance because all that was paid by the university. And of course the job
was interesting and prestigious."[12]

Georgetown medical school in 1947 was housed in the same building
that Coffey had known as a student fifteen years earlier; but much else
had changed. Most students in the freshmen and sophomore classes had
been admitted under the GI Bill; they were seasoned by military service;
many were married; and some were as much as twenty years older than
classmates too young to have served in the war.[13] A few even wore
skirts: this landmark year of 1947 saw women admitted to degree courses
at the medical school for the first time, seven in all.[14] And the school itself
no longer stood in grass-ringed isolation on Reservoir Road. Alongside
was the stark brick block of the new hospital, opened on July 31, 1947.
Among the patients transferred that day by ambulance from the old
hospital at Thirty-fifth Street was the professor who had first instructed
Coffey in surgery, the eighty-eight-year-old former chairman, George
Tully Vaughan.[15] He died there the following April.

The new chairman of surgery made an instant impression on the
medical students. One was John Rose, the future dean of the medical
school, who as a twenty-two-year-old veteran airman had entered
Georgetown on the GI Bill in 1946. "As soon as we encountered Bob
Coffey," he recalled, "everybody said: '*That* is what a doctor should look
like.'" Tall, handsome, and always impeccably dressed, he was a dashing
figure—particularly on those occasions when, called from an evening
engagement, he would sweep into the emergency room in white tie and
tails. "And he wore taps on his shoes. When he came down the corridors
of the hospital, you knew the chief of surgery was coming."

But Robert Coffey impressed the students for more reasons than sarto-
rial elegance. Rose said:

> In lectures, often delivered in his scrubs, he was always a good speaker.
> His level of training was significantly better than most surgeons, and he
> was academic in the true sense. He'd done research, knew the literature,
> and his lectures were substantive. The thing that distinguished him was
> that, perhaps due to his training at the Mayo Clinic, he understood and
> talked about the physiology of illness, not just the pathology and the

surgical techniques. In that sense, he was a cut above the other surgeons who could tell you what they did, but it wasn't always clear they knew why they were doing it. Sophomores and juniors are always impressed by clinicians, and especially by people as impressive as him. Many of my classmates went into surgery and they did it because of Bob Coffey.[16]

The chairman's prestige was further enhanced when, only one month into the academic year on October 6, 1947, he became the first surgeon to perform an operation broadcast by television. His audience consisted of the few hundred people who owned eight-inch black-and-white television sets in the Washington metropolitan area. A few operations had recently been televised by closed-circuit systems for professional education purposes. But this one—an appendectomy on a twenty-three-year-old patient under spinal anesthesia—was, according to press reports, "the first time in history such an event has been broadcast over the airwaves." The camera followed proceedings from the surgical team's scrubbing-up to the patient's removal from the operating room, with a voice-over commentary by Georgetown's professor of surgical anatomy, Philip Caulfield, explaining every step.[17]

While the students were assessing their new professors, Coffey was assessing his department. Many of his views stemmed from his experience at the Mayo Clinic. "From those contacts," he recalled, "I knew what the challenge was and what I should try to attain. There was a conspicuous need for more attention to graduate education in that we wanted to establish the department of surgery nationally."[18] Other ideas derived from a fact-finding trip he had made in the summer of 1947—somewhat similar to Paul McNally's the previous year—when he visited medical schools in New York, Boston, and Canada.[19]

Coffey's immediate priorities were to recruit more full-time faculty, increase clinical teaching and residencies, and encourage more research, more publications, and more involvement in national and regional professional organizations such as American Surgical, Southern Surgical, and Southeastern Surgical, as well the local D.C. Medical Society. The advantages of attending their meetings, presenting papers, and making professional contacts were self-evident: "They provided a platform for

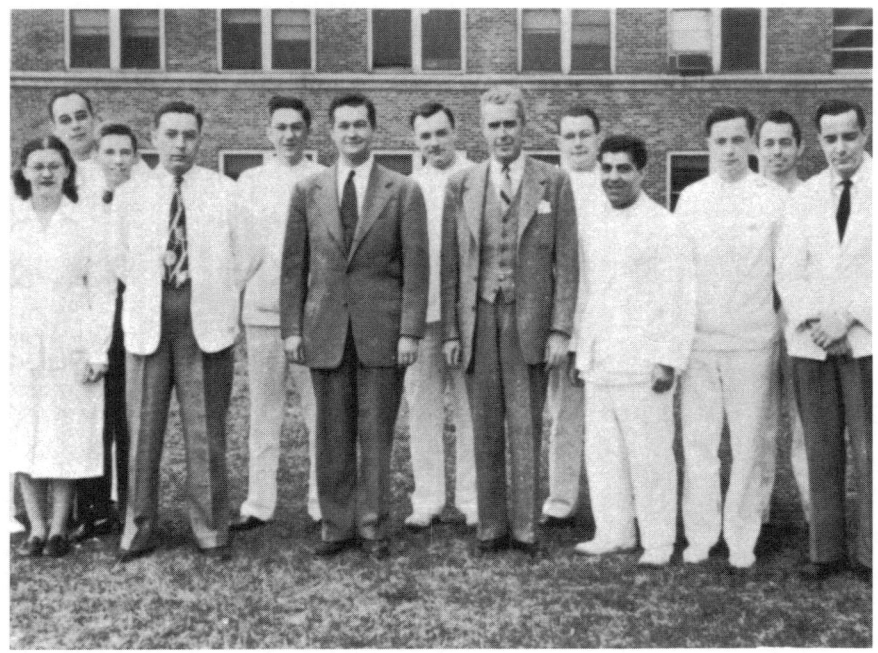

The new chairman of surgery, Robert J. Coffey, with the first full-timer he appointed to the department, Earl Barnes, and surgical residents, 1950. Courtesy of the Georgetown medical school yearbook, "Journey's End," 1950.

Georgetown to display its wares," he said. "And they provided an opportunity to recruit people from other institutions."

The expansion of the surgery department under Coffey's chairmanship was rapid. In 1946, the department had 69 faculty members plus six residents. By 1950, it numbered 132, among them twenty-four residents. It had become the largest of the medical school's seventeen departments.[20]

It included at this time all the then surgical sub-specialties: ophthalmology, neurosurgery, surgical oncology, orthopedics, thoracic surgery, urology, proctology, oral surgery, otorhinolaryngology, pediatric surgery, and plastic and reconstructive surgery. In 1947, some of these were no more than poorly defined units, staffed by private physicians who volunteered time and effort but received little financial or administrative support. In the years to come, however, as the faculty was enlarged and strengthened, these sub-specialties grew into significant divisions; and ultimately (after Coffey's chairmanship) ophthalmology, neurosurgery, orthopedics, and otolaryngology became departments in their own right.

By 1949, the undergraduate curriculum in surgery had evolved to further limit didactic lectures and increase clinical experience. Beginning surgical training in their sophomore year, students attended lectures on the fundamentals of surgery and learned physical diagnosis during ward rounds. One third of their junior year they spent in surgical clerkships at Gallinger Hospital (later renamed D.C. General), where they were responsible for the complete work-up of patients assigned to them and took part in clinical conferences. In the fourth year, assigned to Georgetown University Hospital, they continued their clerkships with greater responsibility for patient care under the supervision of assistant residents in surgery, rotated through the specialties, and assisted in the operating room.[21] Seniors could choose electives in the specialties and in experimental surgery. They were also required to submit a thesis on a surgical subject in competition for the Cahill award, which had been established by the class of 1943 in honor of the former chairman of the department. One of the first students to win this, for a paper on "Aneurysm of the Splenic Artery," was John F. Potter, later a distinguished surgical oncologist and first director of Georgetown's Vincent Lombardi Cancer Center.[22]

To a certain extent, didactic lectures began to be replaced by clinical conferences. Beginning in 1948, third-year students were required to attend conferences where cases of combined medical-surgical interest were demonstrated and discussed.[23] That same year, the Tumor Board was established by the surgery department for similarly dynamic instruction in cancerous and premalignant conditions. Directed by Earl Barnes, Coffey's first full-time appointee, it met every Wednesday at 1:00 P.M. with twenty to thirty students present. "It provided expert diagnostic and therapeutic recommendations for patients who had tumors and, just as importantly, demonstrated to the students the procedure for handling such patients," Coffey recalled. "Patients were brought in by a student

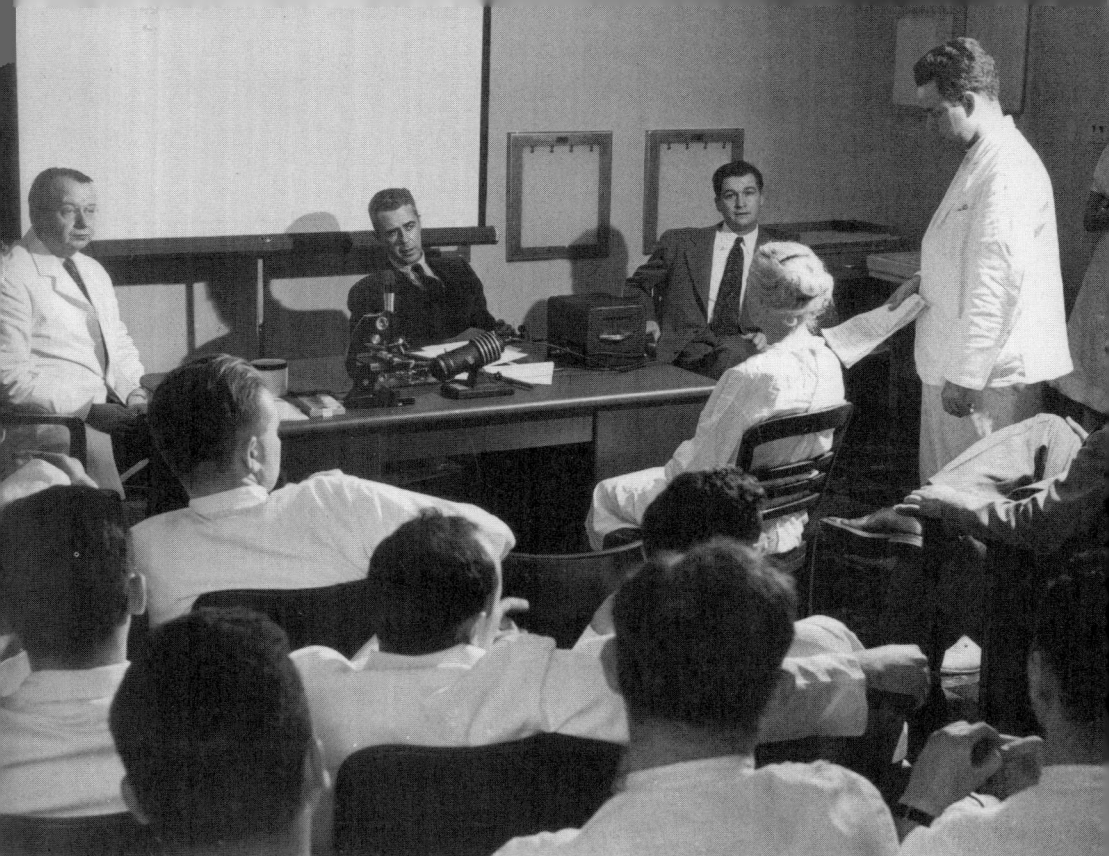

A student presents a case to the Tumor Board in the 1950s. Presiding, left to right: Murray Copeland, chairman of oncology and radiology; Robert J. Coffey; and Earl Barnes. Courtesy of the private collection of Robert J. Coffey.

who would present the case to the whole group—the history, X rays, the physical findings, and the problems involved. Then it would be turned over to Dr. Copeland and myself to discuss."[24]

At the graduate level, Coffey quadrupled the number of surgical residents in his first three years. Nationwide, the late 1940s saw the first sizeable expansion of surgical residency programs. University hospitals had gradually developed them since Halsted's introduction of the system at Johns Hopkins; but for decades they got little recognition and were by no means considered an essential passport to the practice of surgery. No national regulation or certification existed until the American Board of Surgery was established in 1937. But World War II changed all that. It was obvious both to the military medical authorities and to young officers recruited straight out of medical school that the best surgeons were those who had been residency trained. After the war, the demand for residencies rocketed, far exceeding the number of places on offer; and non-university hospitals took advantage of the demand to begin their own programs.[25]

Georgetown accommodated its own expansion by forming affiliations with a number of local community hospitals, starting with Arlington Hospital in 1948 and the Mount Alto Veterans Administration Hospital in 1949. This greatly extended both junior clerkships and graduate training in medicine and surgery beyond the university hospital (then still relatively small) and Gallinger, while also aiding the community hospitals. "These hospitals could not have attracted desirable trainees on their own, but as part of our program they got the kind of residents they wanted," Coffey explained. Under the direction of J. Gordon Lee at Mount Alto, William Dolan and then Frank Cardenas at Arlington, and later William Feller at Sibley Hospital, these affiliates remained for many years an essential part of Georgetown's program. At D.C. General, meanwhile, Georgetown expanded faculty control of its surgical service; Henry Balch became the first full-time director of the service in 1956 and was mainly responsible for developing training programs there for surgical residents and clerks.[26]

Another advance came in the summer of 1949: the surgical residency program was extended from three to four years. Residents were now required to devote at least six months to basic science, either in experimental surgery, pathology, or anatomy. After their first or second year, they could elect to train in the specialties of urologic, thoracic, orthopedic, proctologic surgery, or neurosurgery.[27] "The training experiences required to qualify in surgery could no longer be fitted into three years, and of course later the program was extended further," Coffey explained. "The residents were also given more responsibilities for teaching students and played a much more active role in operative surgery. It was not a hands-off experience. They were part of the team." And expected to behave as such. These early residents attached to Robert Coffey's service soon found themselves on the receiving end of a caustic tongue famous to generations of their successors in the operating room. A note in the 1950 yearbook records how one of that year's residents, attention wandering for a moment, was sharply hauled back to the job in hand by a typically acid Coffey remark: "Feel free to sponge, Howard."[28]

The residents were beneficiaries of another innovation, Surgical Grand Rounds, held in the university hospital for two or three hours every

Saturday morning. Grand Rounds, a concept imported by Jeghers from the Cambridge-Boston schools and instituted in both the medical and surgical departments, was—in the words of Robert Moser, a Georgetown resident in medicine who later became editor of *JAMA*—"postgraduate education at its best."[29] It gave opportunities for faculty members, primarily, to keep up to date—but residents were allowed to watch. "It was the big teaching activity of the week," Coffey said. "Cases were presented and discussed by a panel; we had surgeons visiting who were well-known in certain fields. All the full-time and part-time surgical staff were expected to be there, and the time was divided up equitably in that people in thoracic disease had one Grand Rounds, the gastroenterologists had another, and so on. Of course, these sessions had great educational value and still go on to this day."[30]

The many changes introduced at Georgetown in a mere two and a half years since his appointment as dean gave McNally the confidence to invite inspection by the AMA's Council for Medical Education and Hospitals in March 1949. This was the crucial test. Would the council lift the "confidential probationary" status it had imposed on Georgetown in 1935 and upheld in 1939? Would the school be restored to full accreditation?

Representatives from the AMA's Council and the Association of American Medical Colleges (by now known as the AMA/AAMC liaison committee) arrived at Georgetown on March 14 and for five days inspected the medical school, its teaching programs, finances, and administration. Their report sent two months later was everything the faculty had hoped. "The Georgetown University Medical College has made tremendous strides in improving the quality of its teaching since the last survey in 1939," it concluded. "Great credit should be given the administrative officers who have seen what had to be done and have taken the necessary steps to bring the changes about. The past ten years has been a period of marked progress in most of our medical schools. There are few who have moved more rapidly than has Georgetown."

As "outstanding improvements," they noted specifically the building of the new hospital next to the medical school; the establishing of full-time positions in the clinical departments; the "great improvement and systematic development of the clinical clerkships in the third and fourth years"; the effort "to bring in well-qualified men from a variety of outside institutions"; the improved "spirit of cooperation between members of the staff"; and the foresight displayed in "seeing what had to be done . . . and then doing it." The inspectors suggested further improvements, among them the need for a formal medical school budget, annual reports and budgets from the departmental chairmen, the freshman class cut to one hundred by a more stringent admissions policy, a better library, higher salaries for mid-level faculty members, and a planned retirement and pensions program. In the surgery department, "ably headed" by Robert Coffey, they reported favorably on the improved clinical teaching in junior and senior clerkships, but cautioned: "This department is in need of additional full-time teachers. Dr. Coffey hopes to put on an additional full-time man each year for the next five years."[31]

Two weeks after receiving this report, McNally took delivery of a Western Union telegram. Dated June 8, 1949, it read: "Pleased to inform you that Council for Medical Education and Hospitals has voted to remove the Georgetown University School of Medicine from its confidential probation. The Council joins me in extending congratulations to you and your faculty on the accomplishments of the past three years."[32] The university president, Reverend Hunter Guthrie, S.J. received congratulations of a more informal kind from one of his predecessors, Coleman Nevils, who of course remembered only too well the troubled times of the early 1930s: "I do not think any lay Dean could have accomplished what Fr. McNally has done in so short a time," Nevils wrote. "As you surely know, the school was in a very precarious situation when he took charge and now I hear on all sides that it is 'tops.' I realize that he has antagonized many and that he is terribly undiplomatic, but he has done a grand job in a real crisis."[33]

It was thus in a mood of genuine celebration that the medical school completed its first one hundred years. It had regained full accreditation. University, medical school, and hospital had at last united on one campus. More than two thousand applicants competed each year for 120 places in the school; and students were doing well in the national board examinations, which had been made a requirement at Georgetown in 1947. Of Georgetown students who took part one of the board exams in 1949, 5 out of 106 failed—slightly better than the average national failure rate of 20 percent.[34] In 1950, all Georgetown candidates passed part two, and four of them placed among the top seven in the country; Bernard F. Peacock Jr., with a perfect score in surgery, came first in the nation.[35] Even the financial situation allowed cautious optimism. At the September 9, 1949, meeting of the executive faculty, Dean McNally announced a balance of income over expenditure of $1,742, and claimed (erroneously) that 1949 was "the first year in the history of the medical school that a transition from one school year to another was made without the necessity of borrowing money."[36]

The centennial was formally celebrated on June 9–10, 1950. In commemorative brochures and speeches, the names of Young, Eliot, Howard, and Liebermann were much recalled. But the event was an academic occasion, designed to highlight Georgetown's contribution to modern medical education. Its centerpiece was a two-day symposium, at which the departments presented papers and exhibits.[37] To honor the centennial, the journal *Postgraduate Medicine* published a special issue featuring articles by the Georgetown faculty on advances in medicine and surgery. The twin journals *The Medical Clinics of North America* and *The Surgical Clinics of North America* also published complete Georgetown issues in which the medicine and surgery faculties presented papers on the diagnosis and treatment of cancer and premalignant conditions.[38]

The choice of subject was significant. In the postwar years, the upsurge of public interest in cancer generated substantial sums of money for research. From 1947 onwards, Georgetown, in common with other medical institutions, began to receive ever larger grants for clinical and research projects on cancer from the federal government, national and local fundraising campaigns, and even bequeathed legacies. Funds from the Public Health Service and the American Cancer Society, for example, enabled Murray Copeland in September 1948 to open the Cancer Detection Clinic, an outpatient unit for early diagnosis of the disease.[39] In January 1950, a twenty-five-thousand-dollar grant from the Alexander and Margaret Stewart Trust Fund enabled Coffey to establish the Home Care Service for cancer patients. The first of its kind in the nation, this provided the equivalent of hospital care in the homes of pre-terminal patients who could not afford hospitalization. The Home Care team comprised a physician, a trained nurse, a physiotherapist, two aides, a stationwagon, and a driver.[40]

Most of the grants supported cancer research undertaken largely by the oncology and pathology departments. Small rooms in the hospital were taken over as laboratories, and in 1949 the old animal house in the grounds was extended to provide more space for experimental surgery and pathology plus a laboratory for the medicine and biochemistry departments.[41] By 1950, with funds stimulated by the conviction that a cure for cancer was just around the corner, Georgetown's first significant medical research program was under way.

When the Medical Center began publishing its own journal—then known simply as the *Bulletin*—in the summer of 1947, the first issue contained an article on "The Surgical Treatment of Cardiovascular Disease" by Bernard J. Walsh. Addressing the very few cardiovascular abnormalities that could then be treated by surgery, he added: "Gross and Hufnagel in 1945 described the first successful correction of coarctation of the aorta . . . [but] we have had no experience ourselves with the surgical treatment of this condition."[42] In fact, in 1947 Georgetown had no cardiac program at all. No one could have predicted that only a few years later Charles Anthony Hufnagel, one of the authors of that cited paper, would join the medical faculty, invent the world's first artificial heart valves, and establish Georgetown as a leading international center for cardiovascular research and surgery.

By 1950, Robert Coffey had realized that his increasing administrative and clinical duties left little time for investigative work of his own. He needed someone else to direct the surgical research program. "So I went up to Peter Bent Brigham Hospital, the teaching hospital for Harvard Medical School. A friend of mine, Carl Walter, ran the research program there. I told him my problem and he immediately said, 'I have just the man for you.' He called someplace and a minute or two later this young feller came in, very boyish looking, and we were introduced: Charlie Hufnagel."[43]

For all his youthful appearance, Hufnagel was thirty-three years old, married with two daughters, and director of the Laboratory for Surgical Research at Harvard Medical School. Born in Louisville, Kentucky, on August 15, 1916, the son of a general practitioner, he had been educated at Notre Dame (B.S., 1937) and Harvard (M.D., 1941), and was already recognized as one of the nation's most promising medical scientists.[44]

From 1941, throughout his surgical residency at Brigham, he had worked on the Harvard team led by Robert E. Gross which eventually found a way to preserve arterial grafts for human transplantation; the first successful transplants restored the healthy circulation of nine "blue babies" in 1948. The main surgical problem in inserting grafts into arteries near the heart was that while the surgeon needed time for the delicate work of stitching the cut ends of the artery to the graft, the flow of blood could be stopped only for the shortest possible time—under three minutes in the case of the upper aorta—if brain damage were to be averted. It was Hufnagel, experimenting on dogs, who came up with the idea of a Lucite tube, inserted inside the graft section, that allowed the blood to flow while he sewed the donor segment to the host artery; just before the last stitches, the tube was slipped out. This reduced the interruption in blood flow to two breaks of thirty seconds each. Years later, of course, such repairs would easily be performed by diverting the patient's blood through a heart-lung bypass machine; but in the 1940s, this was still being developed through animal research at Philadelphia, Minneapolis, and Stockholm. Until that machine arrived, Hufnagel's tube provided a simple and inexpensive answer.

Lucite was one of the new plastic materials to come out of World War II. Biologically inert and with a surface tension that repelled blood so that clotting did not occur, it offered completely new possibilities for surgery; Hufnagel was the first to recognize this. Could Lucite, he wondered, be used as a permanent replacement for a weakened section of artery? This inspiration, which struck Hufnagel in bed at two in the morning[45], proved successful in experiments after he also invented an ingenious way of joining the rigid tube to the pliable artery by using a ring with multiple teeth around the inside edge: these held the artery firmly enough to prevent bleeding but not so hard as to cut the blood supply and cause necrosis in the cut ends of the artery—a principle which became known as multiple point fixation.[46] The technique was perfected experimentally in 1946. As Hufnagel explained years later, it marked "the first time that it was possible to achieve a permanent replacement of a major artery with a synthetic material."[47] In fact, it was the first time plastics had ever been used inside the human body. The Lucite tube won Hufnagel his first award and national headlines when he was named one of the "Top Ten Outstanding Young Men of 1948" by the National Junior Chamber of Commerce.[48]

Charles Hufnagel's brilliance lay in resolving practical problems of surgery with elegant simplicity. His use of plastics was but one example. Another, unpublicized at the time, came in 1947 when he was experimenting on kidney transplantation. A young woman who had suffered a miscarriage was admitted to Peter Bent Brigham Hospital in a coma after suffering total renal shutdown. She was on the point of death when a donor kidney became available and Hufnagel began operating, around midnight, right there in her hospital bed by the light of gooseneck lamps. He did not attempt to transplant the donor kidney into the normal retroperitoneal space—"We were not that far advanced," he explained in describing the event more than twenty years later—but instead he transplanted it into her arm.

> Not being certain of what would happen, we preferred keeping it in a more accessible location. We did this by establishing an anastomosis between the brachial artery and a large vein in the anticubital fossa to the donor kidney. . . . An attempt to bury the kidney beneath the skin was made, but because of the position of the vessels, a considerable part of the kidney was still uncovered. The entire area was kept warm with the use of the same gooseneck lamps. Immediately the kidney began to secrete urine.

The next day the patient's condition was greatly improved; the day after that she was entirely alert and the kidney in her arm, having fulfilled its purpose, was removed. Her own kidneys began functioning once again and, Hufnagel recalled, "her subsequent recovery was relatively uneventful."[49] This temporary use of a transplanted kidney came three years before the first attempt was made to transplant a kidney into a human being *in situ* (by Richard H. Lawler, Chicago, 1950) and seven years before the first successful transplant was achieved (by John P. Merrill, 1954), also at Brigham Hospital, by using a kidney donated by the patient's twin brother to overcome the problem of immuno-rejection.[50] Hufnagel's landmark operation never made the record books. But in a book on kidney transplantation in 1964, Francis D. Moore, professor of surgery at Harvard, credited it as the "first attempt in man."[51]

After his success with the Lucite tube, Hufnagel in early 1950 was already experimenting with other plastics in the hope of developing replacements for diseased heart valves. It was one of the matters discussed when, after Carl Walter introduced them, Coffey took Hufnagel to lunch. Needless to say, Coffey was "much impressed" and invited Hufnagel to head the surgical research program he wanted to establish at Georgetown.[52] After the usual negotiations and a visit to the capital, which he found "a sleepy little town,"[53] Hufnagel accepted and took up his position on August 1, 1950. Three months later, Coffey was gratified to note the deference paid to Hufnagel at a surgical meeting and to have the chairman of surgery at Emory University confide that, had he known Hufnagel was willing to leave Harvard, he would certainly have tried to lure him to Atlanta.[54]

From that time, Georgetown's developments in cardiovascular surgery were seldom out of the news. Hufnagel himself, a supremely modest man, never courted media attention, disliked giving interviews, and indeed regarded publicity for doctors as unprofessional.[55] But his work on arterial grafts had already featured in a 1948 article in the *Saturday Evening Post*, then the nation's most widely read magazine, and reporters called his office whenever they heard that something newsworthy was afoot.

The first big story came in October 1950, when Hufnagel and Coffey established one of the nation's first blood vessel banks. Fresh animal and human arteries and large veins were to be preserved at a temperature of minus seventy degrees centigrade in a specially constructed deep-freeze unit. The thawed grafts would be used, in conjunction with Hufnagel's synthetic tubes, to replace diseased or crushed vessels. By February 1951, more than thirty vessels had been "banked." The first of these frozen arteries to be used clinically was rushed to Walter Reed Hospital, where it saved the arm of a soldier injured in the Korean War.[56] Similar procedures, used in field hospitals, did represent a significant surgical advance of this war, vastly reducing the incidence of amputations. Hufnagel, always taking the next logical step forward, was further inspired by the needs of the Korean conflict to experiment with freeze-dried grafts that could be more easily transported and would last longer in the field; he presented a paper on the subject to the Clinical Congress of the American College of Surgeons in Chicago in 1953.[57]

In early 1951, the Georgetown *Bulletin* reported another of Hufnagel's inventions: a snap-hook button to repair holes in the wall of the heart. Once again, the idea was simple, though it took the most delicate surgery. One half of the plastic button was pushed by a special instrument through the hole in the septum, then pulled back so that teeth on the flat side of the button caught in the tissue; the other half was snapped into the first and the instrument withdrawn. Hufnagel, aided in this research by his resident, John F. Gillespie, reported the results on animals as "uniformly good," with complete closure of the heart wall verified up to four months later.[58]

But the focus of his investigations, supported initially by a sixteen-thousand-dollar grant from the National Heart Institute, remained the perfecting of an artifical heart valve. Hufnagel had been working through the technical problems for years. He had designed many valves in many materials, constructing most of them himself in his small basement workshop at home. Animal experiments brought constant setbacks. Eventually he decided to insert the valve not at the site of the natural aortic valve ring but lower in the descending aorta. This reduced the risk of thrombosis (blood clots) and lessened the likelihood of the valve obstructing the flow of blood. Finally, after many modifications, Hufnagel designed a ball-valve of hollow Plexiglas (polyethylene) that brought excellent results. In more than one hundred consecutive insertions in dogs, the ball-valve worked without failing or causing death, and it presented very few problems of thrombosis or rupture of the aorta. At this point, Dean McNally went public with news of the perfected valve. Now, he told the press, Hufnagel was waiting to install one in a human patient.[59]

That historic event came on September 11, 1952, when thirty-year-old Martina Hall became the first human to live with an artificial heart valve.[60] She had been afflicted with rheumatic fever as a seven-year-old in Fairfax, Virginia. The disease had left scarred tissue around her heart valve, so that it failed to close properly; instead of blood pulsing one-way through the valve, some flowed backward, forcing the heart to work harder; over time it enlarged, causing anginal pain and severe fatigue. Martina had been obliged to give up her work as a nurse; the only relief then possible was prolonged rest and digitalis.[61]

The operation that changed her life—and, subsequently, those of thousands of other victims of rheumatic fever—was performed at Georgetown

University Hospital. When Hufnagel opened her chest, he discovered an unexpected problem: the descending aorta was greatly narrowed by coarctation—a thickening of the artery wall. He chose the smallest of his ball-valves, but only with great difficulty was he able to insert it and secure it with nylon ring clamps.[62] But the procedure was successful and Martina recovered. She said afterwards: "I never realized just how bad I had felt most of my life until about two weeks after the operation." Three months later, she was working again, this time as an X-ray technician in the hospital's radiology department, close by Hufnagel's office.

The operation—performed before the advent of by-pass machines made possible many more radical ventures into open-heart surgery—created headlines everywhere, and in the years that followed surgeons visiting Georgetown frequently stopped by to examine Martina. "They were fascinated," she said. She also made a point of talking to new patients about to get heart valves from Hufnagel; she became so knowledgeable that she often explained the operation to medical students. Martina Hall died in 1960, from further complications of her disease, but the artificial valve had given her eight productive years—each marked by Hufnagel every September 11, when he presented her with a cake decorated with one candle for every year since the landmark operation.

A characteristic of this first ball-valve was that the cherry-sized ball inside it clicked softly but audibly with every heartbeat. The noise did not bother Martina—"You know, I find it even comforting," she remarked wryly—but some patients were disconcerted. One man, a poker player, complained that his heart raced so strongly whenever he drew a good hand that the accelerated clicking gave his cards away. But the noise had one advantage. Cardiac arrythmia was a common problem in these patients, and when they returned to their homes far away, they often called Hufnagel if they developed symptoms. By instructing them to open their mouths close to the telephone, Hufnagel could hear the faint clicking of the valve and was frequently able to diagnose an irregular heartbeat and refer them to their local doctors. Eventually he eliminated the noise by devising a hollow nylon valve coated in silicon rubber.[63]

The ball-valve was not perfect, and its insertion required delicate surgery, but as he improved the technique, Hufnagel achieved remarkable success. His first ten valve insertions saw one operative death (occurring

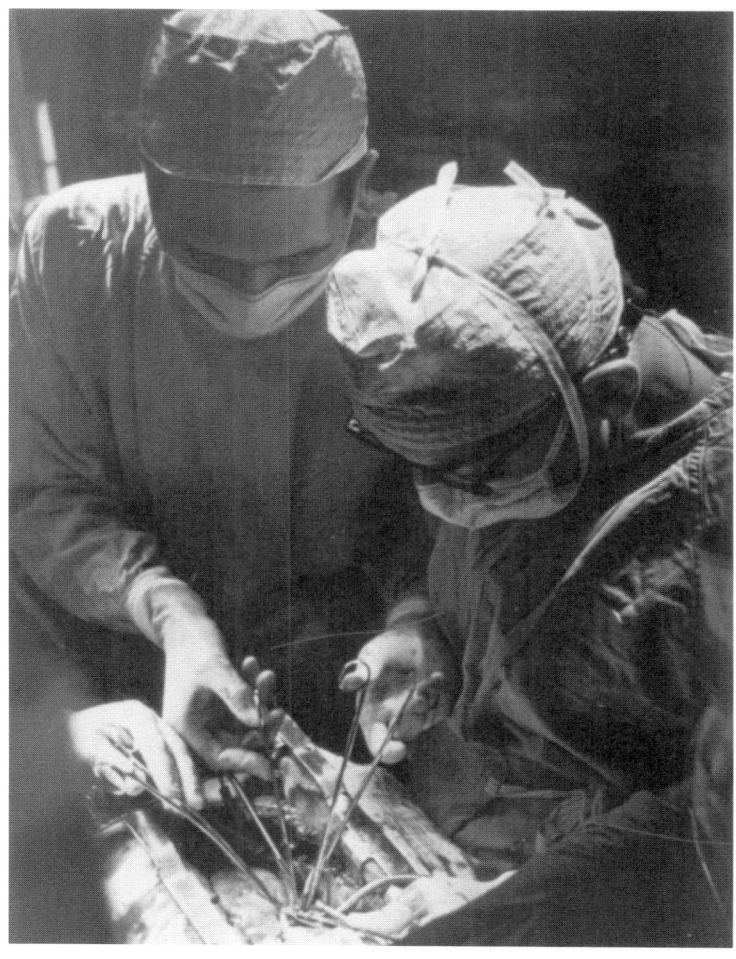

Charles Hufnagel (right) replaces a defective heart valve with one of the artificial valves he pioneered in the 1950s. Courtesy of Georgetown University Archives.

before the valve was put in place) and three patients dying postoperatively (of pneumonitis, acute right heart failure, and ventricular fibrillation respectively). In his second series of ten patients, one died.[64] But thereafter, throughout the 1950s, Hufnagel continued to develop many models of heart valves, fitting them into hundreds of patients who streamed to Georgetown from all over the world.

Hufnagel's inventiveness never flagged. His researches into freeze-dried animal arterial grafts suggested to him that, after sterilization with ethylene oxide, they might be tolerated in the body of a human being. He was right. Early in 1953, he successfully transplanted segments of arteries from calves and a pig into four men. The animal grafts replaced the dangerously hardened and narrowed arteries of two older men and several arteries crushed by accidents in two younger men. This was another first for Hufnagel and for medical science. Announcing the news at the annual meeting of the American College of Surgeons in Chicago that October, Hufnagel explained that the human body cannot grow the fresh elastic tissue needed to keep an artery from swelling or bursting from the pressure of pulsating blood flow. The new technique solved that problem. The animal segments—having been frozen, dried, sterilized, preserved in sealed containers in a vacuum, and finally soaked in water to prepare them for surgery—still retained their elasticity and provided structure for new human tissue to grow over. The problem of rejection in transplants, he said, had been overcome for the first time.[65]

Twenty years before fiber optics, Hufnagel was using in his lab a clear plastic rod to peer inside dogs' hearts. The rod channelled light so effectively that one could read the date and denomination of a coin at the bottom of a tumblerful of blood. Prophetically, Coffey told the press that surgeons hoped to find a way to attach a sewing device so they could see and repair holes in the heart at the same time.[66]

In 1954, Hufnagel turned to another new synthetic material, Orlon. Most people were making shirts out of it. Hufnagel had the idea of using it to fashion the first artificial aorta. He thought the strength and close weave of the fabric would prove more flexible than animal grafts in replacing awkwardly shaped segments of natural arteries. Lois Reed, one of his technicians, bought a length of Orlon at a Washington sewing store known as G Street Fabrics. She took it home and on her sewing machine ran up a prototype, using a dog's artery as a model. Shaped like a tiny pair of pants to reproduce the bifurcation of the aorta, her handiwork was inserted successfully into the abdomen of a forty-three-year-old laborer to replace a hardened section of his aorta. After that, Lois Reed and Hufnagel's wife, Kay, created virtually a cottage industry in artificial arteries, sewing them first in Orlon and later in Dacron, fiberglass, and Teflon. "Right now," a 1956 newspaper report commented, "150 people are walking around with a section of artery stitched up by Miss Reed or Mrs. Hufnagel."[67]

His experience with all these prostheses—the Lucite tube, the Plexiglas valve, the Orlon artery—led Hufnagel to believe that spare parts made from biologically inert and specially treated materials might hold out more hope for success in surgery than live transplants. In the late 1950s, he took this conviction to its logical conclusion by designing an artificial heart of Dacron and silicone rubber.[68] The device was never developed sufficiently for use in man, but it kept dogs alive for several weeks—predating the insertion of the first artificial heart into a human being (by William de Freis, Salt Lake City, in 1982) by twenty-four years.[69]

At the same time, Hufnagel continued his researches into the problem of immuno-rejection in live organ transplants, which he had begun with the Harvard team at Peter Bent Brigham Hospital in the 1940s. Here he had a stroke of luck. His cardiac success had won the attention of the widow of Alexis Carrel, the French-born scientist who had worked for many years at the Rockefeller Institute in New York and whose pioneering experiments on transplantation in animals had won him a Nobel Prize in 1912. Because of Hufnagel, Mrs. Carrel donated her late husband's voluminous papers to Georgetown. They arrived in a large truck in 1953, and from then on Hufnagel had access to Carrel's original notes, which no one had seen since his death in 1944.[70] The gift also sparked a close friendship between Hufnagel and Charles Lindbergh, the aviation pioneer, who in the 1930s had invented a perfusion pump for Carrel's tissue experiments and later collaborated on his classic work, *The Culture of Organs*. Whenever Lindbergh came to Washington, he would visit Hufnagel, often donning scrubs to watch him at work in the operating room.[71]

In the 1950s, organ transplantation was still regarded as so fantastic a notion that funding was hard to find. But in 1955, Hugh A. Grant, one of Coffey's surgical patients, became the surgery department's long-time benefactor. Grant, a millionaire oil producer from Bradford, Pennsylvania, gave one hundred thousand dollars to the department for a ten-year study of organ culture. The first of many gifts by Grant, this funding was designated specifically to continue Carrel's researches in the attempt to fulfill his prediction that one day surgeons would establish organ banks for spare part surgery. This was, as Coffey said in announcing the project, still in "the dreams classification of ideas." He told reporters: "I hope no one gets the idea that we'll be through with this thing tomorrow."[72] But at least a start could be made. "If Mr. Grant had not contributed to this work year after year," Hufnagel said long afterwards, "Georgetown would not have been able to continue research in this direction."[73]

Hufnagel's workload was so heavy—operating, teaching, doing research, going to professional meetings—that he never published many of his experimental findings. By the end of the 1950s, however, his fame had established Georgetown as an internationally-renowned center for cardiac research and surgery—and had brought him personally numerous awards. But what Hufnagel cared for most was thinking through and trying out the next step. "As long as disease exists, doctors must find a way to cure it," he said. "What has already been done really just points the way to what can be done."[74]

The relationship between Robert Coffey and Charles Hufnagel was amicable from the start. It might so easily have proved otherwise: two big-fish surgeons in a relatively small pond is not the likeliest formula for harmony. Yet the relationship worked exceedingly well, perhaps because the two men had such different personalities and because their roles were so distinct and well defined. As one colleague remarked: "They were both great surgeons; but Coffey was the chairman and administrator and Charlie was the inventor and brainy genius. It was a symbiotic relationship."[75]

Apart from surgery, they had only one thing in common. Both were devout Catholics who attended mass regularly. Coffey was active in several Irish-Catholic organizations, was made a Knight Commander of the Order of St. Gregory and a Knight of the Holy Sepulchre, and had two brothers-in-law who were priests. To the mystification of their fellow scientists, both Coffey and Hufnagel kept vials of Lourdes' holy water in their homes, remaining unmoved when a mischievous colleague tested a sample in the lab and found it teeming with bacteria: faith was distinguishable from science. In almost every other way, though, the two were opposites.

Coffey was a take-charge extrovert: highly self-confident, fiercely competitive, socially outgoing. At home, he and Mary Catherine entertained in style, often hosting dinner parties and throwing a Christmas celebration each year to which all the surgical staff and their spouses were invited. Every Christmas, too, Coffey would unearth his treasured Lionel train set, collected over many years and worth thousands of dollars. Spread across an entire basement room—and containing such prized items as real smoke, a rocket launcher, and a recorded conductor's voice announcing the arrival of the Santa Fe—the collection was regarded as "magical" by Coffey's children, who of course were rarely allowed to touch it. They merely watched wide-eyed as their father, cursing and throwing screwdrivers when parts failed to work, revelled in orchestrating his miniature mechanical world. For the rest of the year, Coffey found relaxation in hunting and endless games of golf, pool, skeets, darts, and bowling. He bowled the last as one of a Georgetown surgeons' team known as "the Bloods," who wore white satin jackets with scarlet lettering. Every sport he played to win. He could hit two catapulted skeets with a single shot; out on the marshes of the Chesapeake Bay, he could argue interminably whether it was he, or his companion, who had brought down that final duck. It seemed appropriate that his friend and patient, the millionaire Hugh A. Grant, named a racehorse after him; and equally appropriate when that "Dr. Coffey" came in first at Hialeah racetrack, Florida.

Hufnagel, in contrast, was the classic introvert: self-effacing, devoid of interest in competition or socializing, and replete with paradoxes. "Everybody loved Charlie," was a constant refrain of those who knew him, as they recalled his warmth toward everyone he met and his willingness to listen to anyone's problems. Yet he disliked parties and seldom invited even close friends and colleagues to his home. Hufnagel too enjoyed hunting, in particular deep-sea fishing for marlin off Panama and Belize. But all his other leisure pursuits were solitary and based on the same fine motor skills he used every day in the operating room. He made jewelry, hand-cutting semi-precious stones and setting them in gold; he created ceramic pots and sculptures; and he propagated a fine collection of rare orchids. Sometimes even these pastimes spurred Hufnagel's urge to invent. Faced with leaving his beloved orchids untended for a couple of weeks, he devised an elaborate method of watering them automatically, decades before such systems became commercially available.

The contrasts were clear in the two men's work. Hufnagel never yelled in the operating room, as Coffey did. Coffey never worried or obsessed over details, as Hufnagel did. Coffey organized his time with ruthless efficiency, to the extent of scheduling afternoon consultations with private patients so that they all arrived in his office at the same time, 2:00 P.M. Moving along— not having to wait for anyone who might show up late—was his style. Hufnagel, on the other hand, spent hours talking to patients and their visitors, often explaining the same thing several times to different family members. "Rounds with Charlie were interminable," one former resident recalled. "I used to take a magazine along." This same resident tried to set up a system to extricate Hufnagel from overlong sessions in a patient's room. The plan called for him to go in and say, "Dr. Hufnagel, you have a long-distance telephone call from Pittsburgh," as a signal for Hufnagel to excuse himself gracefully. The first time they tried it, Hufnagel responded: "Who is it? What does he want? Tell him I'll call him back." The experiment was never repeated. The world-famous surgeon continued explaining every detail of the diet and exercise regime a cardiac patient should follow after leaving the hospital. Hufnagel's concern for patients was legendary, but delegation was not his strong point.

Coffey delegated superbly. Never relishing the pedestrian business of paperwork, he largely disposed of it in the early 1960s by appointing a departmental chief executive officer to "get the trains running on time," as John Potter, the first chief, put it. Yet as an administrator, Coffey could be briskly creative. The director of the emergency room, Tom Lee, once complained that whenever an accident victim was admitted with a smashed face, every specialist—plastic, oral, ear-nose-and-throat, and general—would claim the case, with inevitable and frequent arguments. Coffey called a meeting of the division heads. Lee took notes and later drafted an advisory to post on the emergency room wall. He took it to the chairman's office. "Dr. Coffey, here's the result of the meeting." Coffey glanced at the paper, grunted, and tossed it in the waste basket. "What are you doing?" Lee protested. "They only needed to get it off their chests," Coffey said. "You won't have any more problems." Recalling this incident, Lee added: "And actually he was correct. Never another bitch about it. That was a typical Coffey ploy."

Complex and charismatic in their own idiosyncratic ways, Coffey and Hufnagel complemented each other, and they had the wit to know it. Despite

Hufnagel's growing fame and Coffey's growing power, neither envied the other nor ever challenged the other's jurisdiction. It pleased them, for instance, when both were elected to the elite 250-member American Surgical Association in the same year, 1956.[76] For nearly twenty years under Coffey's leadership, Hufnagel remained content to run his research laboratory and found his deepest satisfaction in solving intellectual conundrums. Coffey in turn gave Hufnagel time and space—and often helped find the funds. They remained close friends for thirty-nine years until Hufnagel's death in 1989. To the end of his own life six years later, Coffey talked of Hufnagel with nothing but affection and admiration: "He was very modest, physically attractive, good sense of humor, very hard-working, and he had a wonderful research mind. Nothing was impossible in his opinion."

If Hufnagel was the surgery department's star player, Robert Coffey was its manager, coach, and principal cheerleader. Throughout his chairmanship, Coffey acted as a kind of super-salesman, selling the department to national, regional, and local audiences. He regularly drove to meetings of county medical societies in Maryland and Virginia—as often as twice a month in the early years—to give evening lectures and hand his card to local physicians. In those days, when good surgeons were rarer in rural areas, that was the accepted way of ensuring that complicated cases were referred to Georgetown. He traveled longer distances to meetings of all the regional surgical associations, again to make contacts and present papers. That too was a sign of the times: in those days before peer review, a paper read to the Southern Surgical Association would automatically be published in *The Annals of Surgery*, just as another read to Southeastern Surgical would duly appear in *American Surgeon.*[77]

As Coffey's academic stature grew, honors and appointments came his way; each one added to Georgetown's reputation. Locally, in 1966 he became the ninety-ninth president of the Medical Society of D.C., following in the footsteps of a series of Georgetown surgery professors going back to Charles Liebermann. Coffey devoted his term to encouraging in the metropolitan area the implemention of Medicare, the national health program for older Americans, an advance long resisted nationally by the AMA and still opposed by many members.[78] At the regional level, he served as president of the Southern Surgical Congress (1966) and of the Southern Surgical Association (1967).[79] Nationally, Coffey was deeply involved in the activities of the American College of Surgeons, serving two terms (1965–71) on the national Joint Conference Committee on Graduate Training in Surgery, which reviewed surgical residency programs throughout the country.[80] He edited *Surgical Digest* and was a consulting editor to *Clinical Medicine* and *JAMA*.[81] He was also active in innumerable national and international surgical associations. One was the prestigious Surgeons' Travel Club, an exclusive group of leading American surgeons who meet each year for an academic and social program in one member's city. Coffey was one of the eight surgeons, all former Mayo Clinic fellows, who founded the club in 1941; he hosted its meetings in Washington in 1949 and 1966.[82] At this latter meet, Coffey took the unusual step of inviting his eminent peers to watch him operate on a case of pancreatic cancer using the Whipple procedure—the most technically demanding operation that a general surgeon could then perform—in record time.[83] He never did lack self-confidence, nor an instinct for showmanship.

None of this was mere vanity. Coffey was deliberately fulfilling his original intent "to establish the department nationally." And through the vast network of contacts he made on his travels he was able steadily to build the department by attracting new talent.

The faculty he had inherited had some excellent surgeons. Ralph LeComte was an outstanding urologist whose *Manual of Urology* was the accepted text in many schools.[84] Robert "Pete" Moran had taught at Georgetown since 1929; a colorful character, his legendary practical jokes and profanity in the hospital—this at a time when it was still staffed by nuns—had caused the faculty to fire him more than once; but he was an eminent plastic surgeon who in 1958 was elected president of the American Association of Plastic Surgeons.[85] Edgar Davis, a leading thoracic surgeon known for his challenging operations—once removing razor blades from the esophagus of a drunken would-be suicide; on another occasion excising an esophagal tumor from a one hundred-year-old woman—was famous among students and residents because one finger was missing. It was rumored he had amputated it himself to avoid the spread of an infection in the days before antibiotics; but no one could know for sure. Every time a resident made a false move in an operation, he'd say, in his Southern drawl: "That's how I lost my finger, son."[85]

These, and many others in the department, were fine clinicians; but all were private practitioners who taught students on a voluntary unpaid basis, as Georgetown surgeons always had. From 1947, Coffey radically changed this system. He began to recruit full-timers. By 1968, his last year as chairman, there were thirty-five people working full time in the department.[87] Several, appointed to head divisions, transformed Georgetown's training and research programs in the surgical specialties.

Roger Baker, recruited in 1953 as the first full-time chief of urology, came from the University of Chicago, where he had worked with the Nobel laureate Charles Huggins, a pioneer in the use of hormones to treat prostate cancer. Though still a young man, Baker had already headed the urology division at Chicago and established a reputation for innovative research in kidney disease, winning the American Urological Association's 1950 award.[88] An ebullient, gregarious character, Baker played medical school politics with verve. He also had a flair for making money: he dabbled in real estate; raised Arabian thoroughbreds on his estate at Leesburg, Virginia; and eventually settled in a mansion in McLean, Virginia, next door to the then attorney general, Robert Kennedy.[89]

Baker became Washington's leading urologist. Continuing laboratory research he had begun in Chicago, he developed a technique of open-kidney surgery—"long considered too tricky to perform," according to the medical press—which allowed the surgeon to explore inside a kidney for suspected cancers and staghorn calculi without damaging the kidney itself. By early 1965, he had performed this "bivalve" procedure, so-called because the kidney was split open like a clam, on fifty-one patients (one in the fifth month of pregnancy) with great success. It required tiny needles and sutures to ligate as many as twenty blood vessels in a single operation, a painstaking technique in those days before microsurgery, but not beyond the powers of any competent surgeon, Baker insisted. "Twenty-five percent of my patients were operated on by my residents, with me as assistant," he said.[90]

Baker attracted further attention in the summer of 1965 when he reported in the *Journal of Urology* findings showing that, contrary to conventional wisdom, human bladders could regenerate new, healthy linings after cancerous linings had been surgically stripped away.[91] That same year he was the only urologist appointed to serve on the Surgeon General's Kidney Disease Project and Program Review Committee.[92] At Georgetown, he established a successful teaching and research program in urology, ably assisted by William C. Maxted, who succeeded him as chief of the division in 1976 and later became academic dean of the medical school.

In March 1957, Coffey appointed James F. O'Rourke as the first full-time chief of the division of ophthalmology. A Georgetown medical graduate of 1949, O'Rourke had earned his master's degree in ophthalmology from the University of Pennsylvania Graduate School of Medicine and since 1955 had been chief of clinical eye research at the National Institutes of Health. With Coffey's eager encouragement, O'Rourke quickly established Georgetown's first residency program in ophthalmology. His application was approved by the AMA's Residency Review Committee in October 1957, but it still took much time, effort, and determination to build the program from scratch. By 1960, twelve residents were enrolled in a curriculum offering either three years of basic science, research, and clinical experience, or a four-year program that included a final year of research. This curriculum was accepted by Georgetown as leading to a master of science degree in ophthalmology. "O'Rourke's experience and interest in basic research, immunology, and biophysics, and his uncompromising dedication to education, resulted in an unusually strong academic orientation of the program," noted Peter Y. Evans, who joined the ophthalmology division as a teaching fellow in 1958.

It was Evans himself who in 1963 initiated the pioneering project at Georgetown which later served as a model for similar courses worldwide: the Ophthalmic Technician Training Program. It was designed to relieve over-burdened ophthalmologists by training assistants to perform routine technical tasks such as history taking, pressure measurements, and visual field tests. This project began in a poignant way. In 1961, Charles Douglas, a local police officer who had become a chronic alcoholic, was assigned to the ophthalmology clinic at D.C. General for work therapy and rehabilitation. He enjoyed the work so much that, after some weeks of routine chores, he asked if he could do vision tests and other work with patients. "Gradually," Evans recalled, "nurses and residents began to rely on him and missed him on his off-days. When finally discharged, he promptly relapsed, since he was not yet ready to cope with personal family problems and the outside world. He wanted to return to his 'job' in the Eye Clinic." Evans gave Douglas not only the job but also room and board in his home, books to study, and tutoring discussions in the car to and from the hospital. From this simple beginning, Evans and his chief, O'Rourke, developed the OTT pilot program at Georgetown and later, at the national level, worked to set standards for the training, examination, and certification of technicians. Their efforts resulted in 1969 in the Joint Commission on Allied Health Personnel in Ophthalmology. Charles Douglas himself, after many lapses, triumphed over alcoholism, completed the Georgetown program, passed the national certification examinations, worked as an ophthalmic technician for many years, and became a sought-after national speaker for Alcoholics Anonymous. He and Evans had created, in effect, a whole new healthcare career. Peter Yoshio Evans—born in Tokyo of Japanese, German, and English ancestry and raised in Berlin and Austria—went on to become chief of the ophthalmology division in 1970 and secured its long-awaited elevation to departmental status in 1973. He served as its first chairman until 1982 and established Georgetown's highly successful Center for Sight.[93]

The military was another source of recruits for the surgery department. As consulting surgeon to the Bethesda Naval Hospital—he operated there most weeks—Robert Coffey maintained strong links with the U.S. Navy and brought several naval surgeons to Georgetown. One was George W. Hyatt, who in 1960 became the first full-time chief of the orthopedic division. Hyatt had been a consultant to the U.S. surgeon general, had attended many navy brass, and was director of the Tissue Bank at the Navy Medical School in Bethesda. His pioneering researches on human bone and tissue transplants, and, in particular, the extraction, storage, and reconstruction of tissues for surgical use, brought him international recognition.[94] At Georgetown, Hyatt continued this research and enlarged the training program. Years later, he was the specialist who treated Teddy Kennedy, Senator Edward Kennedy's twelve-year-old son, for chondrosarcoma, a rare form of bone cancer. In an hour-long operation, he amputated the boy's right leg above the knee.[95]

In 1960, Coffey appointed John F. Potter to head the new division of surgical oncology. (This division had been created after Murray Copeland left Georgetown for the University of Texas. Thereafter cancer treatment was divided between the surgery and radiology departments.) Potter, a 1949 Georgetown graduate, had trained in surgery with Coffey after a spell in the navy during the Korean War. After three years of clinical and basic research at the National Cancer Institute, he returned to Georgetown to head the new division.[96]

By now, there was less cancer research at Georgetown than there had been in the immediate postwar period. So Potter, outside his clinical and teaching duties, set up a laboratory to study the way cancer cells spread in the body. But he quickly became convinced that what Georgetown needed was a comprehensive cancer center, where research and treatment would go hand in hand.[97] The problem to be overcome, he felt, was the lack of communication and understanding between clinicians and basic scientists. "Even in the clinical realm," he wrote, "surgeons, chemotherapists, and irradiation therapists frequently do not understand the techniques, problems, successes, and failures of their fellow oncologists." He envisaged a facility where beds were not distant from laboratories, and where patient care was guided by the latest research.[98]

In the mid-1960s, the National Cancer Institute was encouraging the development of just such facilities. Consequently, Potter was able to obtain federal planning and operational grants to create a center at Georgetown. Staff were recruited and the project progressed long before there was a specific building to house it.[99] Then, one afternoon in June 1970, while the Washington Redskins football team was training, as it had for years, on the field behind Georgetown medical school, its coach complained of abdominal pains and was taken to the university hospital. That coach was the legendary Vince Lombardi. Coffey diagnosed cancer of the sigmoid colon and in June and July performed two operations. But the cancer spread rapidly through Lombardi's abdomen. He knew his fate. In late August, against Coffey's advice, the iron-willed coach checked out of the hospital and went to New York to help settle a players' strike. A few days later, on September 3, 1970 he died at age fifty-seven.[100]

As a nation of football fans mourned, John Potter was struck by a shrewd idea. "I suggested to Dr. Coffey that we might name the cancer center after Lombardi," he recalled. "The man was an American hero. His name would attract the support we needed, and in turn the center would perpetuate his name." Lombardi's widow, Marie, was enthusiastic and agreed to be honorary chair of a national fundraising campaign. Over the next few years, $12.5 million were raised, including a $1 million donation from the National Football League. The Vince Lombardi Comprehensive Cancer Center was built at the back of the medical center, overlooking the field where the coach had once trained the Redskins. It became enormously successful, attracting not only oncologists and other scientists of repute but also—in the twenty years that John Potter served as its first director—$95 million in research grants.[101]

In 1965, Coffey appointed Alfred J. Luessenhop as the first full-time chief of the division of neurosurgery. He replaced Hugh Fulcher, who as part-time head of the division had already established a neurosurgery residency program at Georgetown. Luessenhop had trained at Harvard medical school and then held a teaching fellowship there in 1958–59, which was also the last year of his residency in neurological surgery at Massachusetts General Hospital.[102] It was in September 1959—newly arrived at Georgetown as a junior instructor in surgery and two years before he took his boards in neurological surgery—that Luessenhop made a great contribution to the field. He pioneered a wholly new approach to the treatment of aneurysms and arteriovenous malformations (AVMs) of the brain—a procedure now recognized as the beginning of endovascular surgery.

It was during his residency at Massachusetts General that Luessenhop had first focussed on the AVM, an abnormal tangle of cerebral arteries and veins coalesced into a dense mass, highly likely to rupture under arterial pressure. The only treatment known in the 1950s was to remove the AVM surgically; but this was a high-risk operation directly into the brain. Only one in five cases was considered operable. Luessenhop took a lateral approach, reasoning that as most large AVMs were fed by blood from the main cerebral artery it might be possible to block that blood supply without affecting other parts of the brain. He further conceived the

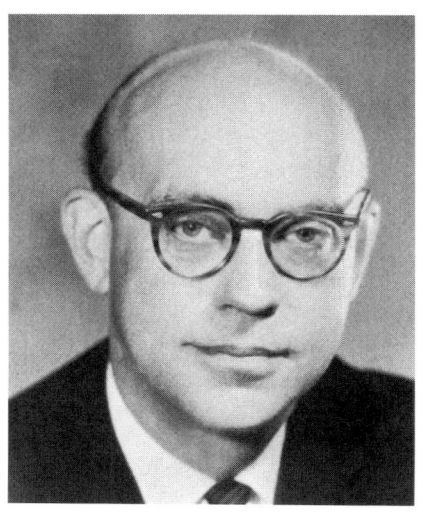

Alfred J. Luessenhop, M.D., pioneer of endovascular surgery. Courtesy of Georgetown University Archives.

radical idea that this blood supply might be blocked artificially: a blockage (in technical terms an *embolism*) introduced into the vascular system some distance from the brain might travel naturally to the site and lodge there, preempting the need for direct brain surgery.

Luessenhop put his theory into practice on September 18, 1959, at Georgetown University Hospital, when he performed the world's first artificial embolization on a forty-seven-year-old woman with an inoperable AVM. Using local anesthesia and working through an incision in her neck, he opened the left common carotid artery and put into it four plastic balls, each up to 4.2 mm in diameter. Postoperative X rays clearly showed that these emboli had traveled to, and lodged at, the beginning of the malformation, as he had predicted. Blood flow to the other cerebral arteries returned to normal; the patient's symptoms of fainting, numbness in the limbs, and loss of movement in her right fingers disappeared; seven weeks after surgery, she was able to write legibly once more with her right hand.

This was the first time that anyone had thought of using the arteries as a surgical channel. Luessenhop described his procedure in a paper published in *JAMA* in March 1960.[103] "Everyone thought me crazy," he recalled. "There was no real criticism, but it wasn't accepted. It just seemed too wild then."[104]

In that paper, he had raised the further possibility of treating saccular brain aneurysms in the same way, sealing them with artificial emboli until the blood clotted naturally. Within two years, Luessenhop had refined his procedure into a technique in which catheters, floated through the intracranial arteries, again from an incision in the neck, released various kinds of emboli (including balloons inflated at the target site) to seal both AVMs and aneurysms of the brain.[105] This also was generally regarded as "too wild," despite Luessenhop's considerable clinical successes. After a few years, though, the problems of getting the tiny catheters manufactured became too onerous and Luessenhop turned to other fields of neurosurgery. "I was a neurosurgeon. I couldn't spend all my time in the lab making these things myself," he said.

But in the 1970s, when the Cold War was thawing and Soviet medical research was first published in the West, Luessenhop discovered that the Russians had picked up his technique and developed to high sophistication the instrumentation it needed. From then onwards, Western European and

American medicine took a serious interest in what soon became known as *intraventional* and, later, *endovascular* therapy and finally produced the necessary instruments. His catheter technique was taken up in the U.S. first by radiologists and, in the mid-1980s, by neurosurgeons once more. It did not solve all problems of AVMs, Luessenhop said, "but it can now eliminate 20 percent of lesions and make the rest much smaller, so bringing most within the realm of operability."[106]

Today, endovascular surgery is an important and expanding discipline, used for a variety of cardiovascular as well as brain conditions. The Harvard department of neurosurgery, on its fiftieth anniversary, presented Luessenhop with a medal, citing his "introduction of endovascular surgery for arteriovenous malformations and aneurysms" as one of the significant contributions of its alumni.[107] In 1997, the American Association of Neurological Surgeons (jointly with two other national organizations) established in his honor the annual Alfred J. Luessenhop Lectureship in Neuroendovascular Therapy and a one-thousand-dollar prize for the resident or fellow who submits the best paper on the subject.[108] "But the important thing to me," Luessenhop said, "is that endovascular surgery was totally a Georgetown product and is now standard treatment throughout the world, with its own experts and professional societies." It ranks with Hufnagel's aortic heart valves and the three-dimensional whole-body CAT scan, invented by Robert Ledley of the department of physiology[109], as one of Georgetown's lasting contributions to twentieth century medicine.

These years of progress in the surgery department had also seen significant changes in the administration of the medical school. In June 1953, the Reverend Edward Bunn, S.J., who had been Georgetown's president for four years, insisted that Paul McNally resign his position as dean and regent to save his health.[110] McNally was not universally liked—some on the faculty found him pompous and dictatorial—but all admired what he had done for the school. In Coffey's words: "He was a little bantam rooster: an abrasive, peppery individual, who easily created enemies as well as making many sincere friends, but full of vigor and diligence. He was the one person most responsible for converting Georgetown from a Class B to a Class A school."[111] The task had taken its toll. McNally had already suffered two heart attacks before his resignation, and he died of another at age sixty-four in March 1955.[112]

In McNally's place, the Reverend Thomas O'Donnell, S.J. was appointed regent, but not dean. For the first time since 1931, the new dean was a medical man: Francis M. Forster, the chairman of neurology. He had arrived at Georgetown three years earlier from Jefferson Medical College in Philadelphia, where he had taught for seven years after holding research fellowships at Harvard and Yale. He was one of the best-known neurologists in the country, having already served as vice president of the American Academy of Neurology—only one of many offices in national and international organizations. Not surprisingly, Forster did not wish to give up his career at the age of forty-one, so he accepted the deanship, at a modest fifteen thousand dollars a year, only with the understanding that he could continue as chairman of neurology.[113]

Forster had little taste for administration—once remarking, it is said, that he liked being dean but didn't like "deaning."[114] Nevertheless, he strove for five years to do justice to both positions—as well as serving in 1955 as president of the American Academy of Neurology. From early in the morning to late at night he worked at his desk, in the hospital, or in the laboratory, sometimes stopping only to take communion with the students. He set up a committee system within the executive faculty so that other departmental heads could share the administrative load.[115] He helped raise the funds for a proposed new $3 million building, now the Gorman Diagnostic and Research Center.[116] And he presided single-handedly over a huge expansion in the research program—from $356,000 in grants in 1953 to more than $1.3 million in 1958—before a new office was belatedly created to coordinate it.[117]

In March 1958, however, the AMA-AAMC liaison committee came back to inspect Georgetown, and concluded "with reluctance" that the school should again be placed on confidential probation.[118] Once more, as it had in 1935, the committee objected to the presence of a Jesuit regent and commented that the dean should "exert more control" over administration. It criticized the lack of annual departmental reports, the "over-didactic" nature of the curriculum, the inadequate library, and the shortage of office and laboratory space, by now so acute that one internationally known professor used a former broom closet for an office, and corridors were lined with the desks of secretaries, technicians, and research fellows.[119] Of the school's sixteen departments, nine were found in some respect below par, with only the department of medicine receiving unqualified praise. The committee's lengthy report on the surgery department commended its "extensive research program" and the "large number of publications" it had produced. The report predicted that the department, with eight full-time faculty now employed, had "the potentiality to carry on an extremely well-rounded program." But that potential was "seriously handicapped by the lack of supervision of the students" during their hospital clerkships, the committee said. It concluded: "The committee was led to speculate whether a number of the full-time members of the department were devoting so much of their time to private practice that they were not able to give as much attention as necessary to the teaching program."[120] This comment proved to be the first shot in a prolonged and acrimonious battle over private practice which came to a head a few years later.

The result of the report was that Forster resigned the deanship and, more significantly, the office of regent was abolished. O'Donnell had always taken a realistic view of his position—insisting that "the regent should in no way interfere with the dean's direct access to and contact with the university president in the administration of the school,"[121]—but the university finally bowed to the AMA/AAMC's enduring suspicion of this uniquely Jesuitical arrangement.[122] For the first time since the early 1920s, the new dean was a medical man who ran the school full-time and alone.

Hugh Hudson Hussey, given to signing himself H3, had been connected with Georgetown all his adult life. A brilliant student, he had graduated *magna cum laude* in 1934, had served his residency with Wallace Yater, and then rose through the faculty ranks until, in 1956, he succeeded Harold Jeghers as full-time chairman of medicine when Jeghers departed to the new Seton Hall College of Medicine in New Jersey. Hussey had also acquired national stature in medical politics: throughout his tenure as dean, he was chairman of the Board of Trustees of the AMA.[123]

Even before the liaison committee's criticisms of Georgetown's "over-didactic" teaching, the faculty had already begun planning an overhaul of the curriculum. Hussey got a three-hundred-thousand-dollar grant from the Commonwealth Fund and chaired the committee. The idea was to devise a more holistic program by integrating overlapping areas of instruction, and to replace most lectures in the second year and all in the third year with multi-disciplinary "conferences" of the type already employed in the medicine and surgery departments.[124]

The new curriculum, introduced in the 1958—59 school year, was not entirely successful in the long run: based on small-group teaching, it took more faculty than Georgetown could afford. But in the short term, it helped the school win back full accreditation when the AMA/AAMC liaison committee returned for another inspection in April 1960. Other factors contributed to the reinstatement, among them the opening of the Gorman building in 1959, the introduction of regular departmental reports, and improved organization of the surgical clerkships. But the committee commended, in particular, Hussey's "vigorous and imaginative leadership" as dean and was pleased to note that, with the abolition of the regent, he had been acknowledged as "the responsible administrator for the medical school in line of authority from the president." The dean's position had been further strengthened, it commented, by his being given greater control of finances and appointed director of the hospital.[125]

It did not last. In November 1960, President Bunn created a new position, vice president for medical center affairs, which brought a Jesuit back into the medical arena.[126] And the following year the dean lost control of the hospital when an executive director was appointed who reported directly to the president.[127] Unhappy with both developments, Hussey left Georgetown in February of 1963 to serve as scientific director of the American Medical Association in Chicago. He later became a distinguished editor of the *JAMA* and a powerful figure in the AMA.[128]

With Hussey's departure, the school appointed a search committee for the first time to find a new dean. The man selected was, at age thirty-eight, the youngest to hold the office since Francis Ashford in the 1870s. John Rose had always been a young achiever: born in New York City in December 1924, he graduated from high school and began college at fifteen; at twenty he was flying combat missions over Europe as a B-24 navigator, for which he was decorated; at twenty-five he graduated from Georgetown medical school *magna cum laude*; at twenty-nine he joined the faculty; and at thirty-four he was appointed chairman of the department of physiology. An inveterate committee man, Rose had masterminded the development of the new curriculum during the 1957–58 academic year. When he took over as dean, on July 1, 1963, he was also medical editor of *GP*, the nation's third largest medical journal, and had authored more than sixty papers, most on his main field of research, the physiology of the circulatory system.[129]

John Rose's term as dean from 1963 to 1973 was the tumultuous decade which saw the assassinations of President John F. Kennedy, Robert Kennedy, and Martin Luther King Jr.; civil rights strife at home and the Vietnam War abroad; Neil Armstrong's walk on the moon; and the gathering scandal of Watergate. It was also a decade that brought unprecedented expansion on all fronts at Georgetown. The government had come to believe that the nation needed more doctors; the result was a massive infusion of federal funds into medical schools. Georgetown benefitted from national legislation such as the Health Professions Education Assistance Act of 1964 ($6 million) and the Physicians Augmentation Program ($8.8 million in 1970–75). For several years it also received five thousand dollars for each medical student and three thousand dollars for each dental student, starting with a grant of $3.3 million for 1970–71, under an act of Congress which at last made special provision for private medical schools in the District of Columbia.[130]

Over that same ten-year period, Georgetown's revenues climbed from $5.6 million to nearly $18 million; enrollment from 430 students to 705; full-time faculty members from 198 to 325; and research grants from $3.6 million to $9.2 million.[131] By 1971, Georgetown had become the nation's second largest private medical school (after Jefferson), and held the record for admission applications.[132]

The medical center itself metastasized, acquiring a badly-needed new medical library, a basic science building, a classroom-auditorium complex, and student laboratories. Reservoir Road throbbed with bulldozers, concrete mixers, and complaints from neighboring residents; and the joke circulated that Georgetown's emblematic bird (actually, the American eagle on its official seal) was now "the construction crane."[133] The medical school's budget deficit, which in 1970 had reached $1.4 million, was wiped out;[134] and John Rose announced that "solvency and security have been attained." He added: "We will continue to pursue financial resources based on the principle that, over and above federal assistance available to all medical schools, the U.S. Congress has an obligation to act as a state legislature with regard to the private medical schools of the District of Columbia."[135] What Congress can give, of course, Congress can also take away—as it would do at the end of the 1970s, bringing new problems to the school. In the meantime, Rose presided over a prosperity which Georgetown had never known before, nor has enjoyed since.

The governance of the medical school in the 1960s was in style much closer to the nineteenth century than to today's system. The executive faculty—dean and departmental chairmen—still ran the school, as they had in the distant days of Eliot and Liebermann. They met once a month in the executive faculty room, on the second floor of the school building directly above the lobby, with former deans staring down at them from gilt-framed portraits on the walls. John Rose took the chair at one end of the long, polished table; Robert Coffey always sat at the other end. "It was as if," recalled Rose, who had been a student of Coffey's fifteen years earlier, "he wanted to make sure things were handled properly."

Coffey was now the most powerful figure on the faculty—not only by dint of seniority and academic stature, but also because of his forceful personality and his skill in medical school politics. By the mid-1960s, the school's administration was becoming more complicated as departments and divisions expanded, building projects were begun, and budgets ballooned. Rose appreciated Coffey's experience and, not least, his financial acumen. "Bob was always smart about money and it was helpful to have somebody on the faculty with common sense about the allocation of resources," he recalled. "Many academics couldn't reconcile their own checkbooks, much less run budgets of the size they were getting to become."[136]

Yet the major controversy which erupted at this time centered on money and the surgery department; in a larger sense it also defined the old and new ways of running a medical school. Rose and Coffey found themselves not only facing each other down the conference table but going head to head on the thorny issue of the faculty practice plan.

Shortly after becoming dean, Rose had decided to take the first cautious steps toward establishing a strict full-time salary structure in the clinical departments: surgery, medicine, obstetrics and gynecology, psychiatry, neurology, and pediatrics. His goal was to change appointments in these departments from the "geographic" full-time system, introduced at Georgetown in 1947, to the "absolute" or "strict" full-time system. This would mean paying clinicians fixed salaries; the fees they generated from private patients in the university hospital would no longer be theirs to keep but would instead revert to the school. Many medical schools had already changed, or were changing, to this system—not least because in those days, unlike today, tuition fees were relatively low ($1,450 a year at Georgetown in 1965) and university hospitals were cash cows. Profits from private patients' fees could therefore be used to subsidize the ever-increasing costs

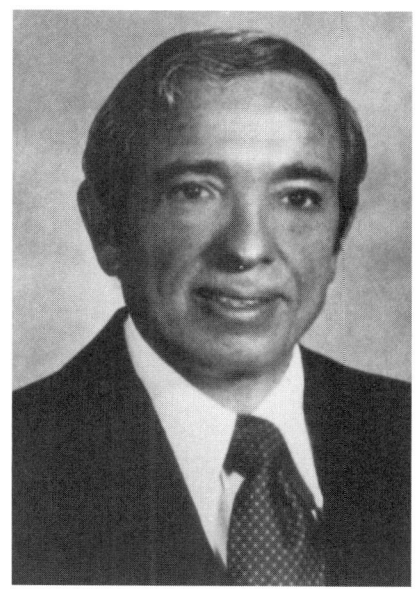

John Rose, M.D., dean of the medical school, 1963–73. Courtesy of Georgetown University Archives.

of medical education. At Georgetown, of ten clinical departments, only four—radiology, anesthesiology, physical medicine and rehabilitation, and clinical pathology—were operating on this strict full-time basis. Rose felt the time had come to bring the others into line.

Moreover, he was under some pressure to do so. The AMA and AAMC, having debated the "full-time" issue without total agreement since the early 1950s, had now begun to endorse the concept. The AAMC, the more university-oriented of the two organizations, insisted that "proper limits" be established on income from private fees "to insure that the care of paying patients does not detract from the primary teaching and research functions of the full-time medical faculty."[137] Pointedly, the licensing authorities were already asking medical schools to report the incomes of their full-time professors.

This put Rose in a quandary: no one at Georgetown knew how much the clinical full-timers were earning beyond the often nominal salaries they received from the university. "It was embarrassing to have to report that a surgeon was receiving twelve thousand dollars or twenty thousand dollars when his actual income was many times that amount," Rose recalled. "It made us look a very peculiar institution." Other schools still on the geographic system had the same problem, but Rose was aware that the issue of private practice—and the absence of some kind of control exerted by the school—would loom large when the AMA-AAMC liaison committee next inspected Georgetown. The point had already been raised, particularly in relation to the department of surgery, in the committee's previous visits in 1958 and 1960.[138]

So as a first step taken in 1964, Rose requested the clinical full-timers to file confidential annual estimates of the time they spent on private patient care in the university hospital and the earnings they derived from it.[139] "And of course," he recalled, "there were big ructions."

Speaking thirty years later, John Potter vividly remembered the surgery department's reaction. "We fought it tooth and nail," he said. Other departments held mixed views, but surgery was the one most wholeheartedly opposed to the notion of income reporting and led the fight. Roger Baker even organized the "Tuesday Club," a social get-together ostensibly to encourage communication between departments after the regular faculty meetings, but actually, Potter said, "to set up a bloc to out-maneuver John Rose."[140]

In long memos to Coffey, Rose tried to explain his rationale and invite the cooperation of members of the surgery department. "They do not see," he wrote, "that in fact this represents a protective mechanism against the mounting criticism of completely uncontrolled private practice in the full-time faculty of a medical school, both on the local and national scene."[141] But the surgeons, and most of the other clinicians, would have none of it. Many of them made large incomes from private fees and they could see which way the wind was blowing. "Income reporting was regarded as an intrusion by Rose who would be using it as a wedge to establish a strict full-time system," Potter recalled. "That's why it was objected to, very vehemently."

Details varied from person to person, but all clinical full-timers had contracts guaranteeing them a certain number of hours or days of private practice each week. Most regarded the income from that, whether three thousand dollars a year or three hundred thousand dollars, as their own business; and they viewed any attempt to change the system as a breach of faith by the university.[142] So financial interest was a major factor. But the surgeons were also fighting a rearguard action in the battle begun in the days of Flexner and Halsted: they saw themselves as upholding a long clinical tradition as independent operators; whereas the administrators, personified in this case by Dean Rose, saw them as employees of the university. "Surgeons are a notoriously independent lot—if they weren't, they wouldn't be surgeons," Potter said. "You're standing on your own two feet literally and figuratively in this business, and you don't want anyone else telling you what to do. So what we objected to, more than anything else, was loss of control. I think that was the most cogent issue in the whole thing, at least for surgeons."

Coffey shared these sentiments. But for him, as chairman, there was another compelling reason to oppose anything leading to an absolute salaried system. He was fully aware that the magnet which had attracted so many first-class people to Georgetown—first the clinical departmental chairmen in 1947, and later the full-time surgeons in his own department—was the geographic system itself. As other schools switched to fixed salaries, opportunities to combine university appointments with private practice were dwindling. Georgetown's aloofness to the trend had helped it recruit and keep some of its best people: Baker, almost certainly for this reason, had turned down a prestigious post at Harvard in 1954.[143] Rose himself recognized the strength of the argument: "I have stated to you and to others my firm belief in this freedom as the reason for our development of a top-notch Department of Surgery," he wrote Coffey, adding reassuringly: "We have a need for the geographic system and could not succeed without it."[144]

Coffey was not reassured. He did not believe that Rose wished to perpetuate the geographic system, nor did he trust the university to offer reasonable salaries if an absolute system was introduced.[145] So he hedged. When his full-timers refused to file individual private income reports, he offered a compromise: a single estimate of the income generated by the department as a whole. Rose countered with another: "divisional" estimates.[146] But as some divisions comprised only one or two full-timers, that idea too was rejected.[147]

Stalemate followed; but Rose soon brought up bigger guns. Armed with an opinion from the university's law firm that the dean had a legal right to insist on income information,[148] he persuaded Georgetown's Medical Center Council that the university should exert control over the faculty's private practice activities.[149] Then he convinced the new university president, Reverend Gerard Campbell, S.J., and the new vice president for medical center affairs, Mark Bauer, that a practice plan was the right way to go. In March 1965, he even took Campbell and Bauer to Chicago, to hear firsthand the views of the AMA and AAMC.[150] Soon after they returned, the university's board of directors agreed to the plan.[151]

Now that he had the full backing of the university, Rose raised the stakes. He presented the clinical full-timers with a choice: either file income reports by April 15, 1965, or agree to "explore intensively" the creation of a faculty practice plan.[152] His memos to Coffey became more forthright: "Just as there are no more horse and buggy doctors, the horse and buggy medical school will soon be out of existence," he wrote. "The individual members of your department must now face these issues squarely, orienting themselves in all of their professional activities towards the university."[153]

Coffey, his worst fears confirmed, was furious at this development, which he perceived as an ultimatum. John Dillon, then a junior member of the department, remembered the atmosphere: "It was like a Balkan revolution." Surgeons whispered together in corners. They were hauled back from social engagements to late-night meetings in the department. Coffey was seen striding off to confront the dean, intimidatingly dressed in bloodstained scrubs—or, worse, was heard shouting at him in the corridor.[154] For both men it was a painful situation, for in every other respect they liked and admired each other—and, indeed, remained friends until the end of Coffey's life.

The climax came one evening at an emergency meeting in the executive faculty room where John Rose faced, in his own recollection, "the whole hostile department of surgery." The issues were once again heatedly discussed, but the bottom line was stark: if the dean insisted on the income-reporting deadline, most of the full-time surgery faculty would resign. To press the point, Coffey went round the table asking each surgeon in turn whether he would stay or quit. Coffey himself, though he had earlier told colleagues he would support their decisions but not himself resign, now sadly changed his mind: if it came to the crunch, he would quit, too.[155]

This was the crisis point, for the surgeons were not alone: several senior professors of medicine and obstetrics/gynecology had told Rose they felt the same way.[156] The dean was thus faced with the unpleasant truth that his best-intentioned effort to bring Georgetown into the modern era had brought instead the threat of crippling defections from the largest departments in the school. The impasse was broken when Coffey agreed to set up a committee to "consider" the question of a faculty practice plan. To Rose, this seemed like progress toward the goal he wanted. To everyone else, the move came as a relief because it shelved the income reporting deadline and removed the imminent prospect of having to resign. The agreement was enshrined in a directive from Campbell, ordering the committee to devise a "regulatory mechanism" for private practice that could apply uniformly to all clinical departments.[157]

The Faculty Practice Plan Committee, set up in June 1965, had twelve members, three of them from the surgery department. Robert Coffey was elected chairman; Roger Baker, John Potter, and George Schreiner, professor of medicine—all vocal opponents of Rose's proposals—headed the three subcommittees. It took nineteen months for the committee to produce "a preliminary proposal" which astounded Rose when it arrived on his desk in January 1967. The document, a scant seven pages long, was a masterpiece of evasion. Fewer than three pages dwelt on any kind of recommendations, and half of those amounted to a detailed demand for better fringe benefits from the university. The "plan" merely endorsed the status quo: "It is envisioned that the large majority of faculty members of the clinical departments will be geographic full-time; pre-existing arrangements will not be abrogated unless agreed by both involved parties."[158]

"Of course," Potter said, recalling the committee's deliberations, "it was a stalling operation. Coffey's political adroitness was in getting Rose and Campbell to believe he was doing something for them, when he was really stalling the issue. In the end, it was stalled to death." Phrasing their frustration in the most restrained language, Rose and Campbell ordered the committee back to work, requesting that in devising a workable plan they also consider how the hospital should handle the new Medicare payments which were about to come into effect.[159] But this second effort, too, brought no more than a three-page paper in May 1968, recommending that a new office be set up to collect federal payments and ignoring the main agenda.[160]

After that, the issue died. Campbell was a president with no taste for confrontation, and by this time he was a sick man.[161] Rose also recognized that his goal was for now out of reach. But if he had lost a four-year battle, he did not concede the war. Abandoning his campaign on the clinical departments, Rose worked on the divisions and persuaded several of the younger divisional heads in both medicine and surgery to change to strict full-time.[162] In 1977 the university finally insisted on the implementing of departmental practice plans. Not until 1980, however, did the surgery department as a whole capitulate; it was the last at Georgetown, and one of the last in the country, to adopt the strict full-time system.[163]

Robert Coffey's handling of the faculty practice plan crisis was much admired within the department, and it summed up his qualities as chairman. His commanding presence, his unquestioned authority as the chief, often inspired fear but always earned respect. Nobody on his staff—not even those who remained close personal friends to the end of his life; not even Hufnagel—ever called him anything but Doctor Coffey.

Though famous for chewing people out, he had a talent for fostering a sense of community within the department. "Coffey was always loyal to his people," John Potter remembered. "He expected loyalty up, and he got it. But also, by God, if anyone tried to trample on his people, he'd hear about it from Coffey. It was one of the salient characteristics of the guy: a tough dude, but if you were on his team, you were on his team, and everybody knew it."

Residents were on his team, but they generally approached the duty with trepidation. Three residents in a row developed ulcers during their months with him, so it became the "tradition" that everyone would. Like gladiators about to enter the arena, newcomers girded themselves by consulting their predecessors and taking copious notes on exactly how Coffey liked things done. There was an inflexible daily ritual. His resident would arrive at the hospital around 6:00 A.M., make rounds to check on Coffey's patients, then look at the day's schedule for operations. At 7:45 A.M. *precisely*—not 7:40 or 7:50—the resident would call Coffey at his home, ten minutes away on Loughborough Road NW, sometimes waking him. "Good morning, Dr. Coffey, we have four cases today . . ." A quick run-down of the schedule, a few terse instructions, and then Coffey would say: "Okay, get 'em prepped." At the hospital, the team would scrub and gown; the first patient would be brought to the operating room and anesthetized. Meanwhile at Loughborough Road, Coffey was snatching breakfast, getting into his car, and dropping off his children at school. At around 8:15, the resident would be making the incision, hoping it was in the right place, hoping it was big enough for Coffey to get his hand in, hoping Coffey would arrive on time. He habitually turned up ten minutes late. (When someone once got up the nerve to point this out, he declared it was important to be on time, but even more important to get the kids to school.) He'd scrub, enter the operating room, peer at the incision through his glasses. "Goddamn it, I told you to make it big enough for *my* hand . . ." Another morning in the OR had begun.[164]

Almost all his residents regarded him as a "bear" or a "tyrant" while operating. The tension of the event—the need to focus all his skill on whatever problem lay exposed beneath the incision, so that the draped figure on the table got the best chance—would explode in curses, cutting remarks, and what one assistant described as the "blue-eyed laser glare" blazing from above the surgical mask.[165] At such times there was no trace of the courteous demeanor known to family, friends, and adoring patients. Coffey's wife was once invited to watch him operating. She stood there, unnoticed by him, and then walked out. "That is *not* my husband," she insisted.[166]

At lunchtime in the cafeteria, residents endlessly recycled "Coffey stories," thereby reassuring each other that their experiences were not unique. One of the most famous illustrated not so much Coffey's bearishness as the state to which a resident could be reduced in anticipation of his wrath. It happened to a resident who wore what he referred to as "spectacles." As he bent over the patient with a retractor, his glasses fell off into the wound. As the others held their breath and Coffey glared, the mortified resident blurted out: "Will someone please place my testicles back on my nose?"[167]

Residents on Coffey's service were always in their third year of training in general surgery, and each usually spent three to six months with him. Tom Lee, in 1959, served a record nine months, and at the end formally thanked Coffey for everything he had learned. "You've taught me something, too," Coffey responded. "I have?" said Lee, surprised. "Yeah, never to have a resident with me nine months again." Coffey was rarely perceived to be joking when he made such comments—Lee did not think so, even though he later became closer to Coffey than anyone both as his surgical partner and life-long friend. Lee attributed Coffey's asperity and the aloofness he cultivated as chairman to his naval training: he was the commander, keeping the men on their toes. Yet in the wardroom, as it were, he could be generous: every three months he entertained every resident and student on the rotation to dinner at the Army Navy Club. "No other chairman of surgery did that, before or since," said Lee.

The underlying reason for the trainees' perennial anxiety over their performance on Coffey's watch was that, throughout his chairmanship, residencies were run on the pyramid system. Of the ten or twelve residents who began together in their first year, only two or three would remain by the last year to serve as chief residents at Georgetown or the affiliated hospitals. It was a policy of attrition, designed to promote the strongest candidates through the gruelling period of training. Those weeded out switched to a specialty or completed their training elsewhere, or, in some cases, decided that surgery was not for them. This Darwinian process later gave way nationally to the block system, in which a group of residents rose together, with a virtual guarantee of all becoming chiefs in their final year. But in his day, Coffey said, "Surgical residencies were highly competitive, and many didn't make it." To Coffey, intensely competitive himself, this was right and proper: the urge to compete was a measure of drive and ambition, a test of one's fitness to attain the goal.[168]

If Coffey was rough on his residents, it was because he demanded excellence. Turning out well-trained surgeons absorbed him more deeply than any other aspect of medical education. His chairmanship coincided with a general raising of training standards, a process that had begun in 1950 when the American College of Surgeons, the American Board of Surgery, and the American Medical Association established the Joint Conference Committee on Graduate Training in Surgery. This body set national standards, evaluated and approved hospital training programs in general surgery and the specialties, and considered medical trends that affected residency—such as the advent of health insurance, Medicare, and Medicaid, which by the late 1960s were all rapidly reducing the pool of "charity patients" on whom medical education had always depended. Between 1965 and 1971, Coffey was one of the leading surgeons who took part in the committee's deliberations at the national level, and for the last two years of that time he served as its chairman.[169]

Coffey's commitment to graduate training had been demonstrated more locally, but in a striking way, early in his years as chairman of surgery when he agreed to take surgical residents from Howard University into the Georgetown service at Gallinger Hospital. This was in 1950, at a time when black students were still not admitted to either Georgetown or George Washington medical schools, and no black physicians had ever been employed on the staff of any major hospital in Washington other than Freedmen's. Charles R. Drew, the celebrated blood bank pioneer and chairman of surgery at Howard, was concerned that his best residents needed wider experience than Freedmen's could offer and so he turned to Coffey for help. The two chairmen enjoyed an amicable relationship. In 1945, Drew had been turned down for membership in the then nearly all-white American College of Surgeons, and in January 1950 he asked if Coffey would support his renewed application. Coffey, who regarded Drew as "a magnificent, outstanding surgeon," said he would be delighted. Three months later Drew was killed in an automobile accident, but the ACS awarded him membership posthumously—a rare occurrence—in 1951. And Coffey honored his agreement to take one Howard resident each year at Gallinger.

The fourth resident selected for this rotation, in 1954–55, was La Salle D. Lefall Jr., who himself later became chairman of surgery at Howard. He

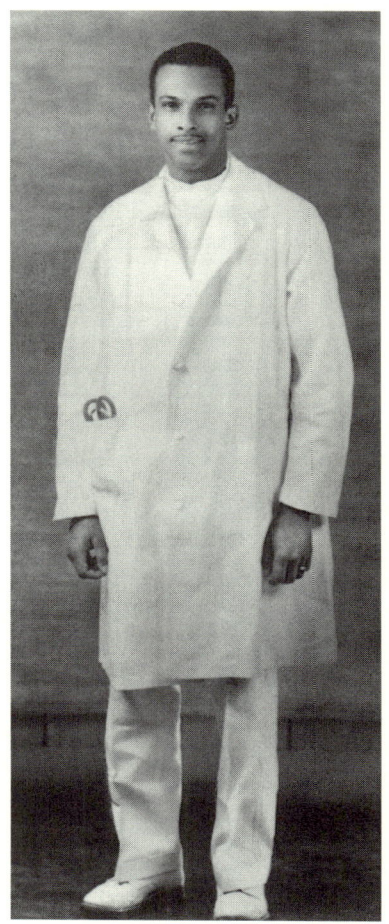

La Salle D. Lefall Jr., who would later become president of the American College of Surgeons, is here shown as a surgical resident on Robert Coffey's service at Gallinger Hospital (later D.C. General) in 1955. Courtesy of La Salle D. Lefall Jr., M.D., chairman of surgery, Howard University College of Medicine.

recalled: "The good chemistry that existed between the two men was important, because if Dr. Coffey had not felt so inclined, particularly at that time in our history, he could have just said no." Those early Howard residents at Gallinger were trailblazers, carefully selected from the most able trainees; perhaps as a result, Lefall said, they were accepted onto the Georgetown team and experienced no discrimination. "But first the door had to open, and Dr. Coffey played an important role there. He had a major impact on the training program at Howard. What he did for minorities might not seem like so much today, but at that time it was a tremendous thing." Coffey later followed, with interest and pride, Lefall's spectacular career in surgery and oncology which brought him a succession of honors until, in October 1995, he became the first black president of the American College of Surgeons.[170]

Coffey was equally ahead of his time in another respect. Of the many Coffey-trained residents who later went on to notable careers in surgery, several were women. Statistics show how unusual this was: in 1966, women comprised only 6.7 percent of American physicians—one of the lowest ratios in the world—and only 0.9 percent of general surgeons.[171] "One of my big challenges in the early days was to get more women into surgery," Coffey recalled. "And we did."

At Georgetown, women medical students were a relatively recent phenomenon: apart from two who in 1881 had been allowed to enroll for a year at the school,[172] Georgetown did not admit women until 1947, exactly one hundred years after the first woman was accepted into an American medical school.[173] Yet of the five women who began as freshmen that year and stayed the course, one graduated *magna cum laude* as the valedictorian of 1951, won the gold medal for the highest four-year scholastic average, and became a surgeon.[174] She was Sister Frederic (Eileen) Niedfield, a nun of the order of the Medical Mission Sisters, who also served six months as Coffey's resident in 1954. Soon after receiving her MS in surgery from Georgetown, she left for India and spent the next thirty-seven years as a surgeon in poor, rural areas always acutely short of medical supplies and trained staff. For two years, she worked in Bhutan on the Indo-Chinese frontier, a region so remote that she trained local school teachers, agricultural workers, and even a borderpost radio operator in rudimentary medicine and surgery since no professionals could reach some areas in the snows of winter. It was in Bhutan, too, that she once had to stop operating in order to draw a unit of her own type O blood to transfuse the patient. Sister Niedfield never forgot her training from Coffey. "He was strict but fair, and an excellent practical teacher," she recalled. "As his assistant, I was able to participate in other-than-ordinary operations, like

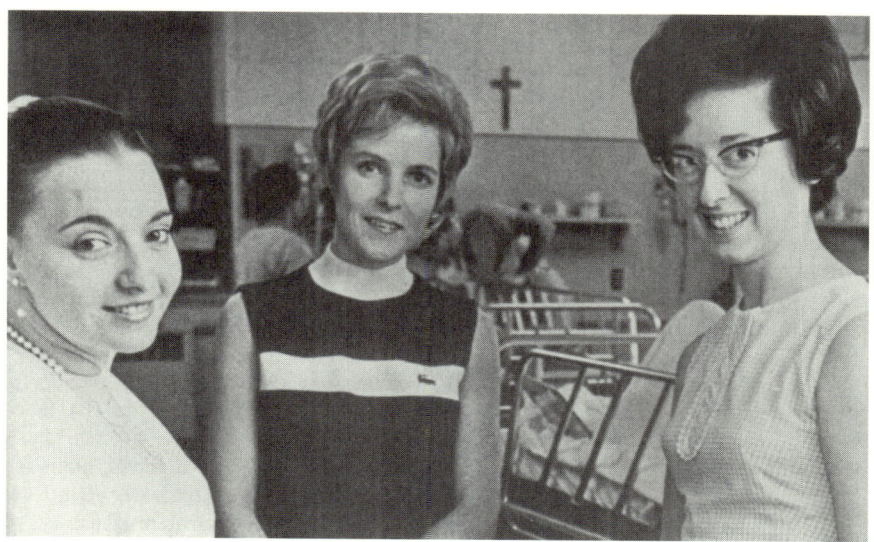

At a time when women doctors were still a tiny minority in American medicine, three women were chief residents of surgery divisions at Georgetown in 1970. From left to right: Carol Shapiro, M.D., chief in plastic surgery; Kathryn Anderson, M.D., chief in surgery; and Barbara Black, M.D., chief in urology. Courtesy of Georgetown University Medical Bulletin.

Whipple procedures and adrenalectomies, that I would never do, but the principles of which stood me in good stead when I was surgically alone in a village hospital."[175] Coffey, for his part, regarded her as "a remarkable woman and an outstanding surgeon"; and he sometimes sent medical supplies and funds to whichever hospital she was working at.[176] In 1992, she returned to the United States to care for AIDS patients in San Diego, California.

Perhaps because Sister Niedfield had led the way in so exemplary a manner, Coffey encouraged other women to specialize in surgery. In a single year (1970), the chief residents of three Georgetown surgery divisions were women—a record unlikely to have been matched in any other graduate surgical program of the time. They were Kathryn D. Anderson (general surgery), Barbara O. Black (urology), and Carol S. Shapiro (plastic surgery).[177] Black and Shapiro went on to become successful private practitioners in their specialties in Maryland and Virginia respectively.[178] Anderson, a pediatric surgeon, became a professor of surgery at the University of Southern

California School of Medicine and Chief Surgeon at Children's Hospital in Los Angeles. In 1986, she was one of the first two women to be elected simultaneously to the Board of Governors of the American College of Surgeons. In 1992, she became the third woman to be elected to the American Surgical Association. That same year, she took office as the first female secretary of the American College of Surgeons, and by 2000 had served eight straight years in that role.[179]

The women also came in for their share of yelled and growled Coffeyisms. Kathryn Anderson remembered his comments on her hands ("too goddamned small") and her interest in pediatric surgery ("all you need is small sutures"). But when Coffey backed her judgment against that of a senior professor of medicine—to the extent of telling the professor that he, Coffey, would not operate on the professor's cases if he ever again overruled a chief surgical resident—she became, she said simply, "his slave." She was on Coffey's team, and he let everybody know it. "He was very demanding. He demanded total, *total* care of his patients," she recalled. "But once he trusted your competence, he let you get on with your job." This trust did not extend to letting residents perform operations on private patients. They assisted in those procedures, opened and closed incisions, but the actual surgery was always performed by the surgeon. Anderson could remember only one occasion during her residency with Coffey that he allowed her to perform an operation (a routine hernia repair) alone; it was the morning after the 1968 presidential election when Coffey—a staunch Republican, despite his long friendship with Robert Kennedy[180]—arrived in the OR uncharacteristically bleary-eyed, having stayed up all night to see Nixon win. Yet looking back, Anderson considered even this a plus: learning to be a good assistant oneself, she felt, shaped the training of one's own assistants when the time came.[181]

Through the 1960s medical research boomed at Georgetown, pulling in more than $47 million in grants and prompting John Rose to announce in 1966 that "over the past three years, Georgetown University stands sixth among all of the medical schools and teaching hospitals in the United States in the number of research abstracts submitted to *Clinical Research*, one of the principal reporters of clinical investigation."[182]

It was a fruitful decade. Members of the surgery department published some five hundred articles, presented more than six hundred papers, and had on average twenty-seven research projects running in any year.[183] These included not only clinical investigations in general surgery and the specialties, but basic studies designed to advance the practice of surgery. Henry Balch studied factors in the development of infection in surgical patients. Earl Barnes investigated the chemistry of wound repair and the rate of healing. John Dillon, director of the Surgical Metabolic Laboratory, investigated changes in metabolism and body fluids after shock and hemorrhage, and conducted a long-term study on the efficacy of salt solution in the treatment of shock.[184]

Robert Coffey, who in the course of his career published over one hundred scientific articles and contributed to four textbooks on surgery, reported clinical investigations into many aspects of general surgery, among them early work on resection of the liver to treat cancer,[185] and the development of a new surgical technique for duodenal ulcers which greatly reduced the risk of their recurrence.[186] Coffey's primary research interest remained, however, disorders of the endocrine system: pancreatic disease, thyroid disease, and hyperparathyroidism.

The pancreas has always presented difficulties for the surgeon: it is a large gland buried in the abdomen—tightly surrounded by the stomach, liver, colon, spleen, gallbladder, kidneys, and duodenum—and it controls complex digestive and glandular mechanisms affecting the whole body. The thyroid gland in the neck is more accessible, but similarly critical to multiple body functions, including heart rate, energy level, muscle strength, vision, menstruation, and emotional state. The parathyroid glands, each the size of a lentil and joined to the thyroid, regulate specifically the balance of calcium and phosphorus in the body. Even today, surgical procedures on these three organs, most often to remove tumors, require considerable skill. Coffey, who performed hundreds from the 1940s on, remembered: "To me, these were some of the most exciting and rewarding operations."

Coffey was fortunate. Through the 1950s and 1960s, the Georgetown endocrinologists Laurence Kyle (chairman of medicine, 1958–71) and John Canary (chief of the endocrinology division) made much headway in the diagnosis of primary hyperparathyroidism. This condition, which arises when the gland secretes too much hormone, causes the bones to release excessive calcium into the blood, leading in some cases to kidney stones, pancreatitis, peptic ulcers, hypertension, and a loss of bone strength. Even today, with sophisticated blood tests, diagnosis of the disorder is problematic; many of those affected suffer either mild or generalized symptoms, such as fatigue or depression, or sometimes none at all. But Kyle's and Canary's early work on diagnosis was notable enough to attract hyperparathyroid patients to Georgetown from across the nation.[187] As most cases were caused by a benign tumor on one of the glands, it was Coffey who cured them with surgery. So, as he noted in 1971, "I have been in the enviable position of being involved in the surgical care of well over one hundred cases of primary hyperparathyroidism since 1958, whereas only one case had been operated on [at Georgetown] prior to that time."[188] By 1977, he and his partner Tom Lee had treated a further one hundred cases, bringing their series to more than two hundred—in sharp contrast to most surgeons who saw few, if any, cases in their whole careers.[189] Coffey was in consequence able to publish and lecture extensively on hyperparathyroidism, and he became recognized as an authority on the subject.

But Coffey's and Lee's most significant contribution to endocrine surgery was in the treatment of hyperthyroidism (or thyrotoxicosis). Because it drives so many physical and mental functions, the thyroid has been called the body's "accelerator." When the accelerator sticks, pumping out uncontrolled quantities of hormone, body functions can go haywire, precipitating a crisis—known as a thyroid storm—which, unchecked, can bring swift deterioration into delirium, coma, and death. Before the 1920s, surgery on the thyroid had high mortality, because the operation itself could and did precipitate a storm. The use of iodine (from 1923) and antithyroid drugs (from 1946) to prepare patients for operation drastically reduced mortality, revolutionizing the surgical treatment of thyroid disease. But these drugs still took weeks or months to ready the patient. Lee and Coffey found that oral doses of propranolol, a beta-adrenergic blocking agent, could prepare a patient for elective surgery within twenty-four hours, or, in an emergency, by injection in an hour. Reporting in 1973 on their first 20 cases, they found that propranolol effectively neutralized hyperactivity without significantly affecting thyroid functon.[190] Eight years later, they reported a further 140 cases of their own, and reviewed 174 others worldwide, in which propranolol had been given alone, without iodine: the results were uniformly good, and no patient suffered thyroid storm.[191] One published history of hyperthyroidism noted that with this advance by Lee and Coffey—which is still used today—"the preoperative preparation of patients with thyrotoxicosis took a quantum leap to contemporary times."[192]

Charles Hufnagel, meanwhile, was making further advances in cardio-vascular surgery. Hufnagel began his second decade at Georgetown in 1960 by introducing a new artificial heart valve to replace the diseased aortic valve itself. His earlier ball-valves had been inserted further down the aorta. His new "tri-leaflet" devices replicated the action of real valves in their natural location and were more successful.[193] Later, to counter the occasional blood clots, Hufnagel further improved his device by coating it in silicone impregnated with an anticlotting agent, which he trademarked as "Hepicone."[194]

The operation to insert this tri-leaflet valve was far trickier than the old ball-valve in the aorta and took more time. Hufnagel continually experimented with different ways of stopping the heart for as much as two hours. He tried various kinds of surgical hypothermia: sometimes immersing the patient in a bath of ice chips to lower body temperature enough to induce cardiac arrest; sometimes applying a cooling slush directly to the aorta.[195] So fascinated did Hufnagel become by natural mechanisms for juggling body temperature that his office was soon lined with aquaria full of African lungfish, whose only known feature of interest is that they can hibernate for long periods.[196]

But it was the heart-lung bypass machines which made possible the new era of open-heart surgery. These brilliant devices to circulate and oxygenate blood outside the body were developed by several surgeons worldwide in the 1950s and 1960s, starting with John H. Gibbon Jr. of Philadelphia, who developed the first pump oxygenator and was the first to use it successfully on a human patient in May 1953.[197] Hufnagel's earliest contribution, invented in 1958, was a pneumatic pump—the part of the bypass machine that pushes blood back into the body—that simulated the pulsating action of the heart.[198] In 1959, to cool a patient's temperature further, he devised a heart-lung unit still known as the Hufnagel Heat Exchanger. Rerouted through this machine, the patient's blood was purified, oxygenated, and passed over a refrigerated surface to cool it twelve degrees below normal before it was pumped back into the aorta.[199] Hufnagel used his exchanger for many open-heart operations, including one of his more bizarre cases. In March 1962, he extracted a bullet from the heart of a Washington grocer, fourteen days after the man had been shot in the leg. It had taken that long,

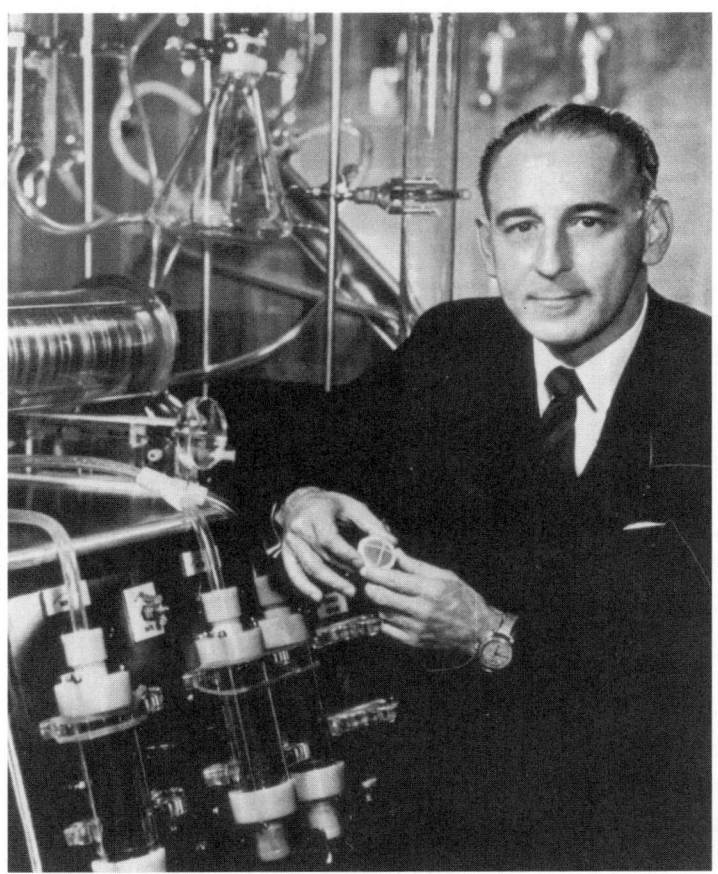

Charles Hufnagel holds the tri-leaflet version of
his artificial heart valve in front of a heart-lung
machine he invented in the 1960s. Courtesy of
Georgetown University Archives.

and a series of X rays, to figure out that the elusive bullet had traveled three
feet up a vein to lodge in the right ventricle of the heart.[200]

Bypass methods brought giant leaps in cardiac surgery. But in its early
days, the pioneering nature of this technology was matched by the make-do
quality of its technical support. There were no trained perfusionists:
Hufnagel's team—his nurse Pat Conway, his surgical assistants John

Gillespie and Peter Conrad, and his research assistant Linda Langan Kildea (later director of Georgetown's experimental surgery laboratories)—all took turns at the pump. After October 1965, when Hufnagel performed Washington's first successful kidney transplant,[201] it was Kildea who drove around the emergency rooms of area hospitals to collect donor kidneys, perfusing them with coolants in perforated steel canisters to keep them fresh for transplantation. "Now, they use specially equipped planes and vehicles to transport organs," she recalled. "Then, I just put them in the trunk of my car."

Similarly, Hufnagel was able to design and use his inventions in remarkable freedom, unencumbered by later laws regulating medical devices. Hufnagel would sketch a new design for a heart valve. Linda Kildea would pop the drawing in an envelope and send it by special air delivery to Rudolph R. Shulte, the manufacturer in California, He, in turn, would swiftly craft a prototype and ship it back to Washington by plane, frequently the following day, in the safekeeping of a stewardess. "So if Dr. Hufnagel had an idea on Tuesday, quite feasibly we'd have the new valve by Thursday night," Kildea recalled. "And if Dr. Hufnagel liked it, I'd sterilize it and he'd use it there and then—on an animal or a human patient. You couldn't do that today."

Hufnagel focussed throughout the 1960s on refinements to his heart valves and on the recurring problem of the rejection of transplants. Honors and awards accumulated—among them the Mendel Medal of Science[202] and the American Heart Association's distinguished service award.[203] In 1966, his contribution to medical history was formally recognized when the Smithsonian Institution's Museum of American History and Technology put his family of valves on permanent display in its exhibit tracing landmarks in the development of heart surgery.[204]

In Washington, Hufnagel was lauded as the great man of cardiac surgery—so much so that the local press felt cheated when on December 3, 1967, Christiaan Barnard of South Africa did the first transplant of a human heart. *Washingtonian* magazine ran an article defiantly headed: "Dr. Charles A. Hufnagel Could Have Performed the First Heart Transplant: When He Does Do One, Expect the Patient to Live."[205] In the days and weeks after Barnard's landmark operation on Louis Washkansky, who died seventeen days later, both local and national media sought Hufnagel's opinion. Tactfully, he acknowledged that any research team had the right to decide when the time had come to apply an experimental procedure to human treatment. But he did not hide his own conviction that Barnard's attempt had been premature.

Indeed, his immediate response, issued the next day, was to describe it as "very interesting, but not too significant. The problem is not in doing a heart transplant but in keeping the heart functional for a long term."[206] He elaborated later: "We have done many animal heart transplants. But we feel that the evidence for long-term acceptance of a transplanted heart is not good enough as yet to justify the operation." Transplanting a heart, he explained, was technically no more difficult than that of a kidney (and considerably less complex than inserting a heart valve); nor was the immune reaction any greater. The difference was that "if the [kidney] operation fails, the results are not so serious." A patient could be maintained indefinitely on an artificial kidney machine while awaiting a new transplant; whereas an artificial heart could keep a patient going for at most two or three days. Doctors had known for many years, he pointed out, that a heart transplant *could* be done: "The only question has been whether the immune-reaction and infection problems have been solved to a degree which would hold promise of prolonged survival in a reasonable percentage of cases."[207]

This was the issue that, at the time of Barnard's operation, Hufnagel was confronting in his own research at Georgetown. Other investigators were approaching the problem by trying to develop drugs to suppress the body's normal immune reaction so as to prevent rejection. The drawback was that this would also make the patient highly vulnerable to infection. So Hufnagel worked on a different approach, one he called "induction of tolerance." His idea was to pre-condition the donor organ with injections of drugs and tissue types to make it more acceptable after transplantation—"so that the recipient is not aware that it is foreign," he explained, "or so that you can specifically change his immune response *only* to the transplant." This approach, Hufnagel thought, had the potential to work most effectively in the transplanting of animal hearts into humans, an option he believed would eventually prove preferable to human-to-human transplants. "It solves all the moral problems; it solves all the logistical problems of supply and demand; it solves the tremendously difficult problems of securing a [human] heart immediately after death," he said in 1969.[208]

As events turned out, medical science moved not in the direction of tolerance induction but toward better immunosuppressive drugs and more controlled protocols; survival rates of human heart transplants improved more rapidly than Hufnagel had expected. In late 1969, his reservations seemed justified, because few patients had then lived longer than three months—indeed, cardiologists worldwide who had rushed to perform hundreds of heart transplants after Barnard led the way, soon gave up doing them for that reason. But from 1970 onwards, the number of long-term survivals began to increase dramatically. And although Christiaan Barnard had been heavily criticized for "superego surgery" after his early failures, it was he who in 1971 transplanted a heart which kept its recipient living until 1994—a total of twenty-three years and fifty-seven days, to date the longest survival on record.[209] By the end of the twentieth century, the operation that once seemed the ultimate surgical triumph had come to be regarded as virtually routine.

Hufnagel himself never performed a heart transplant on a human being, though his early ideas for mechanical hearts and animal-human transplants were later put into practice by others. Hufnagel abstained in part from lack of resources—organizing a heart transplant team required huge funding—and partly because his clinical workload was largely taken up with artificial heart valve insertions. He performed an average of four a day, four days a week, for more than twenty-five years. But at least one element in Hufnagel's disinclination was simple concern for his patients: he would not attempt a heart transplant without reasonable confidence in long-term survival. Hufnagel was famously a "people person," unfailingly interested in someone's new job, car, or hairstyle, and showing the same affability toward the hospital maintenance workers as toward the president of the university or the president of the United States. "I never saw him leave the hospital, late at night, without saying something to the cleaning staff," Linda Kildea remembered. "And his patients just worshipped him."

Throughout the 1960s, Hufnagel was rarely away from the hospital, except for professional meetings. His working day routinely began at 6:00 A.M. and finished around 11:00 P.M. He spent as much time as possible in the laboratory, even took an early speed-reading course to keep up with the latest research. But many, many hours he gave to patients. His notorious insistence on conducting late rounds personally, unusual for so eminent a surgeon, saw him walking the corridors to check on patients and talk with their families until far into the night, to the despair of weary residents.[210] It was, however, these treks that finally got Hufnagel's agile brain thinking about the problem of the hospital.

⊷

Surgical and hospital practices in the 1960s, before the advent of today's sophisticated technological procedures, seem in retrospect almost primitive. No CAT or MRI scans; no ultrasound; no fiberoptics or laparoscopies; few of the monitoring screens now used routinely. The electronic revolution was yet to come.

In the operating room, ether was still the predominant anesthetic; its smell pervaded the medical center, and its volatility brought inevitable accidents. In 1945, Coffey was performing an abdominal operation when a cylinder of ether exploded, shattering the glass skylight above; Coffey reacted instantly, throwing a sheet over his patient to keep falling glass out of the wound.[211] No one was injured, but a similar incident more than twenty years later, in February 1969, ended tragically. Coffey had just removed a patient's thyroid gland and was preparing to close the incision when the gas cylinder exploded. Coffey and his resident were both hurled across the room; surgeons from the adjacent operating room rushed in and smashed the windows to let out fumes and smoke. But the patient had taken the full force in her lungs: she died. There were about forty such accidents every year in hospitals around the country, caused mainly by electrical short circuits.[212]

Hospital rules now taken for granted had not yet even been contemplated. In 1960, for example, the dean sent around a memo suggesting that house staff and clinical clerks refrain from smoking in the wards, on the grounds that some patients were "annoyed, if not made actually uncomfortable, by tobacco smoke on the corridors and in their rooms."[213] Before that, it was common for both doctors and patients to smoke everywhere in the hospital. Doing ward rounds with students, Roger Baker was often seen puffing on a large cigar grasped in one hand while performing a rectal examination with the other.[214] Coffey, too, was a heavy smoker—until he was stricken with cancer of the larynx in 1963. Refusing surgery, he chose to be treated by radiation therapy at the National Cancer Institute and made

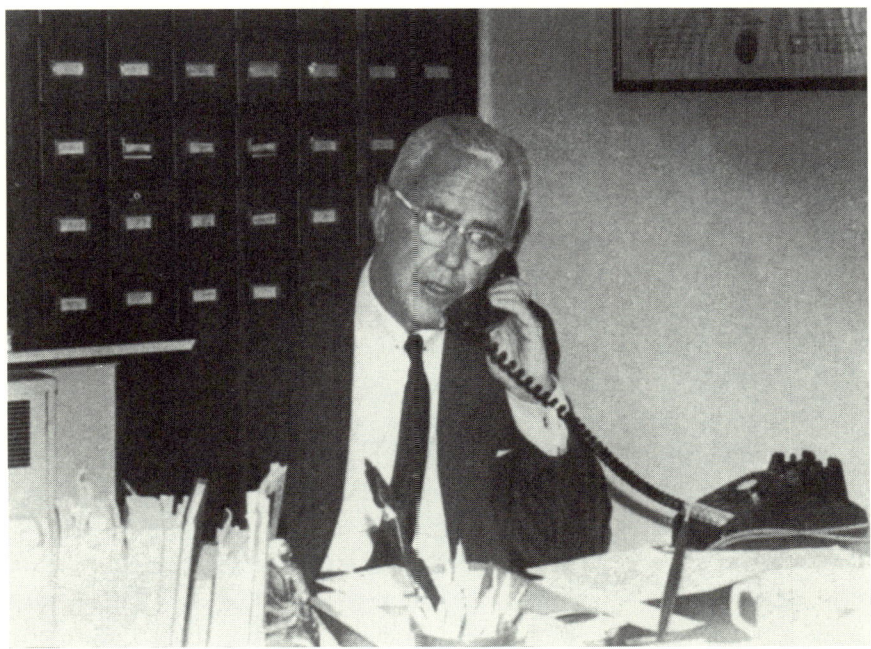

Robert J. Coffey is seen here at his desk in regular clothes—but his habit between operations was to catch up on paperwork, still in bloodstained scrubs, while his assistants closed one procedure and prepared his next patient for surgery. Courtesy of Georgetown University Archives.

a full recovery. Giving up cigarettes made him even more bearish; he got through the withdrawal period by chewing on a toothpick—even in the operating room, where it stuck through the front of his surgical mask like an alien's antenna.[215]

Those were the days before hospital regulations were tightened under the pressures of managed care—and, later, by the risks of the HIV virus. It was Coffey's habit to spend the time between operations at his desk, on the phone or dealing with paperwork, still dressed in cap, mask, and blood-stained gown and gloves. It was his way of organizing his time efficiently, no matter how much his secretary protested. By leaving his assistant to close the incision of one patient and start up the next (and by changing into fresh scrubs only on returning to the OR), he could reduce his role in a whole morning's routine case-load to about ninety minutes.[216]

By 1962, it was clear that Georgetown University Hospital, then fifteen years old, was "already obsolete and much too small to provide the necessary space for the education and patient care that a first class University medical center requires."[217] Not only too small but, by today's standards, badly organized. Like all hospitals of the day, Georgetown's layout resembled that of a hotel: rooms opening off long corridors with a nurses' station at the end. Charles Hufnagel pondered this arrangement, concluded it was inefficient, and came up with a novel design that was to revolutionize intensive care worldwide. He invented, as it were, the wheel: a layout in which the nurses' station was the hub, surrounded on the circumference by patients' rooms with inward-facing walls of glass so that nurses could keep an eye on critical cases as well as monitoring them on computer screens— another innovation—linked to those by the patients' beds.[218]

But which patients needed such care? Hufnagel and his assistant John Gillespie reviewed hospital statistics and found that at any moment only 20 percent of patients were in need of intensive care while being treated for life-threatening conditions, undergoing surgery or recovering from it. The overwhelming 80 percent were in hospital for chronic conditions, or to have diagnostic tests, or to convalesce. Yet both sorts of patients were mixed in together; Georgetown's special facilities for postoperative care was one small recovery room; the equipment needed in an emergency was not always at hand. As Gillespie dramatically described it: "The patient's life hangs in the balance while highly skilled medical talent demonstrates its *galloping* ability, and expensive equipment is dragged bodily through the halls." Their solution: separate critical patients from the non-critical, and organize intensive-care resources to maximize speed in a crisis.[219] But that meant designing a new kind of hospital.

The team of four chosen to tackle this ambitious task comprised Hufnagel, Gillespie, Proctor Harvey, professor of medicine, and Charles Geschickter, chairman of pathology. In April 1964, they secured a $230,000 planning grant from the Public Health Service and went to work.[220] They spent three years developing some extraordinary ideas. One, much publicized at the time, was a hyperbaric surgical unit: entire operating suites enclosed within huge pressurized tanks, under ocean-depth pressures much greater than that of the normal atmosphere, so that a patient's tissues and blood could be saturated in oxygen during operations for certain conditions, such as coronary thrombosis. Another idea was a mass disaster unit, to be built underground, with the capability to treat up to one thousand casualties of any local disaster—natural or otherwise—at a time.[221]

These were dramatic concepts. Underlying them was the need to persuade Congress to appropriate funds for the new hospital. By any standards, it was an expensive project: those hyperbaric surgical suites alone would each cost more than $250,000. Hufnagel, Gillespie, and Geschickter duly went to Capitol Hill to plead for money, as generations of Georgetown faculty had done before them. Unlike their predecessors, however, they used the mid-twentieth-century tool of national publicity to good effect. Breathless articles on "The Hospital of the Future" duly appeared in *Life* magazine and *Readers' Digest*. Millions of people read about the Georgetown proposals for sci-fi hospital reform, spiced by Gillespie's provocative quotes. "New methods and devices pull many people through today who otherwise would be without hope," he proclaimed. "But the basic vehicle, the hospital, is holding us back. It's time to design an entirely new model."[222]

Unusually, Congress responded: in 1966 it voted $6.9 million towards the Georgetown project—unprecedented for a private hospital— to be matched by privately-raised funds.[223] At the height of the Cold War, the idea of a mass casualty unit perhaps appealed to congressmen fearful that Washington was vulnerable to nuclear attack. It helped, too, that Geschickter had influential friends on Capitol Hill,[224] and that a senior member of the House appropriations committee had suffered cancer of the esophagus until Hufnagel performed the operation that had saved his life.[225]

But as the design team's ideas expanded, so did the cost. "It grew, and grew, and grew—from a few million at the outset to about $25 million," John Rose recalled. "That was an awful lot of money." By 1967, the projected total so alarmed the university's Board of Directors that they decided to distance themselves by severing the university and medical center into two legally distinct corporations.[226] This move, they hoped, would protect the university from liability if the medical center ran into financial difficulties with the new hospital. In the end, the idea was abandoned; lawyers insisted that separate incorporation would not, in fact, necessarily protect the university.[227] "It was the old lawyers' expression that, in a case where a corporation creates another and any liability develops, the 'corporate veil can be pierced,'" Rose said.

For many anxious months, though, while the notion of separation was explored, it looked as if the medical center would have to endure either the unthinkable fate of divorce from the university, or the indignity of abandoning its dreams for the "hospital of the future" which it had advertised so successfully across the nation—to the receptive ears of, among others, rival medical centers. Finally in 1973, Congress once more agreed to pick up the tab, voting a further $8.3 million in grants and $6.7 million in loans, raising total federal support to $22 million.[228] Even so, plans for the new hospital were substantially scaled back. Out went the hyperbaric pressure chambers and the mass disaster unit. But Hufnagel's original ideas for reorganizing surgical and intensive care, including his designs for the central nurses' station and computerized monitoring and record-keeping systems, survived. The Concentrated Care Center, built next to the existing hospital, opened in 1976.[229] It served as a model for many other such centers around the world.

On November 14, 1967, Robert Coffey composed a letter to the university president. "Inasmuch as this is my 59th birthday, I am anticipating the next one," he began, then told Campbell he wished to resign the chair of surgery a year hence, on his sixtieth birthday. "This decision, after much soul-searching, was not an easy one to make," he wrote. "However, I am convinced that after twenty years as Chairman I no longer have the imagination, verve, and enthusiastic leadership that is required. Furthermore, I feel that on being relieved, I can contribute much more effectively by devoting more time to writing, teaching, clinical surgery and national organizational activities."[230]

The announcement surprised everyone. As Campbell replied: "It is in fact rather unusual that a person in your position would have the foresight and generosity to take such a step at this particular point in your career." But, after complimenting Coffey on his accomplishments as chairman, Campbell added: "I certainly believe that you are entitled to some relief . . . to devote your full time and talents to your excellent work as a surgeon."[231]

To the department, the news that this man, quintessentially the chairman after two decades in office, intended to step down came as an immense shock. Who would take his place? The job had grown monumentally in Coffey's tenure. "The chairmanship of an academic department is no mean chore," John Rose wrote after a search committee had been appointed.[232] "Departmental budgets run into seven figures. Interpersonal relationships among dozens of talented and ambitious physicians and scientists can become quite trying. Each of the many complex teaching and research programs has difficult and often vexing problems of finance, space, and personnel . . . Department chairmen are the key figures in modern medical schools."[233] The search committee reviewed candidates from across the nation. But it was Coffey's own nominee, the person he felt had graced the department for eighteen years and now deserved the chair, whom they finally named his successor. Charles Hufnagel became chairman of the department, the eleventh head of surgery at Georgetown, in 1969, at age fifty-two.[234]

Laying down his administrative load, Coffey continued teaching, research, and clinical surgery at Georgetown for another dozen years, travelling to lecture at surgical conferences and visiting professorship programs at home and abroad. At commencement in June of 1969, the university conferred on him the John Carroll Medal of Merit, its highest alumni award. At a dinner held in his honor, the guest speaker was Mark Russell, the Washington entertainer and wit. He had done his homework: Coffey roared with laughter as Russell likened Coffey's cuss-ladened operating style to "Vince Lombardi at half-time in the locker room with the Redskins behind 50 to nothing."[235]

Coffey's classmates of 1932 gave to the school a formal portrait of him by the painter Egli.[236] A more piercing likeness—a head almost concealed by surgical mask and cap, yet unmistakeably Coffey—was etched by Tom Lee to illustrate a cover-story profile in the *Georgetown Medical Bulletin*.[237] In the professional arena, Coffey received the Southeastern Surgical Congress's Distinguished Service Award (1972) and was elected president of the Mayo Clinic Alumni Association (1973). In 1971, he delivered Georgetown's forty-seventh annual Kober Lecture, speaking on the management of hyperparathyroidism—as he remarked, an appropriate subject: John Abel, the first Kober lecturer in 1925, had reviewed existing knowledge of the ductless glands; that year too had marked the first surgical procedure for parathyroidism.[238]

Of his many honors, the one which most surprised and elated Coffey was the establishing of a Georgetown chair of surgery in his name. The Robert J. Coffey Distinguished Chair of Surgery was endowed in 1972–73 by the surgery department's long-time benefactor Hugh A. Grant, who pledged seven hundred thousand dollars over five years to fund it.[239] As his first instalment, Grant sent two thousand shares in Gulf Oil Corporation stock.[240] The income of the endowment, Coffey suggested, should go to support the salary and research of the chairman of the department of surgery; thus Charles Hufnagel was named the first incumbent of the new chair. To increase the funding, Coffey also pledged ten thousand dollars a year of his own.[241] This was only the third endowed chair to be established at Georgetown medical center.[242] "It will be a memorial to a physician, scholar and gentleman who is admired and loved by all of his colleagues," wrote Matthew F. McNulty Jr., executive vice president for medical center affairs, in his thanks to Grant. "It is a fitting recognition of Bob's years of capable leadership."[243]

Coffey retired altogether from teaching and practice in 1982, at age seventy-three. He had survived several bouts of ill health—not only cancer of the larynx in 1963 but subsequently two heart attacks, glomerulonephritis, a kidney stone operation, and hip surgery[244]—but he finally succumbed to pneumonia in the early hours of January 26, 1995, at Georgetown University Hospital. He was eighty-six. Later that day, a medical student who had been on the team taking care of Coffey returned home visibly upset. Her mother, surprised, asked why this patient in particular had so moved her. "You don't understand," the young woman replied. "This man was a legend."

In his long years with Georgetown, Robert Coffey had seen the medical school grow from a small and time-worn building in downtown Washington to the huge medical complex that occupies four blocks on Reservoir Road today. He was there when the school was at the nadir of its fortunes, financially disabled, academically impoverished, vulnerable to closure; he had contributed to its transformation into a medical institution of high rank. He lived long enough to see Georgetown beset once again by financial problems, due in part to the changing economics of medicine but also, as ever, to its stateless geographical position. In the meantime, he had personally raised its department of surgery to the national stature his predecessors had only dreamed of; he had trained more young surgeons than they had done collectively; and he had presided over surgical successes that would have awed them.

꿍

Only 120 years passed between Charles Liebermann's appointment as Georgetown's first professor of surgery and the end of Robert Coffey's chairmanship—a blip in history. Yet in that time, the art and science of surgery came of age, moving jerkily but inexorably from bloodletting to heart transplants, from nostrums to antibiotics, from lancets to lasers, from vague diagnoses to the precision of electronics.

Georgetown medical school not only established a few landmarks along the way but illustrated through its whole history a deeper truth: that progress was driven by the personalities of those who worked for it. People who observed, wondered, and were not afraid to look at the human body as a work of sublime engineering that could yet be repaired. People who labored, often without payment, to train the next generation. And whose struggles sometimes brought advances by paths that had nothing to do with surgical skill. Who would have thought that the mighty National Institutes of Health came into being in part because of John Hamilton's political vendettas? Or that Georgetown University Hospital was launched in reaction to James Kerr's ill-temper?

History constantly surprises us with an ironic twist here, an unexpected turn of events there. For Georgetown, the latest and greatest of these came in 1997. Just as the medical school faced another crisis, precipitated this time by cutbacks in federal funding for research, the school learned that it would receive a bequest of more than $60 million—by far the largest private donation in the school's history and the fourth largest for medical research in the history of the United States—from a fund set up by the grandson of its first graduate, Warwick Evans.

Evans himself never became a rich man; but one of his children, Rosamond, married Harry Toulmin, the lawyer who negotiated patent rights for the Wright Brothers' first airplane. Their son, Harry Jr., also a patent lawyer, started a pharmaceutical company which, after his death in 1965, continued to prosper under the direction of his widow, Virginia. Harry Jr. had bequeathed to Georgetown a trust fund in honor of his grandfather, Warwick Evans. The bequest was some of his company's shares, then worth a few thousand dollars. Over the following thirty years, these grew in value until 1995, when Virginia Toulmin sold the company for $178 million.

The $60 million bequest will continue to grow until it becomes available to Georgetown on Mrs. Toulmin's death. But the news was announced in June of 1997 because, as the university president, Reverend Leo J. O'Donovan, S.J. explained: "Given the decline in federal support for medical research, we want to underscore the larger need for private donors whose generosity will enable medical research institutions such as Georgetown's to remain in the vanguard of newer and better ways of treating diseases and saving lives."[245]

The echoes of this remark resonate back nearly 150 years: all those pleas for the wherewithal to do the job. Somehow, Georgetown University School of Medicine has always found the means to provide education and medical care, not only in hard-won cash but, more importantly, in the personal currency of people who gave their all and refused to give up. It is an honorable heritage. Warwick Evans could not have dreamed that his $150 tuition fee, with which he helped start the medical school in 1851, would be transformed by his progeny into a harvest of riches that will benefit Georgetown in the twenty-first century. Nor can we imagine what that century will bring to Georgetown, to medicine, and to surgery.

NOTES

CHAPTER 1

1. *National Daily Intelligencer*, 5, 12–14 May 1851. The Great Exhibition in London, housed in the Crystal Palace (a building constructed mainly of glass) opened 1 May 1851.

2. Byron Sunderland, "Washington As I First Knew It: 1852–1855," *Records of the Columbia Historical Society* (Washington, D.C., 1902), 195–211.

3. The Smithsonian Institution was chartered by Congress in 1846 to fulfill the wishes of James Smithson, a British scientist, who had bequeathed more than five hundred thousand dollars to the United States "to found at Washington, under the name of the Smithsonian Institution, an Establishment for the increase and diffusion of knowledge among men." The building was originally designed to house a museum, art gallery, library, and lecture hall, and to make it a center for scientific research. Cynthia R. Field, Richard E. Stamm, and Heather P. Ewing, *The Castle: An Illustrated History of the Smithsonian Building* (Washington, D.C., and London, 1993).

4. Constance McLaughlin Green, *Washington: A History of the Capital, 1800–1950* (Princeton, 1962), 1:212, 255. Also: Douglas E. Evelyn and Paul Dickson, *On This Spot: Pinpointing the Past in Washington, D.C.* (Washington, D.C., 1992), 84–86.

5. Field, Stamm, and Ewing, 26. This description of the Smithsonian lecture hall comes from a sketch made by Joseph Henry, the institution's first secretary, in his diary, 16 May 1849 (Smithsonian Institution Archives). The room was used for lectures and ceremonies from 1850 to 1855, then converted into living quarters for Henry and his family.

6. "City Matters: Medical Department of Georgetown College," *National Daily Intelligencer*, 13 May 1851. The only other known reference to this ceremony is contained in a letter written by a Georgetown Jesuit, who wrote: "The Rector delivered the opening address of the Medical Appartement [*sic*] of Georgetown College yesterday afternoon to a large audience in Washington, they say it was very beautiful but that he was not as happy as usual." P. Aloysius Jordan to Samuel Barber, 13 May 1851, Maryland Provincial Archives, Georgetown University, 219 T 14.

7. Elmer Louis Kayser, *A Medical Center: The Institutional Development of Medical Education in George Washington University* (Washington, D.C., 1973), 54. Columbian medical school was also known as the "National Medical College," but was referred to as Columbian by local physicians throughout the nineteenth century and thus is so used here.

8. Samuel C. Busey, *Personal Reminiscences and Recollections* (Washington, D.C., 1895), 216. Kayser notes that the Columbian faculty, aware of the antagonism, resolved to place an advertisement in two local newspapers announcing that "any physician may place a patient in this Infirmary and have the entire management of the case." There is no evidence, however, that the notice was published.

9. Kayser, 58–59.

10. *History of the Medical Society of the District of Columbia, 1817–1909* (Washington, D.C., 1909), 25.

11. W. W. Johnston, "History of the Medical Society," *Transactions and Proceedings of the Seventy-fifth Aniversary of the Medical Society of the District of Columbia*, 16 February 1894 (Washington, D.C., 1894), 44.

12. *Transactions of the American Medical Association*, (Philadelphia, 1848), 1:21; (Philadelphia, 1849), 2:27.

13. Busey, 162–64.

14. *History of the Medical Society of D.C.* Biographical information on Young, 227. Also: Eliot, 233–34; Howard, 232, 291; and Liebermann, 235.

15. William G. Rothstein, *American Schools and the Practice of Medicine: A History* (New York, 1987), 49.

16. J. Llewellyn Eliot, "The History of the Foundation of the Medical Department of Georgetown University," (paper presented at a meeting of the Medical Society of Georgetown University, Washington, D.C., 11 May 1907), Georgetown University Archives. Llewellyn Eliot was the son of Johnson Eliot, a founder of Georgetown University medical school.

17. Ibid.

18. Young, Howard, Eliot, and Liebermann to James Ryder, 12 October 1849, Georgetown University Archives.

19. Robert Emmett Curran, S.J., *The Bicentennial History of Georgetown University, Vol. I., From Academy to University, 1789–1889* (Washington, D.C., 1993), 5–8, 19, 22, 339 n 91.

20. Green, 64.

21. Curran, 75.

22. Ibid., 109, 122, 180–81. James Ryder served two terms as president of Georgetown College: 1840–45 and 1848–51.

23. Ibid., 111–112, 132, 141.

24. Ibid., 145–46. Also: Minutes, Medical Faculty, 25 October 1849, Georgetown University Archives.

25. Joseph T. Durkin, S.J., *Georgetown University: The Middle Years, 1840–1900*, (Washington, D.C., 1963), 85–86.

26. Mary Llewellyn Eliot to John Whitney, 13 November 1900. Also: Minutes, Medical Faculty, vol. 1, 1849–1876, Georgetown University Archives.

27. Minutes, Medical Faculty, 3, 5 November 1849, Georgetown University Archives.

28. Joseph M. Toner, "Anniversary Oration," (paper presented to the Medical Society of D.C., Washington, D.C., 26 September 1866), 37.

29. Rothstein, 41–42.

30. *History of the Medical Society of D.C.*, 228.

31. Daniel S. Lamb, "Reminiscences of the Old Medical School," *Hoya*, vol. 7, no. 8, (Georgetown University, 1925), 8.

32. *History of the Medical Society of D.C.*, 227, 427, 433. Also: William B. Atkinson, *Physicians and Surgeons of the United States* (Philadelphia, 1878), 537.

33. Bureau of the Census, *Census of the United States, 1850.* Washington, D.C., 1850.

34. Busey, 152.

35. *History of the Medical Society of D.C.*, 232, 430. Also: Atkinson, 34.

36. *History of the Medical Society of D.C.*, 233–34, 429. Also: Atkinson, 85.

37. Biographical information on Charles H. Liebermann in this section, unless otherwise indicated, from:

Samuel H. Holland, "Charles H. Liebermann, M.D.: An Early Russian-born Physician of Washington, D.C." *Medical Annals of the District of Columbia* 38, no. 9, (September 1969), 499–504.

Solomon R. Kagan, *Jewish Contributions to Medicine in America from Colonial Times to the Present* (Boston, 1939), 39–40, 452, 485.

History of the Medical Society of D.C., 235.

Gravestone of C. H. Liebermann, his wife, and children; section E, lot 246, Rock Creek Cemetery, Washington, D.C.

38. W. W. Johnston, 45–46. Johnston, relating this incident in his remarks on the history of the Medical Society of D.C., said that Liebermann had told him the story himself "and [it] is told here as I heard it from him."

39. Howard A. Kelly and Walter L. Burrage, *Dictionary of American Medical Biography: Lives of Eminent Physicians of the United States and Canada from Earliest Times* (1928; reprint, Boston, 1971), 742. (Biographical item on Liebermann, written by George Kober, quotes Dieffenbach's remarks.)

40. Bureau of the Census, *Census of the United States, 1840.* Washington, D.C., 1840. At this time, the District of Columbia included the separate cities of Georgetown and Washington, of which the northern boundary was Florida Avenue. The rest of D.C., largely unpopulated, was known as Washington County.

41. *History of the Medical Society of D.C.*, 432.

42. Eliot, 2.

43. Abraham Flexner, *Medical Education in the United States and Canada: Report of the Carnegie Foundation for the Advancement of Teaching (Bulletin No. 4)*, (1910; reprint, New York, 1960), 3, 8–9.

44. Louis Mackall, (remarks at the memorial ceremony for Charles Liebermann at the Medical Society of D.C., 29 March 1886), Minutes, Medical Society of the District of Columbia. National Library of Medicine.

45. Thomas C. Smith, "History of the Medical Colleges," *Transactions and Proceedings of the Seventy-fifth Anniversary of the Medical Society of the District of Columbia* (Washington, D.C., 1894), 67–68.

46. Minutes, Medical Faculty, 13 November 1849, Georgetown University Archives.

47. Minutes, Medical Faculty, 28 November 1849, Georgetown University Archives. Howard's house and office stood at the corner of F and Tenth Streets, according to the school's first advertisement.

48. Green, 164, 172, 209, 211. Also: Samuel C. Busey, 61–65.

49. Boschke's Map of Washington, D.C., 1857. Also *Atlas of Washington, D.C.: Surveys and Plats of Properties in the City of Washington, D.C.* (Philadelphia, 1887). Lot 9, square 321, on which Seaver's corner house and the first Georgetown medical school were built, remained a double lot until well into the twentieth century. Under Washington's early street numbering system, the corner house and the medical school were designated together as 303 F Street, but were later

numbered separately as 1116 and 1114 F Street respectively. In 1887, the two buildings were owned by Dr. James E. Morgan, who had been a Georgetown medical professor from 1852 to 1876.

50. Minutes, Medical Faculty, 31 December 1849 and 1 February 1850, Georgetown University Archives.

51. Minutes, Medical Faculty, 14 March 1850, Georgetown University Archives.

52. Busey, 64–65.

53. Minutes, Medical Faculty, 14 March 1850, Georgetown University Archives.

54. Minutes, Medical Faculty, 8, 12, 15, 26 April, 6 May, 3 June, and 7 October 1850, Georgetown University Archives.

55. Minutes, Medical Faculty, 16, 24 September 1850, Georgetown University Archives.

56. Minutes, Medical Faculty, 7, 15 October 1850, Georgetown University Archives.

57. Minutes, Medical Faculty, 5 August and 3, 16 September 1850; 25 February and 3, 24 March 1851, Georgetown University Archives.

58. Curran, 148.

59. Ritchie to Lynch, 20 July 1852, Medical School Files 1851–1874, Georgetown University Archives.

60. Curran, 122.

61. Joseph Henry, Diary, 4 July 1849, Smithsonian Institution Archives. Also: Field, Stamm, and Ewing, 26, 161 *n* 4.

62. Curran, 122.

63. Minutes, Medical Faculty, 31 December 1849, Georgetown University Archives. Also: Smith in *Transactions and Proceedings of the Seventy-fifth Anniversary of the Medical Society of D.C.*, 69–70.

64. Gaslight, only recently arrived in Washington, was not installed at the school until the following year. Minutes, Medical Faculty, 21 October 1852, Georgetown University Archives.

65. Minutes, Medical Faculty, 29 March and 5, 7 April 1852, Georgetown University Archives.

66. "Medical Department of Georgetown College," advertisement in *National Daily Intelligencer*, 5 May 1851, 4.

67. Green, 213.

68. Kayser, 51, 54.

69. Kayser, 63. Also: Smith, 61.

70. Rothstein, 53.

71. Minutes, Medical Faculty, 29 March and 5, 7 April 1852, Georgetown University Archives.

72. Georgetown College commencement program, 1852, Georgetown University Archives.

73. Minutes, Medical Faculty, 15 March 1852, Georgetown University Archives.

74. Ritchie to Lynch, 20 July 1852, Medical School Files, 1851–1874, Georgetown University Archives.

75. Biographical information on Warwick Evans from: *History of the Medical Society of D.C.*, 266; Obituary, *Catholic Times*, 1 October 1915; John C. Rose, "Remarks on Warwick Evans Night" *Georgetown Medical Bulletin* 42, no. 1 (fall 1989): 43.

76. Biographical information on Samuel J. Radcliffe from: *History of the Medical Society of D.C.*, 251–252; James Easby-Smith, *Georgetown University in the District of Columbia*, (New York and Chicago, 1907), 2:163.

77. Harold D. Eberlein and Cortlandt Van Dyke Hubbard, *Historic Houses of Georgetown and Washington City* (Richmond, 1958), 68–71.

78. *History of the Medical Society of D.C.*, 252.

79. *Census of the United States*, 1850.

80. Biographical information on Henry Kalussowski in this section, unless otherwise indicated, from: Marian Tyrowicz, "Henryk Korwin Kalussowski," *Polski Slownik Biograficzny* (Warsaw and Krakow, 1964–5), 9:505–7; "Died a Patriot Exile," *Washington Post*, 26 December 1984; "Death of a Patriot," *Washington Star*, 26 December 1894.

81. Bogdan Grzelonski, *Poles In the United States, 1776–1865* (Warsaw, 1976), 142.

82. Kalussowski's copybook of correspondence, 13 May 1851, 125; *Korespondencja Henryka Kalussowskiego z lat 1838–1891* (Biblioteka Naradowa, Warsaw); microfilm copy in Library of Congress.

83. Boyd's Street Directories of Washington D.C., 1883, 1884, 1884.

84. *Alumni Directory, George Washington University, 1824–1937* (Washington, D.C., 1938), 114.

85. American Polish Civil War Centennial Committee, *A Civil War Centennial Tribute to Dr. Henry Corwin Kalussowski in Observance of the Seventieth Anniversary of His Death* (Washington, D.C., 1964).

86. Medical school catalogues, 1851–1875, Georgetown University Archives. Also: Duplication of courses specifically described by C. H. A. Kleinschmidt, "The Necessity for a Higher Standard of Medical Education," (introductory address to the thirtieth session of the Medical Department of Georgetown University, 2 September 1878).

87. Smith, 58.

88. Thomas Woody, "Medical Views of a Pennsylvania Doctor in 1850 (James Hamer)," *Bulletin of the History of Medicine* 17 (April 1945): 385–414.

89. Wendy Buehr, ed., *American Manners and Morals* (New York, 1969), 148.

90. Owen H. Wangensteen and Sarah D. Wangensteen, *The Rise of Surgery: From Empiric Craft to Scientific Discipline* (Minneapolis, 1978), 456–57.

91. Ibid., 139.

92. Ephraim McDowell, "Three Cases of Extirpation of Diseased Ovaria," *Eclectic Repertory and Analytical Review* 7 (1817): 242–44. Also: David C. Sabiston Jr., "Major Contributions of Surgery from the South," *Annals of Surgery* (May 1975): 487–90.

93. Busey, 41.

94. Fielding H. Garrison, *An Introduction to the History of Medicine*, 4th ed. (Philadelphia and London, 1929), 505. Also: Wangensteen and Wangensteen, 275–7, 283. Also: Roy Porter, *The Greatest Benefit to Mankind: A Medical History of Humanity* (New York and London, 1997), 366–67.

95. Quoted in Rothstein, 40.

96. Busey, 337.

97. Guy Williams, *The Age of Miracles: Medicine and Surgery in the Nineteenth Century* (London, 1981; Chicago, 1987), 57–59. Also: Wangensteen and Wangensteen, 353, 403–5.

98. Remarks made by Joseph M. Toner and Louis Mackall at memorial ceremony for Charles Liebermann, 29 March 1886, Minutes, Medical Society of the District of Columbia.

99. Busey, 153–55. Also: Johnston, 46.

100. Minutes, Medical Faculty, 17 October 1853, Georgetown University Archives.

101. Georgetown Medical Department Catalogue, 1852–53, Georgetown University Archives.

102. Minutes, Medical Faculty, 7, 14 March 1853, Georgetown University Archives.

103. Minutes, Medical Faculty, 4 April and 24 May 1853, Georgetown University Archives.

104. Minutes, Medical Faculty, 21 October 1852 and 4 April 1853, Georgetown University Archives.

105. Wangersteen and Wangersteen, 455, 461, 465–66. Also: Porter, 360–61.

106. Kayser, 65.

107. Busey, 216.

108. Quoted by James E. Morgan, "Commencement Address" (presented at the twelfth annual commencement of the Georgetown College Medical Department, Washington, D.C., 2 March 1869).

109. Minutes, Medical Faculty, 16 January 1859, Georgetown University Archives.

110. Letter from Columbian medical students, referring to a resolution they had adopted on 19 January, Minutes, Georgetown Medical Faculty, 7 February 1859, Georgetown University Archives.

111. *History of the Medical Society of D.C.*, 253.

112. Minutes, Medical Faculty, 23 May 1860, Georgetown University Archives.

113. Minutes, Medical Faculty, 10 June 1857, Georgetown University Archives. Also: Busey, 152.

114. Curran, 400.

115. Minutes, Medical Faculty, 2, 5 March 1860, Georgetown University Archives.

116. Toner, 33–34.

117. Ibid., 31–33.

118. Douglas E. Evelyn and Paul Dickson, *On This Spot: Pinpointing the Past in Washington, D.C.* (Washington, D.C., 1992), 109–10.

119. Minutes, Medical Faculty, 23 March and 5 April 1858; 19 March 1859, Georgetown University Archives.

120. Minutes, Medical Faculty, 7 February 1859, Georgetown University Archives.

121. Minutes, Medical Faculty, 7 September 1860, Georgetown University Archives.

122. Minutes, Medical Faculty, 18 November 1857, Georgetown University Archives.

123. Minutes, Medical Faculty, 9, 15 September 1859 and 15 July 1861, Georgetown University Archives. This degree, purchased by J. Morgan Evans of Radnorshire, was rescinded in 1912 by George Kober, then dean of the medical school. Kober Papers, box 11, National Library of Medicine.

124. Smith, 58–66.

125. Noble Young, "Valedictory Address" (presented to the graduating class of the Georgetown College Medical Department, Washington, D.C., 1857).

126. Minutes, Medical Faculty, 13 November 1858, Georgetown University Archives.

127. Minutes, Medical Faculty, 19 March and 10 June 1859, Georgetown University Archives.

128. Minutes, Medical Faculty, 9 September 1859, Georgetown University Archives.

129. Minutes, Medical Faculty, 7 February 1859, Georgetown University Archives.

130. Toner, 61–66.

CHAPTER 2

1. *Washington Evening Star*, 1 March 1861. Also: Minutes, Medical Faculty, 28 February 1861, Georgetown University Archives.

2. Of the eight graduates, Arthur R. Barry became a Confederate surgeon; Charles McCormick, W. H. Gardner, John Hampden Porter, W. W. Hayes, and Louis C. Hootee all served on the Union side in medical roles. Charles Allen practiced in Washington, D.C., after graduation and may have assisted in the military hospitals. Of J. M. Binckley, nothing is known.

3. Margaret Leech, *Reveille in Washington, 1861–1865* (1941; reprint, New York, 1986), 34–36, 46.

4. Constance McLaughlin Green, *Washington: A History of the Capital, 1800–1950* (Princeton, 1962) 1:231–32. Also: Kathryn Allamong Jacob, *Capital Elites: High Society in Washington, D.C., after the Civil War* (Washington, D.C., and London, 1995), 41–42, 45. Also: Leech, 48–49.

5. Georgetown Medical Department Catalogue, 1860–61, Georgetown University Archives.

6. *Washington Star*, 16 November 1860.

7. *Washington Star*, 11, 13 March 1861.

8. *Census of the United States, 1850 and 1860.* Washington, D.C., 1860.

9. *Census of the United States, 1860*, Washington, D.C. Also: Boyd's Washington and Georgetown Directory, 1860.

10. *Washington Star*, 14, 15 March 1861.

11. Reuben Cleary, Service Records 1861–65, National Archives.

12. Sworn statement of John B. Foote, formerly lieutenant of Company K, 12th New York Volunteers, quoted in Senate Report no. 827, 57th Congress, 1st session, 24 March 1902.

13. Leech, 66–71.

14. Robert Emmett Curran, S.J., *The Bicentennial History of Georgetown University, Vol. I, From Academy to University, 1789–1889* (Washington, D.C., 1993), 228.

15. Rand to the Secretary of War, 5 January 1899, Rand Papers, National Archives.

16. Memorandum by U.S. Army Record and Pension Office, 18 October 1897, noting that Rand had been awarded the Congressional Medal of Honor "for gallantry at Blackburn's Ford, Virginia, July 18, 1861." Also Rand's letter acknowledging he had received the medal, October 26, 1897. Rand's application for the medal had been denied as recently as September 30, 1897; it was awarded only after Rand contested the decision and his story, as told by his witness John B. Foote, was published in the press. Rand Papers, National Archives.

17. David F. Riggs, *Seventh Virginia Infantry* (Lynchburg, Va., 1982), 2–3.

18. Numbers compiled by the author from following sources:

J. J. Woodward and George A. Otis, eds. *Medical and Surgical History of the Civil War* (Wilmington, N.C., 1990).

Roster of Regimental Surgeons and Assistant Surgeons in the U.S. Medical Department during the Civil War (reprint, Gaithersburg, Md., 1989).

Daniel D. Hartzler, *Medical Doctors of Maryland in the CSA* (Gaithersburg, Md. 1979).

Robert A. Campbell, *Rebellion Register* (Indianapolis, 1867).

Thomas H. S. Hamersly, ed., *Complete Regular Army Register of the United States, 1779–1879* (Washington, D.C., 1880).

William B. Atkinson, *Physicians and Surgeons of the United States* (Philadelphia, 1878).

L. Allison Wilmer, J. H. Jarrett, G. W. F. Vernon, ed., *History and Roster of Maryland Volunteers, War of 1861–65* (Baltimore, 1899).

Thomas V. and Joanne M. Huntsberry, *Maryland in the Civil War* (Baltimore, 1985).

Gregory A. Coco, *A Vast Sea of Misery: A History and Guide to the Union and Confederate Field Hospitals at Gettysburg, July 1–November 20, 1863* (Gettysburg, 1988).

Margaret K. Fresco, *Doctors of St. Mary's County, MD, 1634–1900* (Ridge, Md., 1992).

The Appomattox Roster (1887; reprint, New York, 1962).

James S. Ruby and Thomas E. Prendergast, *Blue and Gray: Georgetown University and the Civil War* (Washington, 1961).

History of the Medical Society of the District of Columbia, 1817–1909 (Washington, D.C., 1909).

19. Margaret Leech, *Reveille in Washington* (1941; reprint, New York, 1969), 95–96.

20. W. S. King, "Report of Surgeon W. S. King," in *Medical and Surgical History of the Civil War* eds. J. J. Woodward and George A. Otis, (Wilmington, N.C., 1990), 2:3.

21. Shelby Foote, *The Civil War, A Narrative: Part 1, Fort Sumter to Perryville* (New York, 1986), 84.

22. King, 6.

23. D. S. Magruder, Assistant Surgeon USA, Report on Battle of Bull Run. Also: Woodward and Otis, 2:6.

24. Report of Assistant Surgeon C. C. Gray, Woodward and Otis, 2:7. Also: Thomas H. S. Hamersly, *The Regular Army Register of the United States, 1779–1879* (Washington, D.C., 1880), 2:370.

25. Riggs, 68.

26. Daniel D. Hartzler, *Medical Doctors of Maryland in the CSA* (Gaithersburg, Md., 1979), 14.

27. "U.S. Army Participation and Casualties in Major Wars," U.S. Army Center of Military History. http://www.army.mil/cmh-pg/war.html. (The number of deaths, from wounds or other causes, of American army personnel in all wars from the Revolution to the Gulf War, excepting the Civil War, totalled 514, 749.)

28. George Worthington Adam, *Doctors in Blue* (New York, 1952), 113–14, 133. Adam notes: "Of the 144,000 cases where the type of missile could be ascertained, the conoidal ball (minié ball) caused 108,000 wounds, the old-fashioned round ball 16,000 wounds, and shell fragments 12,500. Cannon balls were responsible for only 359 cases, and explosive bullets for 130."

29. Trevor N. Dupuy, ed., *International Military and Defense Encyclopedia* (Washington, D.C., 1993), 1213–14. Also: Patricia L. Faust, ed., *Historical Times Illustrated Encyclopedia of the Civil War* (New York, 1986), 497–98.

30. Report of Henry E. Woodbury, Woodward and Otis, 9:465.

31. Adam, 118, 125, 131–37, 139,

32. Adam, 126–27, 133–34.

33. Adam, 130.

34. Frank Hastings Hamilton, *A Treatise on Military Surgery and Hygeine* (New York, 1865), 482–85.

35. Hamilton, 342. Hamilton wrote: "It is unfortunately true that in nine cases out of ten, when a ball has penetrated the abdomen, the patient dies within 24 or 48 hours . . . Be assured, the patient will have a better chance for life if we let him entirely alone, and it surprises us that any good surgeon would think otherwise."

36. Report of Henry E. Woodbury, Woodward and Otis, 9:99.

37. Adams, 129. Late twentieth century use of maggots in European medicine: *British Medical Journal* (1999): 318:807–8.

38. Robert Reyburn, "Fifty Years in the Practice of Medicine and Surgery in Washington, D.C., 1856–1906" (address to the American Therapeutic Society, Washington, D.C., 4 May 1907), 8.

39. J. M. Toner, "Anniversary Oration" (address to the Medical Society of D.C., 26 September 1866; published by the Medical Society, Washington, D.C., 1869), 61–66.

40. Elmer Louis Kayser, *A Medical Center: The Institutional Development of Medical Education in George*

Washington University (Washington, D.C., 1973), 68–69, 76.

41. *Harper's Weekly*, 23 November 1861. The infirmary burned the night of November 3, 1861; some one hundred sick and wounded soldiers were among patients evacuated to local houses and public buildings.

42. Toner, 64.

43. Adam, *Doctors in Blue*, 151, 155. Also: Samuel Zola, John A. Long, and Philip A. Caulfield, *Providence Hospital Centennial Book, 1861–1961* (Washington, D.C., 1961) third chapter. Also: Thompson, 52–53.

44. Adam, 3, 14–21, 197. Also: Albert Gaillard Hart, *The Surgeon and the Hospital in the Civil War* (1902; reprint, Gaithersburg, Md., 1987), 8–9.

45. Walter Lowenfels, ed., *Walt Whitman's Civil War* (New York, 1961; Da Capo reprint), 85–89, 92, 121.

46. Daniel S. Lamb, from an article written in the *Cripple* (a newspaper published weekly at the Third Division U.S. General Hospital, Alexandria, Va.), 3 December 1864.

47. Adam, 67.

48. William K. Beatty, "Daniel Roberts Brower— Neurologist, Psychiatrist and Medico-Legal Expert," *Proceedings of the Institute of Medicine of Chicago* 41 (1988): 97.

49. Minutes, Medical Faculty, 11 December 1862, Georgetown University Archives.

50. Leech, 188–89.

51. Geoffrey C. Ward, Ric Burns, and Ken Burns, *The Civil War, An Illustrated History* (New York, 1994), 147.

52. Eliot's obituary notice, written by J. M. Toner, *Journal of the American Medical Association* (January 1884): 80.

53. *History of the Medical Society of the District of Columbia, 1817–1909* (Washington, D.C., 1909), 234.

54. Ibid., 237–38.

55. Biographical information on Thomas Antisell in this section, unless otherwise indicated, from:

Wyndham D. Miles, "CSW's First President: Thomas Antisell," *Capital Chemist: Journal of the Chemical Society of Washington* 18, no. 1 (January 1968): 7–9.

Wyndham D. Miles, ed., *American Chemists and Chemical Engineers* (Washington, D.C., 1976).

Thomas Antisell Collection, Georgetown University Archives.

Samuel C. Busey, *Personal Reminiscences and Recollections* (Washington, D.C., 1895), 140–41.

William B. Atkinson, *Physicians and Surgeons of the United States* (Philadelphia, 1878), 16–17.

History of the Medical Society of the District of Columbia, 1817–1909 (Washington, D.C., 1909), 261–63.

Obituary, *Washington Star*, 15 June 1893.

56. Owen H. Wangensteen and Sarah D. Wangensteen, *The Rise of Surgery: From Empiric Craft to Scientific Discipline* (Minneapolis, 1978), 418.

57. Minutes, Medical Faculty, 5, 6 April 1858, Georgetown University Archives. Antisell was recommended to the faculty by Charles Liebermann.

58. Bureau of the Census, *Census of the United States*, 1870. Washington, D.C., 1870. Also: Obituary, *Washington Star*, 15 June 1893.

59. U.S. Congress, House Report 389, 52nd Congress, 1st session, 17 February, 1892; and Senate Report 764, 52nd Congress, 1st session, 27 May, 1892.

60. Quoted by Miles, in his article in *Capital Chemist*, attributed to William Seaman, one of Antisell's colleagues in the chemistry division of the U.S. Department of Agriculture after the Civil War.

61. Thomas Antisell, Military Service Record, National Archives. Also: Louis C. Duncan, *The Medical Department of the United States Army in the Civil War* (Medical Corps, U.S. Army, 1987), 95, 171.

62. Surgeon General's Circular No. 2, 21 May 1862. Also: Adam, 31, 34, 37.

63. Minutes, Medical Faculty, 2 February 1863, Georgetown University Archives. Also: J. Havens Richards, Kober Seventieth Anniversary Issue, *Georgetown College Journal* (March 1920): 265.

64. Thomas Antisell, Military Service Records, National Archives.

65. Daniel S. Lamb, "Reminiscences of the Old Medical School," *Hoya*, vol. 7, no. 8, (Washington, D.C.: Georgetown University, 1925), 8, Georgetown University Archives.

66. Frank Hastings Hamilton, *A Treatise on Military Surgery and Hygiene* (New York, 1865), 14–17.

67. Adam, 19–20, 125, 168, 203–5.

68. Adam, 46–47. Hamilton, 38. Hamersly, 373.

69. Thomas Antisell, *Suggestions Towards Improvement of Sanitary Conditions in the Metropolis* (Dublin, 1847).

70. Thomas Antisell, "Extracts from a Narrative of His Services in the Medical Staff during the Summer of 1862," in *Medical and Surgical History of the Civil War* eds. J. J. Woodward and George A. Otis, (Wilmington, N.C., 1990), 2:120.

71. Hamilton, 17.

72. Hart, 10.

73. Hart, 37.

74. Hamilton, 17.

75. Adam, 9–11, 48–49, 54–55.

76. W. F. Tibballs to Georgetown medical faculty, 4 January 1865, Minutes, Medical Faculty, Georgetown University Archives. Tibballs was accepted into the school, then midway through the winter course, and graduated only two months later in March 1865.

77. F. Terry Hambrecht, introduction to *Roster of Regimental Surgeons and Assistant Surgeons in the U.S. Medical Department During the Civil War* (Gaithersburg, Md., 1989), vi.

78. Hamersly, 372. Hart, 45.

79. Jonathan Letterman, "Report on the Operations of the Medical Department of the Army of the Potomac from July 4 to December 31, 1862," in *Medical and Surgical History of the Civil War* eds. J. J. Woodward and George A. Otis, (Wilmington, N.C., 1990), 2:104.

80. Hamersly, 375

81. Hamersly, 374. Also: George A. Otis, List of regular and volunteer officers of Union medical staff killed and wounded, *Medical and Surgical History of the Civil War*, 7:xxx–xxxii. Otis noted that this list should suffice "to correct the popular fallacy that, in time of battle, the post of the medical officer is one of comparative safety . . ."

82. Ibid., xxx.

83. *History of the Medical Society of D.C.*, 243–44.

84. James S. Ruby and Thomas E. Prendergast, *Blue and Gray: Georgetown University and the Civil War* (Washington, D.C., 1961), 157. This source lists the death of another medical school graduate, Lucius B. Smith. Service records show, however, that Lucius B. was the not the same person as the Lucius Smith who studied in the same class as Reuben Cleary and shared rooms with him after their graduation in 1859. It is not known what happened to Georgetown's Smith.

85. Ruby and Prendergast, 30.

86. Margaret K. Fresco, *Doctors of St. Mary's County, Maryland, 1634–1900* (Ridge, Md., 1992), 56–57.

87. Those not mentioned in text are: Dent Burroughs, John T. Digges, and Carl H. A. Kleinschmidt (CSA); and William F. Tibbals (USA). Information on Burroughs and Digges from Ruby and Prendergast, 94, 141. Information on Tibbals and Kleinschmidt from Coco, 184, 186.

88. Riggs, 24–26, 48, 68.

89. Ruby and Prendergast, 142.

90. Information on Barry from Hartzler, 14. Information on Shekell and Walsh from Coco, 184–85. Information on Sylvester from *History of the Medical Society of D.C.*, 270.

91. Jonathan Letterman, "Report on the Operations of the Medical Department during the Battle of Gettysburg, 3 October 1863," in *Medical and Surgical History of the Civil War* eds. J. J. Woodward and George A. Otis, (Wilmington, N.C., 1990), 2:141–42.

92. Ruby and Prendergast, 142.

93. Senate Committee on Veterans Affairs, *In the Name of the Congress of the United States: Medal of Honor Recipients, 1863–1978* (Washington, D.C., 1979).

94. "Surgeon Thompson's Medal," *The (Baltimore) Sun*, 5 December 1870.

95. Brigadier General J. G. Foster to Assistant Adjutant General Lewis Richmond, 20 March 1862. Also: J. H. Thompson to Adjutant General Townsend, 10 November 1970. Thompson's military service records, National Archives.

96. J. H. Thompson, "Report of the Wounded at the Battle of Newbern, N.C.," *American Medical Times* (5 July 1862): 6–8. In this account of 12 amputations performed on the battlefield, Thompson contended that immediate amputation offered a more successful outcome than delayed surgery—a topic much debated in the Civil War.

97. J. H. Thompson to the secretary of war, volunteering his services and detailing his credentials, 17 May 1861.

98. U.S. Army General Order No. 24, on command of Major General Ambrose Burnside, 4 April 1862. Also: Burnside to Hon. E. M. Stanton, Secretary of War, 12 June 1862.

99. J. Harry Thompson, Military Service Records, National Archives.

100. The medal was issued 11 November 1870, with the citation that Thompson had "voluntarily reconnoitred the enemy's position and carried orders under the hottest fire." In the list of Medal of Honor recipients, he is listed as J. (James) Harry Thompson, although in other records (notably the biography included in the *History of the Medical Society of the District of Columbia, 1817–1909*) his first name is given as John. Thompson always signed himself either J. H. Thompson or J. Harry Thompson. At least three J. H.Thompsons served as Union surgeons in the Civil War, leading to some confusion in the military records. But personal details in those records (dates and places of birth and death, and medical education) which match those in the *History of the Medical Society* biography and other sources, plus identical handwriting samples, all confirm that the Medal of Honor recipient was the same J. Harry Thompson who, after the war, founded the Columbia

Lying-in Hospital for Women, Washington, D.C., in 1866 and taught clinical surgery at Georgetown medical school from 1867 to 1876. As the *History of the Medical Society* also lists his son, Dr. John Harry Thompson Jr., it is concluded that his first name was indeed John, and he is so referred to in this book.

101. J. Harry Thompson was the first medical officer to receive a Medal of Honor. But a woman physician, Mary E. Walker, who served on contract as an acting assistant surgeon on several battlefields and was taken prisoner, received the medal by special order of President Andrew Johnson in November 1865.

102. Faust, 659–60.

103. Ruby and Prendergast, 142.

104. Riggs, 68.

105. Hartzler, 14.

106. Howard A. Kelly and Walter L. Burrage, *Dictionary of American Medical Biography: Lives of Eminent Physicians of the United States and Canada from Earliest Times* (1928; reprint, Boston, 1971), 706. Also: Hartzler, 51. Also: *History of the Medical Society of D.C.*, 206.

107. Ruby and Prendergast, 94.

108. Leech, 384.

109. "Tells of Seeing Lincoln Slain 66 Years Ago: Doctor Recalls Tragedy in Ford's Theater," *Chicago Tribune*, 12 April 1931. Also: Shelby Foote, *The Civil War: A Narrative: Red River to Appomattox* (New York: Vintage Books, 1986), 980.

110. Reyburn, 18–20.

111. C. S. Taft, "Last Hours of Abraham Lincoln," *Medical and Surgical Reporter* 12 (1865): 454. M. H. Shutes, *Lincoln and the Doctors* (New York, 1933), 114. Helen R. Purtle, "Lincoln Memorabilia in the Medical Museum of the Armed Forces Institute of Pathology," *Bulletin of the History of Medicine* 32 (1958): 68, 70. According to Purtle, the hair Liebermann removed from around Lincoln's wound was later contributed to the Lincoln collection at the Army Medical Museum (now the National Museum of Health and Medicine, Washington, D.C.).

112. Reyburn, 18–20.

113. Curran, 246–47.

114. Thomas Courtney Lee, "The Role of Georgetown's Dr. Samuel A. Mudd in the Lincoln Conspiracy," *Georgetown Medical Bulletin* 29, no. 4 (May 1976): 5–34.

115. John B. Foote, "How Sergeant Rand Became a Private—a Tale of Self-Sacrifice and Heroism," *National Tribune*, 25 April 1901. Reprinted in Senate Committee of Pensions Report 827, 57th Congress, 1st session, 24 March 1902, 5–6.

116. Charles Franklyn Rand Papers, National Archives.

117. Obituary of Rand, *Washington Medical Annals* 7 (1908–9): 386.

118. Thomas Antisell, Military Pension Records, National Archives.

119. U.S. Congress House Report 3591, 52nd Congress, 1st session, 17 February 1892; and Senate Report 764, 27 May 1892.

120. "Death of Dr. Antisell," *Washington Star*, 15 June 1893.

121. Reuben Cleary, "Chronicas Lageanas," or "A Record of Facts and Observations on Manners and Customs in South Brazil," unpublished manuscript in two drafts; 161–62 (first draft, n.d.); 3, 125, 129, 315–16 (second draft, n.d.); Reuben Cleary Collection, Manuscripts Division, National Library of Congress.

122. *Annual Report of the Supervising Surgeon General of the Marine Hospital Service of the United States for the Fiscal Year 1898* (Washington, D.C. 1899), 651. For several years up to his death, Reuben Cleary served as sanitary inspector for the U.S. Marine Hospital Service in Rio de Janeiro, Brazil. His duty was to inspect all ships and crews bound for the United States, in accordance with U.S. quarantine laws.

123. According to Library of Congress records, one draft was given to the library by Dr. Joseph T. Howard of Washington, D.C., in 1908, and the other by L. M. Gottschalk in 1921.

124. Ruby and Prendergast, 30. Also: *History of the Medical Society of D.C. 1817–1909*, 267.

125. Curran, 398.

126. Minutes, Medical Faculty, 10 January 1865, Georgetown University Archives.

127. Medical school commencement lists, 1862–65, Georgetown University Archives. These lists break down to: three in 1862, fifteen in 1863, seventeen in 1864, and thirty-five in 1865.

128. Medical school commencement programs, 2 March and 1 July 1865; Minutes, Medical Faculty, 23 February 1865, Georgetown University Archives.

129. Minutes, Medical Faculty, 1 September 1863, Georgetown University Archives.

130. Samuel C. Busey, *Personal Reminiscences and Recollections* (Washington, D.C., 1895), 177–78.

131. Kayser, 68–70.

132. Horace H. Cunningham, *Doctors In Gray* (Baton Rouge, 1958), 35.

133. W. W. Johnston, "History of the Medical Society," *Transactions and Proceedings of the Seventy-fifth Anniversary of the Medical Society of the District of Columbia* (Washington, D.C., 1894), 53.

134. J. J. Woodward and George A. Otis, eds., *Medical and Surgical History of the Civil War* (Wilmington, N.C., 1990; originially published as *Medical and Surgical History of the War of Rebellion, 1861–65* (Washington, D.C., 1870).

135. Thomas Antisell, "Introductory Address" (presented to the Medical Department of Georgetown College, Washington, D.C., October 1865), 12.

136. Wangensteen and Wangensteen, 426 and 692 n 37. Lister began his researches on the carbolic irrigation of wounds in March 1865; his earliest paper on the subject was dated July 1866.

CHAPTER 3

1. Reverend Patrick H. Brennan, "The First Quarter Century," *Diamond Jubilee of the Georgetown University School of Medicine, 1850–1925* (Washington, D.C. 1925), 19. Brennan graduated from the medical school in 1867 and later entered the Jesuit order.

2. Noble Young, "Valedictory Address" (presented at the Georgetown University commencement, Washington, D.C., 6 March 1866), 3.

3. Robert Emmett Curran, S.J., *The Bicentennial History of Georgetown University, Vol. I., From Academy to University, 1789–1889* (Washington, D.C., 1993), 398.

4. Minutes, Medical Faculty, 9 March 1867 and 25 March 1868, Georgetown University Archives.

5. Brennan, 19. Also: Boyd's Washington Directory, 1866 onwards. In 1866, the medical school was listed as "over 303 F Street North," according to the street numbering of the time; a hairdresser and ice retailing business occupied the first floor.

6. Thomas C. Smith, "History of the Medical Colleges," *Transactions and Proceedings of the Seventy-fifth Anniversary of the Medical Society of the District of Columbia*, 16 February 1894 (Washington, D.C., 1894), 58–66.

7. Minutes, Medical Faculty, 21, 25 March 1868, Georgetown University Archives.

8. Minutes, Medical Faculty, 28 March 1868, Georgetown University Archives.

9. Minutes, Medical Faculty, 6 September 1864, Georgetown University Archives. Antisell's proposals to amend graduation requirements had earlier been tabled at faculty meetings in September 1863 and May 1864, which suggests that his resolution was not

unopposed. Montgomery Johns, for one, had gone on record ("Valedictory Address," Georgetown Medical commencement, Washington, D.C., 3 March 1862) as saying: "I greatly fear that too early clinical observation subjects the young student to the risk, if not the certainty, of becoming a mere blind routinist, and has tended to retard rather than advance the progress of medical science."

10. Hagner was appointed on 24 March 1865; Thompson on 19 November 1866; and Reyburn on 25 January 1867; Minutes, Medical Faculty, Georgetown University Archives.

11. J. Harry Thompson, *Report of the Columbia Hospital for Women and Lying-In Asylum, Washington, D.C.* (Washington, D.C., 1873), 2–6, 247.

12. Minutes, Medical Faculty, 24 March 1865 and 1 October 1870, Georgetown University Archives.

13. George M. Kober, *A Condensed History of the Medical School of Georgetown University* (typescript, 1914, n.p.), 3; Kober Papers, MS C 315, box 11, National Library of Medicine.

14. Minutes, Medical Faculty, 25 January 1867, Georgetown University Archives.

15. Biographical information on Robert Reyburn in this section, unless otherwise indicated, from:

Robert Reyburn, "Fifty Years in the Practice of Medicine and Surgery, 1856–1906" (presidential address presented to the American Therapeutic Society, Washington, D.C., 4 May 1907), 21–22, 38.

"Robert Reyburn," Resolutions adopted by the Medical Society of the District of Columbia, 31 March 1909, *Washington Medical Annals* 8 (1909–10): 136–43.

Martin Kaufman, Stuart Galishoff, and Todd L. Savitt, eds., *Dictionary of American Medical Biography*, (London, 1984), 2:83–84.

Daniel S. Lamb, *Howard University Medical Department: A Historical, Biographical and Statistical Souvenir* (Washington D.C., 1900), 110.

History of the Medical Society of the District of Columbia, 1817–1909 (Washington, D.C., 1909), 281.

Obituary, "Robert Reyburn," *Washington Evening Star*, 26 March 1909.

16. Constance McLaughlin Green, *Washington: A History of the Capital, Vol. 1, 1800–1878* (Princeton, N.J.,1962), 301.

17. Minutes, Medical Faculty, 28 March 1868, Georgetown University Archives.

18. Minutes, Medical Faculty, 11 June 1868, Georgetown University Archives.

19. Minutes, Medical Faculty, 7 August 1868, Georgetown University Archives.

20. W. Montague Cobb, *The First Negro Medical Society* (Washington, D.C., 1939), 9–10. Also: Lamb, 3–8.

21. Elizabeth Blackwell, *Pioneer Work in Opening the Medical Profession to Women: Autobiographical Sketches* (New York and London, 1895), 58–87. Also: Rayford W. Logan, *Howard University: The First Hundred Years, 1867–1967* (New York, 1967), 5.

22. Minutes, Medical Faculty, 19 August 1868, Georgetown University Archives.

23. Cobb, 9–10.

24. Minutes, Medical Faculty, 16 September 1868, Georgetown University Archives.

25. Quoted in Cobb, 9–10.

26. Minutes, Medical Faculty, 23 September 1868, Georgetown University Archives.

27. Lamb, 3–8. Also: Dwight O. W. Holmes, "Fifty Years of Howard University, Part 2," *Journal of Negro History* 3, no. 4 (1918): 370.

28. Minutes, Medical Faculty, October 1861, Georgetown University Archives.

29. Minutes, Medical Faculty, 11 May 1868, Georgetown University Archives.

30. Minutes, Medical Faculty, 13 February and 24 March 1869, Georgetown University Archives.

31. Wyndham D. Miles, ed., *American Chemists and Chemical Engineers* (Washington, D.C.: American Chemical Society, 1976), 9. Antisell did, however, return to Georgetown in 1880 as professor of chemistry. The following year he was named professor emeritus and was awarded an honorary Ph.D. by Georgetown University.

32. Minutes, Medical Faculty, 10, 24 September and 1 October 1868, Georgetown University Archives. A few months later, Thompson became professor of physiology (which Antisell had taught) as well as clinical surgery. Minutes, 16 February 1869.

33. James S. Easby-Smith, *Georgetown University in the District of Columbia,* (New York and Chicago, 1907), 2:83.

34. George M. Kober, "Daniel S. Lamb, a Man of Science" (presented at the Howard University School of Medicine exercises commemorating the fifty years of service of Dr. Daniel Smith Lamb, 1873–1923, Washington, D.C., 7 June 1923), 16. Also: D. S. Lamb, *History of the United States Army Medical Museum, 1861–1917.* The Army Medical Museum is today known as the National Museum of Health and Medicine, located on the Walter Reed Army Medical Center campus in northwest Washington, D.C.

35. Johnson Eliot, "Commencement Address" (presented at the eighteenth annual commencement of the Georgetown College Medical Department, Washington, D.C., 5 March 1867), 7.

36. Frank Bradway Rogers, *Selected Papers of J. S. Billings*, Medical Library Association, 1965, 5–16. Also: "Skulls and Bones," *Washington Evening Star*, 11 July 1885.

37. William K. Beatty, "Daniel Roberts Brower— Neurologist, Psychiatrist, and Medico-Legal Expert," in *Proceedings of the Institute of Medicine of Chicago* (1988), 41:96.

38. Daniel S. Lamb, "Reminiscences of the Old Medical School," *Hoya*, vol. 7, no. 8 (1925), 8.

39. Frank Hastings Hamilton, *A Treatise on Military Surgery and Hygeine* (New York, 1865), 438–9.

40. Thompson, 2.

41. Thompson left Washington in June 1877 bound for Europe in order to place himself "beyond the reach of investigating committees," according to a published report alleging mismanagement of the Columbia Hospital for Women, lack of accountability for public funds, the admission of women on a fee-paying basis in violation of the hospital's charter, and "the concealment of mistakes and wrong-doing." See letter from "A Citizen of Washington" (attributed to Samuel C. Busey), dated October 1877, entitled "An Exposure: The Columbia Hospital and Lying-In Asylum, a Government Institution, with some account of its past and present Management," *Richmond and Louisville Medical Journal* 24 (1877): 406–22. Thompson continued to practice gynecology in Rome, Italy, where he died 4 November 1896.

42. Note of agreement signed by Flodoardo Howard, for Georgetown, and W. P. Johnston, for Columbian, dated 18 March 1868; and Minutes, Medical Faculty, 14, 21, March 1868, Georgetown University Archives.

43. Samuel C. Busey, *Personal Reminiscences and Recollections* (Washington D.C., 1895), 217. Samuel Zola, John A. Long, and Philip A. Caulfield, *Providence Centennial Book, 1861–1961* (Washington, D.C., 1961), chap. 6.

44. "Arrest of Resurrectionists," *Washington Star*, 11, 12 January 1869.

45. E. L. Kayser, *A Medical Center: George Washington University Medical School* (Washington, D.C., 1973), 84–85.

46. Lamb, "Reminiscences," *Hoya*, vol. 7, no. 8 (1925), 8.

47. Kayser, 84–85.

48. Minutes, Medical Faculty, 19 November and 17 December 1866, and 16 September 1867, Georgetown University Archives.

49. Thomas Dwight, "Anatomy Laws Versus Body-Snatching," *The Forum* 22 (1896): 498.

50. James E. Morgan, "Commencement Address" (presented at the twelfth annual commencement of the Georgetown University Medical Department, Washington, D.C., 2 March 1869), 6.

51. *History of the Medical Society of D.C., 1817–1909*, 116–117. Also: "Letters from the People," *Washington Star*, 18 January 1869.

52. A. M. Lassek, *Human Dissection, Its Drama and Struggle* (Springfield, Ill., 1958), 231.

53. Dwight, 499. Although this source does not identify the two D.C. medical schools which paid for Janssen to leave town, the fact that Georgetown and Columbian had a cooperative relationship and both were antagonistic toward Howard suggests they must have been the schools referred to.

54. Llewellyn Eliot to the faculty, 18 February 1884, Medical School Files, Georgetown University Archives.

55. Green, *Washington*, 1:314.

56. Ibid., 274–77, 295, 306.

57. Ibid., 300, 321–22.

58. *Washington Star*, 3 May 1870. This untitled news item referred to black people being allowed to ride trams in Baltimore. It concluded: "As was the case when the experiment was first made here [in Washington], some indignant Caucasians bounced out of the cars when colored people entered, but for the most part the white passengers seemed to stand the equality business with equanimity."

59. *Washington Star*, 20 June 1869.

60. Green, 322.

61. Ibid., 300.

62. *Washington Star*, 17, 18, 20 June 1869, and near issues.

63. Melvin R. Williams, "A Blueprint for Change: the Black Community in Washington, D.C., 1860–70," in *Records of the D.C. Historical Society* 48: 359–393. According to this source, the issue of black suffrage was the main reason Congress again took over the administration of D.C. in 1871.

64. Green, 323.

65. Lamb, 110. Augusta received his medical degree from the University of Toronto and served as a surgeon in the Civil War, brevetted Lieutenant-Colonel. Purvis graduated in medicine from Western Reserve Medical College, Cleveland, Ohio, and served

as an assistant surgeon in the Civil War. Soon after their applications for membership in the Medical Society were rejected, both became full professors at Howard University College of Medicine.

66. "The Colored Question in the Medical Society," *Washington Star*, 17 June 1869. Also: "The Society and Colored Physicians," *History of the Medical Society of the D.C., 1817–1909*, 100–5. Augusta and Purvis were rejected by votes of 57–12 and 55–11 respectively.

67. Senator Charles Sumner, speech to the U.S. Senate, 9 December 1869, quoted in Cobb, 13–14. Also: *Washington Star*, 9 December 1869.

68. *History of the Medical Society of D.C.*, 422.

69. "Medical Society of the District of Columbia: The Color Question Again," *Washington Star*, 4 January 1870.

70. Busey, *Personal Reminiscences*, 277–78.

71. *An Appeal to Congress* (Washington, D.C., 12 January 1870). Also: Busey, 247; Cobb, 16–17; and *History of the Medical Society of D.C.*, 102.

72. Report of the District of Columbia Committee of the Senate, presented 8 February 1870, to accompany Senate bill 511. Also: "Bill to Repeal the Charter of the Medical Society," *Washington Star*, 8 February 1870; Cobb, 18–21; and *History of the Medical Society of D.C.*, 103–5.

73. "The New Medical Society," *Washington Star*, 5 January 1870. Also: Lamb, *Howard University*, 21. (The first officers of the National Medical Society were: Robert Reyburn, D. W. Bliss, A. T. Augusta, S. A. H. McKim, R. J. Southworth, Henry W. Sawtell, John E. Mason, A. W. Tucker, D. C. Patterson, John G. Stephenson, and Charles H. Bowen.)

74. *Transactions of the American Medical Association, Twenty-first Annual Meeting, May 3–6, 1870*, vol. 21, (Philadelphia, 1870). Also: *Washington Star* reports of the AMA Convention, 3–6 May 1870. The only new organization seeking accreditation that did not include black doctors was the Medical Society of the Alumni of Georgetown College. This society, founded in March 1869 and all white, was recognized as an accredited delegation at the 1870 AMA convention, whereas the other four were not.

75. "American Medical Association: The Color Question: Doctors Differ," *Washington Star*, 3 May 1870.

76. Cobb, 21–35.

77. Cobb, 40–41.

78. Nancy B. Paull, *Capital Medicine: A Tradition of Excellence, an Illustrated History of the Medical Society of*

the *District of Columbia* (Encino, Calif., 1994), 67. It is of interest that, when the MSDC finally voted to admit black doctors in 1952, the resolution put to its members was virtually the same as that proposed by Reyburn eighty-two years earlier: "That no qualified physicians applying for membership in the Society shall be denied membership because of race, creed or color."

79. *History of the Medical Society of D.C.*, 101.

80. James D. Morgan, remarks made in memory of Robert Reyburn, *Washington Medical Annals* 8 (1909–10), 141.

81. Lamb, *Howard University*, 23.

82. *History of the Medical Society of D.C.*, 102 and 427.

83. Cox and Bliss were both founder members of Reyburn's National Medical Society—*Washington Star*, 5 January 1870—and supported his cause at the 1870 AMA Convention.

84. Eugene Fauntleroy Cordell, *The Medical Annals of Maryland, 1799–1899* (Baltimore, 1903), 364.

85. *History of the Medical Society of D.C.*, 277.

86. Ibid., 110–12.

87. Busey, *Personal Reminiscences*, 285–293. Also: *History of the Medical Society of D.C., Part 2, 1833–1944* (Washington, D.C., 1947), 30.

88. John Mercer Langston, *From the Virginia Plantation to the National Capitol* (New York, 1969), 328–29.

89. Busey, 290–91. Also: Comments made in *Howard University School of Medicine: Exercises Commemorating the Fifty Years of Service in this School of Dr. Daniel Smith Lamb, 1873–1923* (Washington, D.C., 7 June 1923), 23, 31, 33.

90. *History of the Medical Society of the District of Columbia, Part 2, 1833–1944*, 24–25, 46–47.

91. Lamb, 29–30.

92. *History of the Medical Society of D.C., 1817–1909*, 281, 284.

93. Minutes, Medical Faculty, 16 March 1874; Medical School Catalogues, 1874–75 and 1875–76, Georgetown University Archives.

94. "Robert Reyburn," Resolutions Adopted by the Medical Society of the District of Columbia, 31 March 1909, following the death of Reyburn on 25 March 1909, *Washington Medical Annals* 8 (1909–10).

95. Albert and Mary Cocke, "Hell-Roaring Mike: A Fall From Grace in the Frozen North," *Smithsonian Magazine* (February 1983): 119–37.

96. Curran, 255–56. Also: Joseph T. Durkin, S.J. *Georgetown University* (New York, 1964), 44–49.

97. Minutes, Medical Faculty, 14 March 1868, Georgetown University Archives.

98. Minutes, Medical Faculty and Medical School Catalogues, 1868–1876, Georgetown University Archives.

99. Curran, 309.

100. *History of the Medical Society of D.C.,* *1817–1909,* 26, 240–42. Also: Howard A. Kelly and Walter L. Burrage, *Dictionary of American Medical Biography: Lives of Eminent Physicians of the United States and Canada from Earliest Times* (1928; reprint, Boston, 1971), 178–79. Also: Busey, *Personal Reminiscences,* 25.

101. *History of the Medical Society of D.C.,* *1817–1909,* 286. Also: Remarks by A. A. Snyder on death of Kleinschmidt, *Washington Medical Annals* 4 (March 1905), 260–61. Also: Kelly and Burrage, 706.

102. C. H. A. Kleinschmidt, *The Necessity for a Higher Standard of Medical Education* (Washington, 1878).

103. Georgetown Medical School Catalogues, 1878–79 onwards, Georgetown University Archives. C. H. A. Kleinschmidt, letter to the editor, *Journal of the American Medical Association* (8 August 1890): 231.

104. William G. Rothstein, *American Medical Schools and the Practice of Medicine: A History* (New York and Oxford, 1987), 104. Also: Kleinschmidt, 19.

105. Curran, 398.

106. Georgetown Medical School Catalogue, 1880–81, Georgetown University Archives.

107. Proceedings of the Association of American Medical Colleges, 1880.

108. Rothstein, 104.

109. Joseph T. Durkin, *Georgetown University: The Middle Years, 1840–1900* (Washington, D.C., 1964), 103–9.

110. Reverend Patrick Healy, S.J., *Addresses Delivered at the Nineteenth Annual Commencement of the Medical Department of the University of Georgetown, 19 March 1878* (Washington, D.C., 1878), 5–6.

111. Kelly and Burrage, 372.

112. Johnson Eliot, "Simultaneous Ligation of the Carotid and Subclavian Arteries for Aneurism of the Arteria Innominata," *American Journal of the Medical Sciences* (April 1877): 374.

113. Rothstein, 102.

114. Biographical information on Francis A. Ashford in this section, unless otherwise indicated, from:

    History of the Medical Society of D.C., 1817–1909, 283–84.

    Washington Obstetric and Gynaecological Society, *In Memoriam: Francis Asbury Ashford, M.D.* (Washington D.C., 1883), 15–20.

    Bailey K. Ashford, *A Soldier in Science* (New York, 1934), 6–7.

    Eminent and Representative Men of Virginia and the District of Columbia in the Nineteenth Century (Madison, Wisconsin, 1893), 39.

    Busey, *Personal Reminiscences,* 188–91.

    Easby-Smith, 327.

115. Virginia Miller, "Dr. Thomas Miller and His Times," *Records of the Columbia Historical Society,* vol. 3 (1900): 315.

116. "Children's Hospital," typewritten statement, maybe press release, 1960; library of Children's National Medical Center, Washington, D.C. Incorporated 5 December 1870, Children's Hospital was the third pediatric hospital in the U.S., chartered "for the gratuitous medical and surgical treatment of indigent children without distinction of race, sex, or creed."

117. *In Memoriam,* 17.

118. Minutes, Medical Faculty, 11 September 1874, Georgetown University Archives.

119. Quoted by Easby-Smith, 327.

120. The District of Columbia's first telephone directory, 1878; copies at the Historical Society of the District of Columbia and the library of the Children's National Medical Center. Only eleven physicians are listed as subscribers—among them Joseph Taber Johnson, another Georgetown medical professor—and no hospitals other than Children's.

121. The Central Dispensary was founded by Georgetown professors G. L. Magruder and H. H. Barker, and opened 1 May 1871 at the school on Tenth and E Streets. In 1880, it moved to another building on Tenth Street (between D and E) where more space permitted a few beds for emergency cases and it became known as the Central Dispensary and Emergency Hospital. See *History of the Medical Society of D.C., 1817–1909,* 36; and Busey, 219–21.

122. Busey, *Personal Reminiscences,* 189, 219–22.

123. *Washington Star,* 3 August 1881.

124. J. Howe Adams, *History of the Life of D. Hayes Agnew* (Philadelphia and London, 1892), 220–36.

125. Kaufman, Galishoff, and Savitt, 8.

126. Reyburn, *Fifty Years in the Practice of Medicine and Surgery,* 25–31. See also: Robert Reyburn, *The Assassination of President Garfield* (Washington, D.C., 1905).

127. Healy to Georgetown Medical Faculty, 17 February 1882, Georgetown University Archives.

128. Curran, 319.

129. *History of the Medical Society of D.C., 1817–1909*, 227. Also: "Death of Dr. Young," *Washington Star*, 12, 14 April 1883.

130. Obituary of Johnson Eliot, *Medical and Surgical Reporter*, vol. L (Philadelphia, 1884): 64.

131. Gravestone of Charles H. Liebermann, his wife, and children; section E, lot 246, Rock Creek Cemetery, Washington, D.C.

132. Montgomery County Historical Society, *Genealogical Abstracts from the Montgomery County Sentinel, 1855–1899* (Rockville, Md., 1986), 189. Also: *History of the Medical Society of D.C., 1817–1909*, 232.

133. Busey to Ashford, 12 May 1883, Georgetown University Archives.

134. *In Memoriam*, 18.

135. Bailey K. Ashford, 6–8.

136. *In Memoriam*, 9. Obituary, *Washington Star*, 22 May 1883.

CHAPTER 4

1. *History of the Medical Society of the District of Columbia, 1817–1909* (Washington, D.C., 1909), 319. Also Francis B. Heitman, *Historical Register and Dictionary of the U.S. Army, 1789–1903* (Washington, D.C., 1903), 1:493.

2. Ralph Chester Williams, *The United States Public Health Service, 1798–1950* (Washington, D.C., 1951), 475–76. Howard A. Kelly and Walter L. Burrage, *Dictionary of American Medical Biography: Lives of Eminent Physicians of the United States and Canada from Earliest Times* (1928; reprint, Boston, 1971), 520.

3. Thomas B. Bailey to Dean J. W. H. Lovejoy, 2 November 1883, Georgetown University Archives.

4. Doonan to Dean J. W. H. Lovejoy, 2 November 1883, Georgetown University Archives.

5. Llewellyn Eliot, "Life and Work of Dr. John B. Hamilton," *Virginia Medical Semi-Monthly* 4 (25 August 1899): 293–94.

6. Williams, 475–76; and Eliot, 293–94. Hamilton succeeded in having the MHS reorganized as a career corps of commissioned officers by Act of Congress, 4 January 1889.

7. Walter A. Wells, "The Beginnings of Otolaryngology in Washington: Some Personal Reminiscences," *Medical Annals of the District of Columbia* 20 (February 1951).

8. *Transactions of the Ninth International Medical Congress, September 5–10, 1887* ed. John B. Hamilton (Washington, D.C., 1888).

9. John B. Hamilton, *Response to the Welcome Given the American Delegates at the Berlin Congress, 1890*, National Library of Medicine. Also: James S. Easby-Smith, *Georgetown University in the District of Columbia* (New York and Chicago, 1907) 2:346. Also: Owen H. and Sarah D. Wangensteen, *The Rise of Surgery, from Empiric Craft to Scientific Discipline* (Minneapolis, 1978), 429, 447–48.

10. Martin Kaufman, Stuart Galishoff, and Todd L. Savitt, eds., *Dictionary of American Medical Biography* (London, 1984) 1:321–22.

11. *Washington Post*, 7 February 1884.

12. Report to the Secretary of the Treasury on the Administration of the National Quarantine Service and the Epidemic Fund, (Washington, D.C., 14, 23 February 1884).

13. Kaufman, Galishoff, and Savitt, 321–32.

14. *Annual Report of Providence Hospital, November 1, 1884—October 31, 1885* (Washington, D.C., 1885), 29.

15. Joseph Taber Johnson, "Recent Advances in Abdominal Surgery" (address presented to the Georgetown University Medical Department, Washington, D.C., 3 October 1887), 16.

16. Samuel Zola, John A. Long, and Philip A. Caulfield, *Providence Centennial Book, 1861–1961* (Washington, D.C., 1961), chapter on doctors at Providence.

17. Johnson, 16–17.

18. John B. Hamilton, *Penetrating Pistol-Shot Wound of the Abdomen*, undated pamphlet, National Library of Medicine.

19. *Transactions of the Ninth International Medical Congress*, September 5–10, 1887 (Washington, D.C., 1888), 424.

20. Wagensteen and Wagensteen, 162–63.

21. Ibid., 387.

22. Ibid., 413–17.

23. Ibid., 426–27, 438–43.

24. Ibid., 420, 424–33, 446.

25. Ibid., 233–34.

26. Ibid., 429.

27. Ibid., 317, 426.

28. Ibid., 693, n 48.

29. Hamilton, *Penetrating Pistol-Shot Wound*.

30. Victoria A. Harden, *Inventing the National Institutes of Health: Federal Biomedical Research Policy, 1887–1937* (Baltimore, 1986), 12.

31. John B. Hamilton, "Our Alumnus and His Medical Environment" (presented to the annual meeting of the Alumni Association of the Medico-Chirurgical College, Philadelphia, Penn., 1888).

32. Harden, 13. Also: Kaufman, Galishoff, and Savitt, 1:415–16.

33. Medical School Catalogues, 1892–99, Georgetown University Archives. Kinyoun became a professor in the summer of 1892, but another source (see note 62) suggests he had already been lecturing at Georgetown during the 1891–92 session. Kinyoun left the school in 1899 when the Marine Hospital Service posted him to California.

34. George Kober, (address presented at a dinner honoring J. J. Kinyoun, Washington, D.C., 20 May 1899), *Georgetown College Journal*, June 1899.

35. See chapter 1 ("A Laboratory of Hygeine") of Harden's history of the National Institutes of Health, which traces their origin to the Marine Hospital Service laboratory, first on Staten Island, N.Y., and later in Washington, D.C. She quotes Hamilton's first announcement in the 1888 MHS Annual Report: "In August, 1887, a bacteriological laboratory was established at the port of New York."

36. John B. Hamilton, (toast presented to the Medical Faculty, Georgetown University Medical Department Alumni Dinner, Arlington Hotel, Washington D.C., 23 June 1886).

37. Joseph T. Durkin, S.J., *Georgetown University: The Middle Years, 1840–1900* (Washington, D.C., 1963), 121.

38. Robert Emmett Curran, S.J., *The Bicentennial History of Georgetown University, Vol. I, From Academy to University, 1789–1889* (Washington, D.C., 1993), 398.

39. *The Washington Post*, 15, 19 November and 18 December 1888. Also: *New York Times*, 17 November 1888.

40. Report of the Committee on Specialties, 1869, *Transactions of the American Medical Association*, vol. 20 (Philadelphia, 1869): 111–13.

41. W. W. Johnson, "History of the Medical Society," *Transactions and Proceedings of the Seventy-fifth Anniversary of the Medical Society of the District of Columbia* (Washington, D.C., 1894): 41.

42. Johnson Eliot, "Commencement Address" (presented at the eighteenth annual commencement of the Georgetown College Medical Department, Washington, D.C., 5 March 1867), 6–7.

43. *Transactions of the American Medical Association*, (Philadelphia, 1869), 20:111–13.

44. W. W. Johnson, 41.

45. William G. Rothstein, *American Medical Schools and the Practice of Medicine: A History* (New York and Oxford, 1987), 72–73.

46. Medical School Catalogues, 1874 onwards, Georgetown University Archives.

47. *History of the Medical Society of the District of Columbia, 1817–1909*, 311.

48. Ibid., 284–85. Also: Daniel S. Lamb, *Howard University Medical Department: A Historical, Biographical and Statistical Souvenir* (Washington, D.C.,1900), 6–7, 22–23, 109. Also: Hiram C. Polk Jr., ed., *Transactions of the Southern Surgical Association"* (Philadelphia, 1987), 99:x, lxiv, 23.

49. *History of the Medical Society of the District of Columbia, 1817–1909*, 308. Also: Kelly and Burrage, 176.

50. Ira M. Rutkow, *The History of Surgery in the United States 1775–1900*, vol. 1: *Textbooks, Monographs, and Treatises* (San Francisco, 1988), 166.

51. Easby-Smith, 1:346.

52. Swann M. Burnett, "Persistent Headache," *Journal of the American Medical Association*, (14 January 1899): 62–65.

53. Vivian Burnett, *The Romantick Lady* (New York/London, 1927), 121, 211, 275–76.

54. George Rothwell Brown, *Washington: A Not Too Serious History* (Baltimore, 1930), 317. Also: Vivian Burnett, 113.

55. "Death of Doctor Swann M. Burnett . . . Lord Fauntleroy's Father," *Washington Times*, 18 January 1906. Also: *History of the Medical Society of the District of Columbia, 1817–1909*, 308.

56. Quoted by Easby-Smith, 334.

57. John B. Hamilton, preface to *Lectures on Tumors from a Clinical Standpoint* (Detroit, 1891). Also: Rutkow, 106.

58. Easby-Smith, 338–39.

59. Minutes of the Association of Medical Students of Georgetown University, 1890–91, Georgetown University Archives.

60. O'Malley to Richards, 8 November 1891, Georgetown University Archives.

61. George M. Kober, Kober Papers, box 11, National Library of Medicine. This undated typescript is a brief account of Kober's stewardship as dean, circa 1928.

62. *Washington Star* and *Washington Post*, 9–13 January 1892.

63. O'Malley to Richards, 10 December 1891, Georgetown University Archives. Also: Durkin, 197–99.

64. Richards to Reverend David Buel, S.J., 30 April 1906, Georgetown University Archives.

65. Magruder to Richards, 20 May 1891, Georgetown University Archives.

66. O'Malley to Richards, 10 December 1891, Georgetown University Archives.

67. Magruder to Richards, 31 May 1891, Georgetown University Archives.

68. Wells, 100–101.

69. Llewellyn Eliot, 293–94.

70. History of the Medical Society of the District of Columbia, 1817–1909, 319. Also: Henry D. Hamilton to Francis Tondorf, S.J., 28 July 1924, Tondorf Papers, box 1, folder 4 (correspondence, 1924), Georgetown University Archives.

71. Richards to Kerr, 2 June 1891. Also: Kerr to Richards, 13 June 1891, Georgetown University Archives.

72. Biographical information on James Kerr in this section, unless otherwise indicated, from:

Ross Mitchell and T. Kenneth Thorlakson, "James Kerr, 1848–1911, and Harry Hyland Kerr, 1881–1963: Pioneer Canadian-American Surgeons," The Canadian Journal of Surgery (July 1966) 9:213–20.

Ross Mitchell, "History of Canadian Surgery. Manitoba Surgical Pioneers: James Kerr and H. H. Chown," The Canadian Journal of Surgery (July 1960) 3:281–83.

Who's Who In America 1908–1909, 1047.

John Clagett Proctor, ed. Washington Past and Present (New York, Lewis Historical Publishing: 1930), vol. 3, 518–9.

History of the Medical Society of the District of Columbia, 1817–1909, 332.

James Kerr, Second Introductory Lecture to Students of the Manitoba Medical College, Session 1884–85 (Winnipeg, 1884).

Obituary, Journal of the American Medical Association 61, no. 8 (25 February 1911): 603.

"Dr. Kerr's Funeral: Death of a Noted Surgeon," Washington Evening Star, 3 February 1911.

73. Evidence of Kerr's visit to Edinburgh comes from a remark Kerr made in a 1892 report (see note 79): "We have had no occasion to use any form of drain in amputation wounds. More than once we have, on removing the dressings at the end of one or two weeks, found at the edge of the flaps the blood clot undergoing organization, just as I have seen it in Lister's wards over twenty years ago. . . ." (emphasis added). In the early 1870s, Lister was professor of surgery at the University of Edinburgh. It is possible, though not confirmed, that Kerr met Lister on this occasion.

74. Joseph Leymann, All Sir Garnet: A Life of Field Marshall Lord Wolseley (London, 1964), 180.

75. "Mrs. Laurie Kerr Succumbs at 97 in Hospital Here," Fauquier (Warrenton, Va.) Democrat, 14 July 1949.

76. Transactions of the International Medical Congress, Philadelphia, 1876, ed. John Ashhurst Jr. (Philadelphia, 1877), 535–44.

77. Transactions of the Ninth International Medical Congress, Washington, D.C., September 5–10, 1887, 122.

78. Bell to Kerr, 23 May (year not given), Alexander Graham Bell Family Papers, box 50, Library of Congress. Bell wrote: "How does Laurie enjoy Winnipeg? I have succeeded in inducing my father to come to Washington and I think it not unlikely that the other members of the Bell family may gradually collect around the nucleus formed here. How about the Curs? Any chance of you coming to the States at any time?" This letter also refers to Bell loaning money to Kerr to build a house in Winnipeg, which suggests it was written in or soon after 1880.

79. Washington Past and Present, 519.

80. James Kerr, Report of Some of the Surgical Work at the New Emergency Hospital During the Past Year, (pamphlet reprinted from the Virginia Medical Monthly, September 1892): 4–6.

81. Ibid., 6–16.

82. "Report of the Committee of the Medical Board for the year ending October 31, 1891," Annual Report of Providence Hospital, 1891, 9–10.

83. Easby-Smith, 1:349.

84. Zola, Long, and Caulfield, chapter on doctors at Providence.

85. Mitchell and Thorlakson, 217.

86. In pursuing its ideal of a full-time faculty, Johns Hopkins attempted from the start to limit the professors' clinical work outside the university hospital. Since the highly-qualified men it sought to recruit earned large incomes from private practice, that policy was unsuccessful for many years. This, almost certainly, was why Kerr declined the chair. Halsted, however, both accepted the appointment and refused to give up private practice throughout his long career at Hopkins.

87. O'Malley to Richards, 17 May 1892, Georgetown University Archives.

88. Editorial, The Medical News, 31 December 1892.

89. Durkin, 199–201.

90. Minutes, Medical Faculty, 13 May 1901, Georgetown University Archives. Also: George M. Kober, "Condensed History of Georgetown University Medical School," 1914, typescript, n.p., Kober Papers, box 11, National Library of Medicine, 11.

91. Durkin, 215–23.

92. Ibid.

93. Magruder to Monsignor Satolli, March 1894, Georgetown University Archives.

94. Bailey K. Ashford, *A Soldier In Science* (New York, 1934), 15.

95. Ashford to Kober, 28 October 1919, Kober Papers Collection, box 3, National Library of Medicine. In this letter, Ashford recalled that he and his two brothers had gone through Georgetown "at greatly reduced rates on account of my father's connection with the medical school." Other letters in the Georgetown University Archives show that it was school policy to charge the sons of faculty members 50 percent of the normal tuition fee.

96. Kober, "Condensed History," 8.

97. John B. Marbury to George L. Magruder, 1 November 1884, Georgetown University Archives.

98. Easby-Smith, 357.

99. Ibid.

100. Information on Kerr's actions and expressed opinions in this section, unless otherwise indicated, from: "Majority Report of the Committee on the Curriculum," Minutes, Medical Faculty, 18 June 1895, Georgetown University Archives.

101. Minutes, Association of Medical Students at Georgetown University, 3, 8, 10, 13 November 1893, Georgetown University Archives.

102. Minutes, Medical Faculty, 29 April and 18 June 1895, Georgetown University Archives.

103. Unidentified press clipping, n.d., Medical School Files, 1928, Georgetown University Archives.

104. Richards to La Place, 16 May 1895, Georgetown University Archives.

105. Richards to La Place, 30 May 1895, Georgetown University Archives.

106. Richards to La Place, 30 May and 1 June 1895, Georgetown University Archives. La Place declined the appointment, but accepted the degree, which he had solicited: La Place to Richards, 28 May 1895, Georgetown University Archives.

107. "Majority Report of the Committee on the Curriculum," Minutes, Medical Faculty, 18 June 1895, Georgetown University Archives.

108. Minutes, Medical Faculty, 18 June 1895, and Kerr's resignation note to Richards, Georgetown University Archives.

109. Richards to Kerr, 27 June and 30 June 1895. Also: Kerr to Richards, 28 June 1895, Georgetown University Archives.

110. Minutes, Medical Faculty, 17 September 1895. Also: Magruder to Richards, 18, 27 September 1895, Georgetown University Archives.

111. Magruder to Richards, 29 November 1895, Georgetown University Archives.

112. "Georgetown Medical School Opens for Another Year," *The Washington Post*, 1 October 1895.

113. Magruder to Richards, 8, 22 October 1895, Georgetown University Archives.

114. Noted in Medical School Catalogues, 1896 onwards, Georgetown University Archives.

115. Magruder to Richards, 23 September 1895, Georgetown University Archives. Magruder wrote: "I find that the loss of Dr. Kerr's clinics is being used against us. Is it not possible to obtain from him the exact conditions upon which he will allow the students of our school to attend?" Subsequent correspondence suggests that the issue of the surgery clinics was not resolved, although Georgetown students continued to attend other clinics not controlled by Kerr at Emergency Hospital.

116. Minutes, Medical Faculty, 11, 16 March 1895, Georgetown University Archives. The special meeting on March 11 was "called as a result of a recent conversation with President Richards in regard to the desirability of establishing a Dispensary or Hospital under the control of the Med. school." At the second meeting, "President Richards called attention to the fact of the desirability of having all the Departments of the University close together and that this would be a beginning of the accomplishment of that aim." This seems to be the first time the goal of a "medical center" was raised.

117. Fund-raising letter signed by J. Havens Richards, 25 February 1897, Georgetown University Archives.

118. Constance McLaughlin Green, *Washington: A History of the Capital, 1800–1950* (Princeton, 1962, 1976), 2:64.

119. Magruder to Richards, 23 September 1895 and 4 March 1896.

120. Magruder to Richards, 10 April 1897.

121. "Dr. Kerr's Funeral: Death of a Noted Surgeon," *Washington Evening Star*, 3 February 1911. Also: Land records, Fauquier County Courthouse, Warrenton, Va. Kerr's mansion, Antrim, later known by other names, still stands at 402 Culpeper Street, Warrenton.

122. *Transactions of the Southern Surgical Association* ed. Hiram C. Polk Jr. (Philadelphia, 1987), 99:xi.

123. Minutes, Medical Faculty, 15 October and 9, 26 December 1896; 2 January 1897, Georgetown University Archives. Also: Fehleisen to Magruder, 31 December 1896, and Magruder to Richards, 12 January 1897, Georgetown University Archives.

124. Minutes, Medical Faculty, 18, 24 March 1897, Georgetown University Archives.

CHAPTER 5

1. Biographical information on George Tully Vaughan in this section, unless otherwise indicated, from:

History of the Medical Society of the District of Columbia, 1817–1909 (Washington, D.C., 1909), 386–87.

Richard French Stone, Biography of Eminent American Physicians and Surgeons (Indianapolis, 1898) 3:683.

J. Easby-Smith, Georgetown University in the District of Columbia, 1789–1907 (New York, 1907) 2:105–6.

Martin Kaufman, Stuart Galishoff, and Todd L. Savitt, eds., Dictionary of American Medical Biography (Westport, Conn., 1984), 2:761–62.

Association of Military Surgeons, "Personal records of members, 1901–1914," National Library of Medicine, Washington, D.C.

University of Virginia: Its History, Influence, Equipment, and Characteristics (Charlottesville, Va., 1904).

University of Virginia Alumni Records, UVA Archives.

"Dr. Vaughan, Distinguished Surgeon, Dies," Washington Post, 27 April 1948.

2. Quoted in an unidentified press report dated 14 May 1948, Medical School Files, Georgetown University Archives.

3. Kaufman, Galishoff, and Savitt, 1: 247–48.

4. "List of Medical Publications of the Faculty of Georgetown University School of Medicine," n.d, n.p., circa 1933, Medical School Files, Georgetown University Archives.

5. Stone, 683.

6. Minutes, Medical Faculty, 18, 24 March 1897, Georgetown University Archives.

7. Personal communication from Robert J. Coffey.

8. "Extension of Death Penalty and Lash Urged By Vaughan," Washington Post, 6 June 1932. Letter to The Washington Post, n.d, republished in Papers on Surgery and Other Subjects, by George Tully Vaughan (Washington, D.C:, 1932), 373.

9. George Tully Vaughan, "The Progress of Surgery During the Last Forty Years" (address presented at Gill Memorial Eye, Ear, and Throat Hospital, Roanoke, Va., 12 April 1934, published in Virginia Medical Monthly, March 1935).

10. George Tully Vaughan, "Address to the Graduating Class of the Training School for Nurses of Georgetown University Hospital," n.d., published in his Papers on Surgery, 375–76.

11. George Tully Vaughan, "Address to the Phi Chi Medical Fraternity, Philadelphia," n.d., published in his Papers on Surgery, 384.

12. Patricia L. Faust, ed., Historical Times Illustrated Encyclopedia of the Civil War (New York, 1986), 461.

13. Edgar Erskine Hume, History of the Association of Military Surgeons of the United States, 1891–41 (Washington, D.C., 1941), 25, 46.

14. Personal Papers of Medical Officers and Physicians, Adjutant General's Office, RG 94, boxes 603 and 666, National Archives, Washington, D.C.

15. Remarks by George Tully Vaughan, Georgetown University Hospital Annual Report, October 1926, Georgetown University Hospital Records, Georgetown University Archives, 85–86.

16. Nellie E. Fealy, "Historic Sketch of Georgetown University Hospital, 1897–1926," Georgetown University Hospital Annual Report, 1926, Georgetown University Hospital Records, Georgetown University Archives.

17. Sister Pauline, "History of Georgetown University Hospital," typescript, n.p., Varia, box 19, folder 355, Georgetown University Archives. This detailed account of the hospital's first months is undated and unsigned, but is unmistakeably the work of Sister Pauline, who refers to herself in the third person, except for one lapse in which she has crossed out the pronoun "I."

18. Remarks by George T. Vaughan, Georgetown University Hospital Annual Report, October 1926, 85–86.

19. The Old Georgetown University Hospital, 1898–1947, unsigned typescript, n.p., n.d., Georgetown University Archives, 15.

20. Joseph T. Durkin, S.J., Georgetown University: The Middle Years, 1840–1900 (Washington, D.C., 1963), 215–23.

21. Remarks by Reverend J. Havens Richards, S.J. reported in the Kober Anniversary issue, Georgetown College Journal (March 1920): 264–65, Georgetown University Archives.

22. George M. Kober, "A Condensed History of the Medical School of Georgetown University,"

typescript, n.p., 1914, Kober Papers, box 11, National Library of Medicine, 7.

23. *The Old Georgetown University Hospital, 1898–1947*, 13. Also: Magruder to Medora Riggs, 31 March 1911, Georgetown University Archives. Also: Minutes, Medical Faculty, 6 June 1911, Georgetown University Archives.

24. "Notes on the History of the Georgetown University Hospital," appendix to *The Old Georgetown University Hospital, 1898–1947*.

25. Sister Pauline, "History of Georgetown University Hospital," Georgetown University Hospital Files, Georgetown University Archives.

26. George Kober to Reverend Joseph Himmel, S.J., 14 March 1910 and 15 June 1912, Medical School File, 1907–12, Georgetown University Archives.

27. Kober, 11.

28. Minutes, Medical Faculty, 22 September 1898, Georgetown University Archives.

29. Minutes, Medical Faculty, 28 May 1898, Georgetown University Archives.

30. Minutes, Medical Faculty, 7 May 1901 and 6 June 1911, Georgetown University Archives.

31. George M. Kober, *Reminiscences of George Martin Kober, M.D., LL.D.* (Washington, D.C., 1930), vol. 1. Also: Francis Tondorf, S.J., ed., *Anniversary Tribute to George Martin Kober in Celebration of his Seventieth Birthday by his Friends and Associates* (Washington, D.C., 1920).

32. Kober, typescript, n.p., n.d., (written as the basis of a biographical sketch), Kober Papers, box 1, National Library of Medicine.

33. Kober, "A Condensed History of the Medical School of Georgetown University," 3.

34. Kober to N. P. Colwell, 22 August 1912. Also: Georgetown University School of Medicine Commencement Catalogue, 1873, Georgetown University Archives.

35. U.S. War Department to Kober, 13 June 1929, listing his military postings; Kober Papers, box 3, National Library of Medicine.

36. Letters from J. S. Billings to Kober, Kober Papers, box 3, National Library of Medicine.

37. "Remarks on the Presentation of the Kober Medal to Dr. William H. Welch," *Science* LXVI, no. 1697 (8 July 1927): 21–25.

38. Ibid. Also: Kober to N. P. Colwell, 22 August 1912, Georgetown University Archives.

39. Kober to President and Members of the General Education Board, Rockefeller Foundation,

15 September 1927, Medical School Files, Georgetown University Archives.

40. Ibid. Also: Medical School Catalogue, 1890–91, Georgetown University Archives.

41. George M. Kober, "Discussion on Milk Bacteria," in the *Transactions of the Medical Society of the District of Columbia* (1896), 99. Also: Kober's *Milk in Relation to Public Health* (Washington, D.C., Government Printing Office, 1902).

42. Fielding H. Garrison, *An Introduction to the History of Medicine* 4th ed. (Philadelphia and London, 1929), 583–84. Also: Kober to Colwell, 22 August 1912. Kober's observations on the connection between flies and typhus, reported in 1892 and published in 1895, were proved by Walter Reed and others in 1898.

43. List of Kober's scientific publications; Kober Papers, box 11 (file labeled "Georgetown University undated"), National Library of Medicine. In all, Kober published more than two hundred papers.

44. Samuel Zola, John A. Long, and Philip A. Caulfield, "Radiology Department," in *Providence Hospital Centennial Book, 1861–1961* (Washington, D.C.: 1961).

45. George Tully Vaughan, "The Progress of Surgery During the Last Forty Years," pamphlet reprinted from *Virginia Medical Monthly* (March 1935): 3–4.

46. George Tully Vaughan, "A Few Cases of Surgery in which the Roentgen Ray was Used," *The Military Surgeon* (May 1899).

47. George Tully Vaughan, *The Principles and Practice of Surgery* (Philadelphia and London, 1903), 132–35.

48. Owen H. Wangensteen and Sarah D. Wangensteen, *The Rise of Surgery: from Empiric Craft to Scientific Discipline* (Minneapolis, 1978), 293–95.

49. George Tully Vaughan, "Anesthesia as produced by Schleich, of Berlin," *Virginia Medical Monthly* (January 1906).

50. Wangensteen and Wangensteen, 476–86.

51. Minutes, Medical Faculty, 10 May 1906, Georgetown University Archives.

52. Buel to Kober, n.d., but verifiably May 1906, Georgetown University Hospital Files, Georgetown University Archives.

53. Vaughan, *Principles and Practice of Surgery*, 36.

54. *Journal of the Association of Military Surgeons* XIII (1903): 406.

55. Vaughan, *Principles and Practice of Surgery*, 207.

56. George H. A. Clowes Jr., "The Historical Development of the Surgical Treatment of Heart

Disease," *Bulletin of the History of Medicine* 34, no. 1 (January–February 1960): 29.

57. Stephen L. Johnson, *History of Cardiac Surgery, 1896–1955*, (Baltimore, 1970), 4–5. Also: Garrison, 596.

58. George Tully Vaughan, "A Case of Suture of a Stab Wound of the Heart with Remarks on, and a Table of, the Cases Previously Reported" (presented to the Medical Society of Virginia, Lynchburg, Va., 5–7, November 1901), published in *Virginia Medical Semi-Monthly* (March 1902).

59. Ibid.

60. Performed by H. L. Neitert, surgeon in charge of St. Louis City Hospital, in April 1901. Published in *Philadelphia Medical Journal* (14 December 1901). Neitert reported another heart operation performed on 17 October 1901 in *Philadelphia Medical Journal* (2 May 1902). This patient recovered, but there was apparently doubt as to whether the wound had actually penetrated the heart; credit for the first successful American heart suture is thus generally given to Luther Hill.

61. Johnson, 6. Hill's operation was performed 14 September 1902, and published in the New York *Medical Record* 29 (29 November 1902). He performed it on a thirteen-year-old boy on a kitchen table by the light of a kerosene lamp.

62. George Tully Vaughan, "Suture of Wounds of the Heart," *Journal of the American Medical Association* 52 (6 February 1909): 429–38. Previously presented as presidential address to Association of Military Surgeons of the United States, Atlanta, Ga., 13 October 1908. Also: "Operation on Heart," *Washington Evening Star*, 3 February 1908.

63. "Dr. George Tully Vaughan Complimented by Judge Kimball on His Wonderful Feat of Surgery," *The (Charlottesville, Va.) Daily Progress*, 20 March 1908.

64. *Journal of the American Medical Association* 50, no. 4 (25 January 1908): 300.

65. Vaughan, "Suture of Wounds of the Heart," *Journal of the American Medical Association* 52 (6 February 1909): 429–38.

66. George Tully Vaughan, "Transplantation of the Left Knee Joint" (presented at the first meeting of the Washington Surgical Society, Washington, D.C., 17 March 1911), published in *Surgery, Gynecology, and Obstetrics* (July 1911). Also: "Visitors Praise Dr. Vaughan's Feat," unnamed newspaper clipping, n.d., circa April 1909, Kober scrapbook, Kober Papers, box 22, National Library of Medicine.

67. George Tully Vaughan, "The Arrest of Hemorrhage from Bone by Plugging with Soft Tissues,"

in *Transactions of the Medical Society of Virginia*, 1905, 359. Also: *New York Medical Journal* (17 February 1906). Also: *Journal of the American Medical Association* (9 November 1907). Also: *(Berlin) Deutsche Medizinische Wochenschrift*, (12 December 1907): 2111. Also: *International Clinics* (1908) 4, no. 18: 110. Also: Da Costa, *Modern Surgery*, 6th ed., 1910, 452.

68. *History of the Medical Society of D.C.*, 302.

69. George M. Kober, "Report of the Committee on National Uniformity of Curricula of the Association of American Medical Colleges" (presented at the AMMC meeting, Chicago, 10 April 1905). Also: Wilfred M. Barton, "Kober as Dean," *Georgetown College Journal* (March 1920): 257–58.

70. Minutes, Medical Faculty, 12 May 1904, Georgetown University Archives.

71. Kober's report to the AMMC.

72. Minutes, Medical Faculty, 11 May 1905, Georgetown University Archives.

73. Awarded at Georgetown University Commencement, July 1906, after university president Reverend David Buel had consulted former president Reverend J. Havens Richards on the propriety of bestowing a doctorate in laws on a medical professor. Richards to Buel, 30 April 1906, Medical School Files, Georgetown University Archives.

74. Minutes, Medical Faculty, 11 May 1905, Georgetown University Archives.

75. Medical Faculty Minutes, 12 October 1905 and 11 October 1906, Georgetown University Archives.

76. Kober to Buel, 17 October 1905, Medical School Files, Georgetown University Archives.

77. Flexner Report, 39. (See note 82.)

78. Lester S. King, "The Flexner Report of 1910," *Journal of the American Medical Association* 251, no. 8 (24 February 1984): 1083.

79. Minutes, Medical Faculty, 11 October 1906, Georgetown University Archives.

80. James A. Gannon, "Address to the Alumni on Medical Alumni Day, 8 June 1957," published in the Georgetown University Medical Center *Bulletin* 11, no. 1 (September 1957): 4–9.

81. King, 1084.

82. Abraham Flexner, *Medical Education in the United States and Canada* (New York: Arno Press, 1972). Originally issued as *A Report of the Carnegie Foundation for the Advancement of Teaching (Bulletin Number Four)* (New York, 1910), xi, 14–18.

83. Ibid., 139, 202–3.

84. Ibid., 82–83, 88, 112, 120, 122, 190, 238.

85. Ibid., 13, 140–41.

86. Flexner himself wrote: "I went to Baltimore—how fortunate for me that I was a Hopkins [University] graduate!—where I talked at length with Drs. Welch, Halsted, Mall, Abel and Howell, and with a few others who knew what a medical school ought to be, for they had created one . . . Without this pattern in the back of my mind, I could have accomplished little." *Abraham Flexner: An Autobiography* (rev. ed. New York, 1960), 74.

87. Flexner Report, 12, 206, 235.

88. King, 1085–86.

89. William G. Rothstein, *American Medical Schools and the Practice of Medicine: A History* (New York and Oxford, 1987), 143.

90. Minutes, Medical Faculty, 10 March 1910, Georgetown University Archives. Also: Kober to Pritchett, 10 March 1910, Georgetown University Archives.

91. In 1904, the faculty had considered establishing an "alcove" of medical books at the Carnegie Public Library in Washington, D.C., to benefit students and physicians "as the Library of the Surgeon General's office is not accessible after 4:30 P.M." Minutes, Medical Faculty, 9 December 1904, Georgetown University Archives.

92. James A. Gannon, "Address to the Alumni on Medical Alumni Day," 8 June 1957, reprinted in the Georgetown University Medical Center *Bulletin* 11, no. 1 (September 1957): 4–9.

93. Kober to Himmel, 14 March 1910, Medical School Files, Georgetown University Archives. Also: Minutes, Medical Faculty, 10 March and 14 April 1910, Georgetown University Archives.

94. Minutes, Medical Faculty, 12 May 1910, Georgetown University Archives.

95. Minutes, Medical Faculty, 9 March 1911, Georgetown University Archives.

96. Report of the Committee on the Curriculum, Minutes, Medical Faculty, 12 October 1911, Georgetown University Archives.

97. Minutes, Medical Faculty, 14 December 1911, Georgetown University Archives.

98. Colwell to Kober, 19 July 1912, Minutes, Medical Faculty, Georgetown University Archives. Also: Kober to Colwell, 6 August 1912, Minutes, Medical Faculty, Georgetown University Archives.

99. Minutes, Medical Faculty, 11 April and 7, 13 May 1901, Georgetown University Archives.

100. Financial report 1909–10, Minutes, Medical Faculty, 15 June 1910, Georgetown University Archives.

101. Minutes, Medical Faculty, 12 October 1911, Georgetown University Archives.

102. Minutes, Medical Faculty, 9 May 1912. Also: Kober to A. S. Downing, Minutes, Medical Faculty, 22 June 1912, Georgetown University Archives.

103. Kober to Himmel, 16 August 1911, Medical School Files. Also: Kober to Downing, 22 June 1912, Minutes, Medical Faculty, Georgetown University Archives.

104. Durkin, 92–94.

105. Transcript of Tondorf's course at Johns Hopkins, Tondorf Papers, box 2, folder 18, Georgetown University Archives.

106. Colwell to Kober, 6 July 1912, Minutes, Medical Faculty, Georgetown University Archives.

107. Kober to Colwell, 8, 24 July and 6, 14 August 1912, Minutes, Medical Faculty, Georgetown University Archives.

108. Colwell to Kober, 5 August 1912, Minutes, Medical Faculty, Georgetown University Archives. Also: Colwell to Kober, 19, 29 July and 9 August 1912.

109. Kober to Colwell, 14 August 1912, in Minutes, Medical Faculty, 12 September 1912, Georgetown University Archives.

110. Kober to Himmel, 25 August 1912, Medical School File, 1907–12, Georgetown University Archives. The CME's list of A schools was published in the educational issue of the *Journal of the American Medical Association* (24 August 1912).

111. Colwell to Kober, 29 July and 5 August 1912, Minutes, Medical Faculty, Georgetown University Archives.

112. In a letter to Colwell, Kober quoted Donlon as saying that the CME was placing itself "in a position of legal accountability" in downgrading Georgetown to class B while allowing George Washington Medical School to remain in class A (Kober to Colwell, 17 August 1912). Woodward drafted a letter to the CME that Donlon signed (Minutes, Medical Faculty, 12 September 1912, Georgetown University Archives).

113. Minutes, Medical Faculty, 30 November 1912, Georgetown University Archives.

114. Kober to Donlon, 28 December 1912, Minutes, Medical Faculty, 9 January 1913, Georgetown University Archives.

115. 9 October 1913, Minutes, Medical Faculty, Georgetown University Archives.

116. Kober to Himmel, 15 June 1912, Medical School Files, Georgetown University Archives. Also: Minutes, Medical Faculty, 25 September 1913,

Georgetown University Archives. In the premedical course's first year, 1913–14, thirty-five students enrolled.

117. Minutes, Medical Faculty, 30 November 1912, Georgetown University Archives.

118. Georgetown University School of Medicine Catalogue, 1913–14, Georgetown University Archives.

119. *Transactions of the Southern Surgical Association: Vol. 99, 1987* ed. Hiram C. Polk Jr. (Philadelphia, 1988), x.

120. Walter A. Wells, "The Beginnings of Otolaryngology in Washington: Some Personal Reminiscences," *Medical Annals of the District of Columbia* 20 (February 1951): 99–103.

121. Rothstein, *American Medical Schools*, 160–69.

122. Minutes, Medical Faculty, 3 June 1910, Georgetown University Archives.

123. Minutes, Medical Faculty, 9 February 1905 and 9 March 1911; 12 February 1914, Georgetown University Archives. Also: Kober to Himmel, 9 March 1911, Georgetown University Hospital Records, Georgetown University Archives.

124. Minutes, Medical Faculty, 9 November 1905, 11 November 1909, and 10 November 1910, Georgetown University Archives.

125. Flexner Report, 116.

126. Rothstein, 110–11, 113–15.

127. Minutes, Medical Faculty, 11 November 1909, Georgetown University Archives.

128. Minutes, Medical Faculty, 12 February 1914, Georgetown University Archives.

129. George Tully Vaughan, "Experience at Vera Cruz," *Washington Medical Annals* (January 1915). Also: D. N. Carpenter, "Report of Work at the Field Hospital of the Marine Brigade, Vera Cruz, Mexico," *U.S. Naval Bulletin* 9, no. 1 (January 1915): 177–78.

130. Minutes, Medical Faculty, 8 October 1914 and 11 February 1915, Georgetown University Archives.

131. George Tully Vaughan, "In Memoriam: Dr. Ernest Pendleton Magruder" (presented to the Medical Society of D.C.), published in Vaughan's *Papers on Surgery and Other Subjects*, 389–392.

132. *Georgetown College Record* 28 (October 1919): 50, Georgetown University Archives.

133. Minutes, Medical Faculty, 4 January 1917, Georgetown University Archives.

134. Minutes, Medical Faculty, 12 April 1917, Georgetown University Archives.

135. Thomas G. Frothingham, *The Naval History of the World War, 1917–1918* (Cambridge, Mass., 1926),

157, 202–3. Also: "Status of Germans on Seized Ships is Fixed," *Washington Evening Star*, 6 April 1917.

136. George Tully Vaughan, "Remarks at Epiphany Church Supper to Soldiers and Sailors," 11 June 1919, published in Vaughan's *Papers on Surgery and Other Subjects*, 387–88.

137. Werner Bamberger, "Crewmen Recall U.S. Leviathan," *New York Times*, 9 April 1967.

138. Wangensteen and Wangensteen, 478.

139. Creeden to Surgeon General, n.d., Medical School Files, 1917–18, Georgetown University Archives.

140. *Georgetown College Journal* 27 no. 3 (December 1918): 133, Georgetown University Archives.

141. Medical School Minutes, 9 January 1919, Georgetown University Archives. "Home After Twenty Overseas Trips," (unidentified press report, n.d., circa January 1919), Medical School Files 1917–18, Georgetown University Archives.

142. *Georgetown College Journal* 28 (October 1919): 17.

143. M. Elliot Randolph, *The Wilmer Ophthalmological Institute: The First Fifty Years, 1925–75* (Baltimore, 1975), 7–8.

144. Minutes, Medical Faculty, 23 June 1919, Georgetown University Archives.

145. George Tully Vaughan, "A Case of Ligation (Partial Occlusion) of the Abdominal Aorta for Aneurysm" (paper presented to the American Surgical Association, Washington, D.C., May 1921), published in Vaughan's *Papers on Surgery and Other Subjects*, 94–99.

146. George Tully Vaughan, "Ligation of the Aorta: Necropsy Two Years and One Month after Operation" (paper presented to the American Surgical Association, Washington, D.C., 2 May 1922), published in *Annals of Surgery* (October 1922).

147. George Tully Vaughan, "Aneurysmorrhaphy: Two Cases Treated by Matas' Method" (paper presented to the American Surgical Association, Washington, D.C., 7 May 1913), published in *Annals of Surgery* (July 1913).

148. Loyal Davis, *Fellowship of Surgeons: A History of the American College of Surgeons* (Springfield, Illinois: Thomas, 1960), 477–81.

149. Minutes, Medical Faculty, 13 March 1919, Georgetown University Archives. Also: Bowman to Creeden, 29 December 1920, Georgetown University Hospital Records, Georgetown University Archives.

150. Robert Y. Sullivan, et. al. "Report of an investigation into Georgetown University Hospital as a

teaching institution," 19 October 1920, Georgetown University Archives.

151. Minutes, Medical Faculty, 13 January 1921. Georgetown University Archives. "Summary of Report of Dispensary, May to December 1921," Varia box 19, Georgetown University Archives.

152. Frederick W. Slobe to Col. W. H. Arthur, 9 June 1923, Georgetown University Hospital Records. Georgetown University Archives.

153. Minutes, Medical Faculty, 12 May 1921. Georgetown University Archives.

154. Gannon to Reverend W. Coleman Nevils, S.J., 8 September 1930, Medical School Files, Georgetown University Archives.

155. Minutes, Medical Faculty, 11 March 1920. Georgetown University Archives.

156. Minutes, Medical Faculty, 18 September 1919. Georgetown University Archives.

157. Personal communication from Robert J. Coffey, who as a student attended Tondorf's physiology lectures in 1929.

158. Durkin, 92–94. After the earthquake, the editor of *National Geographic* decided to change the already-printed October 1923 issue to include material on Japan. He commissioned Tondorf to speedily write an article on the seismology of the region—John O. LaGorge to Tondorf, 5, 12 September 1923, Tondorf Papers, box 1, folder 2, Georgetown University Archives.

159. William G. McEvitt, M.D., *The Hilltop Remembered* (Washington, D.C., 1982), 36–37.

160. Edward Parker Luongo, *A Biography of Wallace Yater, M.D.* (n.p., 1982): 29–31.

161. "Dying Boy Led In Prayers of Crash Victims," *Washington Times*, 29 January 1922. Also: "Four Georgetown Students Give Invaluable Aid," *Washington Times*, 30 January 1922. Also: "Last Rites Today," *Washington Herald*, 1 February 1922. The students who helped rescue victims were Hudson Gruenwald of New Orleans, La., Tom O'Brien of New York City, Chris Dyer of Waterbury, Conn., and Thomas Jackovicz of Passaic, N.J.

162. Personal communication from Dr. Thomas C Lee, whose father, John J. Lee, then a medical student at Georgetown, was present at the memorial service for the Knickerbocker Theater victims.

163. Kober to Creeden, 2 September 1924, Medical School Files, Georgetown University Archives.

164. Minutes, Medical Faculty, 11 March 1920. Georgetown University Archives.

165. Minutes, Medical Faculty, 12 February 1920. Georgetown University Archives.

166. "The Clinic," *Boston Evening Transcript*, 29 September 1920.

167. George Tully Vaughan, "A Vindication of Vivisection" (presented to the Georgetown University School of Medicine, Washington, D.C., 16 May 1920), published in Vaughan's *Papers on Surgery and Other Subjects*, 364–65.

168. Tondorf Papers, box 2, folder 15, Georgetown University Archives.

169. Maxwell Z. Woodhall to Reverend John B. Creeden, S.J., 19 June 1919, Medical School Files, Georgetown University Archives.

170. William C. Braisted to Congress, 21 June 1919, Medical School Files, Georgetown University Archives.

171. "John D. Rockefeller adds $100,000,000 to Funds of Two Boards as Christmas Gift," *New York Herald*, 25 December 1919.

172. Bailey K. Ashford, *A Soldier in Science* (New York:, 1934), 96–98.

173. "Brave Aspirer after Truth," *Georgetown Medical Bulletin* 14, no. 4 (May 1961): 319. Also: William Fitzgerald, "Medical Men of Georgetown," *Georgetown Medical Bulletin* 19, no. 2 (November 1965): 102.

174. Ashford to Kober, 28 October 1919, Kober Papers, box 3, National Library of Medicine.

175. Garrison to Creeden, 1 December 1919, Medical School Files, Georgetown University Archives.

176. "Rockefeller Fund Gives $1,675,000: Scores of Universities, Colleges and Medical Schools are Latest Beneficiaries," *New York Herald*, n.d., Medical School Files, 1919–20, Georgetown University Archives.

177. Minutes, Medical Faculty, 13 July 1920, Georgetown University Archives.

178. Nevils to ?, n.d., circa 1922–23, Medical School Files, 1921–24, Georgetown University Archives.

179. George Kober, account of his stewardship as dean, delivered at faculty meeting, 4 October 1928, Kober Papers, box 11, National Library of Medicine.

180. Randolph, *The Wilmer Ophthalmological Institute*, 8–13.

181. Statement of MSDC Committee, n.d., Kober Papers, box 5, National Library of Medicine.

182. Kober to Wilmer, 17 April 1924, Kober Papers, box 5, National Library of Medicine.

183. "Dr. William Holland Wilmer Returning to Georgetown U." *Washington Star*, 16 September 1934.

184. "Dr. Wilmer Estate Valued at $292,667," *Washington Star*, 10 April 1936.

185 "Georgetown University Medical School Finances," Medical School Files, 1926, Georgetown University Archives.

186. George Kober, remarks made at a dinner to celebrate the fiftieth anniversary of his graduation in medicine, Kober Papers, box 1, National Library of Medicine.

187. Kober to President and Members of the General Education Board, Rockefeller Foundation, 15 September 1927, Medical School Files, Georgetown University Archives.

188. Agar to Kober, 5 October 1927, Medical School Files, Georgetown University Archives.

189. W. W. Brierley to Kober, 25 November 1927, Medical School Files, Georgetown University Archives.

190. Kober, remarks at fiftieth anniversary dinner. The surviving classmate was Charles V. Petteys, who attended the dinner.

191. "Statement of Trust Funds," 1 January 1926, Medical School Files, 1926, Georgetown University Archives.

192. Harold Zehner, "George Martin Kober, 1850–1931," Georgetown University Medical Center Bulletin 7, no. 6 (July 1954): 202.

193. Kober to Donlon, 26 June and 11 July 1917, Medical School Files, Georgetown University Archives.

194. Ashford to Kober, 13 May 1925, Kober Papers, box 3, National Library of Medicine. Also: Kober to Lyons, 15 June 1925, Medical School Files, Georgetown University Archives.

195. Kober to Nevils, 1 September 1928, Medical School Files. Also: Minutes, Medical Faculty, 14 June 1928, Georgetown University Archives.

196. James Gannon, remarks at a fundraising reunion dinner of the medical alumni, held 18 May 1927, A Plea for a Building and Endowment Fund of the Medical and Dental Schools, Georgetown University, May 1927, Medical School Files, Georgetown University Archives.

197. "Father Summers Dies in New York: Perfector of Lie Detector Succumbs to Coronorary Thrombosis," Washington Star, 27 September 1938. Also: "Reverend W. G. Summers of Fordham Dead," New York Times, 26 September 1938.

198. Kober to Lyons, 20 July 1928, Kober Papers, box 4, National Library of Medicine.

199. Lyons to Kober, 26 August 1928, Kober Papers, box 4, National Library of Medicine.

CHAPTER 6

1. Architect's drawing of proposed medical school building on Thirty-seventh Street, Georgetown, Medical School Files, 1926–31, Georgetown University Archives.

2. Minutes, Georgetown University Board of Directors, 27 August 1928. Also: Walter C. Hess, "The History of Georgetown University School of Medicine, 1900–1930," Georgetown Medical Bulletin 17, no. 4 (May 1964): 244.

3. George Kober to Reverend W. Coleman Nevils, 18 October 1928, Medical School Files, Georgetown University Archives.

4. Minutes, Georgetown University Board of Directors, 8 October 1928. Also: Various unidentified press reports, Medical School Files, 1928, Georgetown University Archives.

5. Maryland Provincial to Reverend W. Coleman Nevils, 20 November 1928, Medical School Files, Georgetown University Archives.

6. Account submitted by George A. Didden, architect, to Nevils, 28 January and 10 June 1929, Medical School Files, Georgetown University Archives.

7. Personal communication from Jerome Coffey.

8. This and other reminiscences of the medical school in this section, unless otherwise identified, are from recorded conversations between the author and Robert J. Coffey.

9. Georgetown Medical School Catalogue, 1928–29, Georgetown University Archives.

10. "Many Medical Students Refused by Georgetown U.," Washington Post, 23 August 1928. Different sources give varying numbers for the freshmen enrollment of 1928. The medical faculty minutes (14 June 1928) record that the class would be limited to 140; but the 1928–29 catalogue lists 155 freshmen by name, and the Rypins Report of 1932 (see note 24) lists 160. The latter number is most likely accurate.

11. Edward Parker Luongo, A Biography of Wallace Mason Yater, M.D. (n.p., 1982), 29.

12. Reverend John B. Creeden, S.J. to Madigan, 25 July 1922, Alumni Files, Georgetown University Archives.

13. Document headed "Dr. Gannon's Letter to the Executive Faculty," unsigned, n.d., Medical School Files, 1928, Georgetown University Archives. A letter from the Georgetown Clinical Society, commenting on this controversy and dated 13 January 1928, suggests that Gannon's complaint was made around the same time.

14. Statement of Henry Fletcher and witness statement of faculty members; both dated 30 July 1932, Medical School Files, Georgetown University Archives.

15. Walsh to Madigan, 1 August 1932, Medical School Files and Alumni Files, Georgetown

University Archives. Gipprich and Morgan to Nevils, 12 September 1932, requesting a reference for Madigan, on which Nevils wrote "Not approved," Medical School Files, Georgetown University Archives.

16. Personal communication from Robert J. Coffey

17. Morgan to Nevils, 11 August 1931, Medical School Files, Georgetown University Archives.

18. M. W. Ireland and William D. Cutter, AMA Council on Medical Education and Hospitals' report on Georgetown medical school, inspected 9–11 April, 1933. Also: Fred Zapffe, secretary of the AAMC, to Eugene Whitmore, 18 December 1933, Medical School Files, Georgetown University Archives.

19. Note written on unidentified press report headed "New York January Examination," n.d. Medical School Files, 1931, Georgetown University Archives.

20. "Medical Building to be Used Feb. 3," unidentified press report, Medical Faculty Files, 1930 Georgetown University Archives.

21. Personal communication from Robert J. Coffey

22. Minutes, Medical Faculty, 6 February 1930 Georgetown University Archives. Also: "Financial Statement for the New Medical & Dental Building December 24, 1929." Medical school files, Georgetown University Archives.

23. Medical School Catalogue, 1931–32 Georgetown University Archives.

24. Harold Rypins, *Report on Georgetown University Medical School*, 27 December 1932, Medical School Files, Georgetown University Archives. Rypins, secretary of the New York State Board of Medical Examiners inspected the school 17–19 November 1932.

25. Note on Enrollment, 29 September 1931 Medical School Files, 1931, Georgetown University Archives.

26. William G. Rothstein, *American Medical Schools and the Practice of Medicine: A History* (New York and Oxford, 1987), 148–49.

27. Rypins' Report, for example, pointed out that only a third of the school's income was being spent on instruction. It commented: "Whether the profits from students' fees go into the pockets of the stock-holders as was the case formerly in commercial medical schools, or into the construction of buildings for the improvement of the medical school, makes very little difference to the student so long as in either case he is not given a reasonable return on his investment of time or money."

28. Nevils to William Wilmer, 17 April and 15 May 1929, Medical School Files, Georgetown University Archives. Also: "Dr. Foote heads Medical Society," *Evening Star*, 2 May 1929. Also: Foote to Nevils, 10 November 1930, Medical School Files, Georgetown University Archives.

29. Reverend John L. Gipprich, S.J., curriculum vitae, Varia 1, box 4, Georgetown University Archives.

30. W. J. Morgan to W. Coleman Nevils, 12 July 1930, Medical School Files, Georgetown University Archives.

31. Luongo, 37–55. Also: Wallace Yater to Wilfred Barton, 23 February 1928, Medical School Files, Georgetown University Archives. Also: Minutes, Medical Faculty, 15 February 1928, Georgetown University Archives.

32. Several obituaries, all unidentified press reports, n.d., Medical School Files, 1930, Georgetown University Archives.

33. Minutes, Medical Faculty, 10 April 1930, Georgetown University Archives. Also: "A Preliminary Meeting of the Personnel Committee," 25 May 1931, Medical School Files, Georgetown University Archives. Also: Walter Summers to George Kober, 16 January 1929, Medical School Files, Georgetown University Archives.

34. Luongo, 37–55.

35. Robert J. Coffey, "Experiences of a Surgeon at G.U., 1928–69," History of Medicine Lecture, 22 May 1982, Dahlgren Medical Library, Georgetown University Medical Center, audiotape.

36. Personal communication from Robert J. Coffey.

37. Luongo, 61.

38. *World Who's Who in Science: A Biographical Dictionary of Notable Scientists from Antiquity to the Present* (Hannibal, Mich., 1968), 1113.

39. Luongo, 66. Also: List of the Medical Publications of the Faculty of Georgetown University School of Medicine, pamphlet, n.d., circa 1933, Medical School File January–April 1932, Georgetown University Archives.

40. Walter G. Summers's alumni file, Georgetown University Archives. Tondorf obituary, Associated Press, Washington, 29 November 1929, Tondorf Papers, Georgetown University Archives.

41. Luongo, 54.

42. J. Markowitz to Finance Committee, 8 June 1931, Medical School Files, Georgetown University Archives.

43. Jacob Markowitz, *Textbook of Experimental Surgery* (Baltimore, Md., 1937), chapters 3 and 4. Also: "Societies Gird for Georgetown University Fight on Vivisection," *Washington Herald*, 22 December 1930.

44. Markowitz to Nevils, 31 January 1931, Medical School Files, Georgetown University Archives.

45. "Vivisection Dog Thief Fined $25," *Washington Star*, 4 April 1931.

46. "Transplanted Heart and Dead-Alive Cat are Viewed at Georgetown University," *New York Times*, 29 March 1931. Also: Markowitz's *Textbook*, 430. Also: Luongo, 72. More than thirty years later, when Markowitz returned to Georgetown as a visiting lecturer, the local press recalled the experiment, noting: "Markowitz, Yater, and two Mayo Clinic researchers are now cited as the first to transplant hearts between dogs—and, because of this, as pioneers in the currently important research in human organ transplants." "Markowitz at Georgetown University: Pioneer in Transplants Returns," *Washington Star*, 26 October 1965. This was three years before the first human heart transplant was performed.

47. Markowitz's *Textbook*, 1–5.

48. Luongo, 64, 66–67, 69.

49. Sworn statement by Yater and Markowitz of complaint against Bennett, 31 March 1931. Also: Yater to Nevils, 1 April 1931, Medical School Files, Georgetown University Archives. Also: Minutes, Medical Faculty, 11 March and 10 April 1931, Georgetown University Archives. Also: Luongo, 67.

50. Reverend Edward C. Phillips to Reverend W. Coleman Nevils, 20 July 1932, Medical School Files, Georgetown University Archives.

51. Willson to Nevils, 23 March 1931, Medical School Files, Georgetown University Archives.

52. Statement for publication in the Georgetown *Hoya*, dated 13 February 1933, Medical School Files, Georgetown University Archives. Also: John Rose to Mark Bauer, 23 September 1965, Yater Faculty File, Georgetown University Archives. Also: "Yater Re-elected [Secretary-General, ACP]," *Washington Post*, 4 April 1965.

53. "A Preliminary Meeting of the Personnel Committee," 25 May 1931, and Nevils to Markowitz, 17 June 1931, Medical School Files, Georgetown University Archives.

54. Yater to Nevils, 22 June 1931, Medical School Files, Georgetown University Archives. Also: Luongo, 75–76.

55. Louis Titus (Markowitz's lawyer) to Nevils, 1 July 1931, and Nevils to Markowitz, 6 July 1931, Medical School Files, Georgetown University Archives.

56. Nevils to Willson, 24 June 1932, Nevils to Markowitz, 1 July 1932, and Gannon to Nevils, 31 July 1933, Medical School Files, Georgetown University Archives. Also: Nevils to George E. Hamilton (Georgetown University's lawyer), 28 September 1932, Markowitz Faculty File, Georgetown University Archives.

57. Willson to Nevils, 23 March 1931, Medical School Files, Georgetown University Archives.

58. Nevils to Reverend Hunter Guthrie, 9 July 1949, W. G. Morgan Faculty File, Georgetown University Archives. Hearing of Morgan's death in 1949, Nevils wrote from retirement to the then university president to recount the circumstances of Morgan's appointment as dean in 1931. He recalled that "these same protesting doctors who happened to have been very special friends of mine felt that Fr. G.'s tactics etc. were due to the fact that he had the Provincial's ear etc. which actually happened to be true though I had not even hinted at the same."

59. Louis B. Wilson, director of the Mayo Clinic and president of the AAMC, to an unidentified New York physician, 7, 14 July 1932, Medical School Files, Georgetown University Archives.

60. Phillips to Nevils, 20 July 1932, Medical School Files, Georgetown University Archives.

61. W. G. Morgan Faculty File, Georgetown University Archives. Includes unidentified newspaper report, "Dr. William G. Morgan Heads American Medical Association," 12 July 1929.

62. Nevils to Reverend Hunter Guthrie, 9 July 1949, W. G. Morgan Faculty File, Georgetown University Archives. (See note 58.) Also: Nevils to Phillips, 26 August 1931, Medical School Files, Georgetown University Archives.

63. Wilmer to Nevils, 24 October 1929, W. H. Wilmer Faculty File, Georgetown University Archives. Also: Nevils to George Kober, 19 October 1929, Kober Papers, National Library of Medicine.

64. Nevils to Irvin Abell, 10 February 1932, and Gipprich to Nevils, 6 February 1933, Medical School Files, Georgetown University Archives.

65. Minutes, Medical Faculty, 14 February 1929, Georgetown University Archives.

66. Gannon to Morgan, 12 July 1933, and Gipprich to Nevils, 16 February 1933, Medical School Files, Georgetown University Archives.

67. James Cahill, Report on the Department of Surgery, February 1933, Medical School Files, Georgetown University Archives.

68. John Foote, "Memorandum of Suggested Recommendations to the Faculty," March 1930; "Personal Notes to Father Rector," and Foote to Nevils,

13 March 1930, Medical School Files, Georgetown University Archives.

69. Memorandum headed "Department of Surgery," 1933, Medical School Files, Georgetown University Archives.

70. Morgan to Nevils, 12 July 1933, Medical School Files, Georgetown University Archives.

71. Nevils to Vaughan, 17 July 1933, Medical School Files, Georgetown University Archives.

72. Nevils to Abel, 10 February 1932. Also: Gipprich to Nevils, 6 February 1933. Several letters of this period show that Georgetown was trying to recruit only Catholics for the chair of surgery and other appointments. In a letter to Nevils' successor, the Provincial, Edward Phillips, made it plain that this policy had been decided in Rome: "The ideal of having an all-Catholic staff for our schools, and the mandatory regulation of Very Reverend Father General that no new non-Catholic Deans should be appointed to our schools should be kept in mind and carried into practice as far as our circumstances permit." Phillips to Arthur O'Leary, 20 October 1934, Medical School Files, Georgetown University Archives.

73. *Who's Who in the Nation's Capital, 1938–39* (Washington, D.C., 1939), 134.

74. List of the Medical Publications of the Faculty of Georgetown University School of Medicine, pamphlet, n.d., circa 1933, Medical School File, January–April 1932, Georgetown University Archives.

75. Nevils to Abel, 10 February 1932, Medical School Files, Georgetown University Archives.

76. "Inventor of Artificial Heart Joins Georgetown Faculty," *Washington Star*, 23 July 1933. Also: Gibbs to Morgan, 21 November 1934, Medical School Files, Georgetown University Archives.

77. Gannon to Nevils, 31 July 1933, Medical School Files, Georgetown University Archives.

78. Nevils to Guthrie, 9 July 1949, W. G. Morgan Faculty File, Georgetown University Archives. (See note 58.)

79. Morgan to Nevils, 3 August 1934, and Nevils to Morgan, 11 August 1934, Medical School Files, Georgetown University Archives.

80. Reverend John L. Gipprich, S.J., curriculum vitae, Varia 1, box 4, Georgetown University Archives.

81. Morgan to Nevils, September 14, 1934, Medical School Files, Georgetown University Archives.

82. Read and discussed at a preliminary meeting of the personnel committee, 25 May 1931, Medical School Files, Georgetown University Archives.

83. Harold Rypins, Report on Georgetown Medical School, 16 April 1934, result of inspection performed 3–5 April 1934.

84. Rothstein, 148–49.

85. Phillips to O'Leary, 11 December 1934, Medical School Files, Georgetown University Archives.

86. The report of the 1935 inspection is missing from the medical school records. But the 1949 AMA/AAMC report noted that "on the basis of the survey carried out February 11–13, 1935, Georgetown University medical school was placed on confidential probation" and that another inspection, 10–11 April 1939, "failed to show sufficient improvement to justify removal from the confidential probation status," from "Georgetown University School of Medicine: Outline of Developments Since the 1939 Survey."

87. Morgan to Nevils, 24 February 1935, and Nevils to Morgan, 6 March 1935, Medical School Files, Georgetown University Archives. Morgan's resignation became effective 1 July 1935.

88. Nevils to Guthrie, 9 July 1949, W. G. Morgan faculty file, Georgetown University Archives.

89. Medical faculty (fourteen signatures) to Nevils, 5 June 1935, Medical School Files, Georgetown University Archives.

90. Resolution passed at a meeting of the Department of Surgery, 28 October 1930. Also: Gannon to Nevils, 8 April 1931, Georgetown University Hospital Files, Georgetown University Archives.

91. Report of AAMC inspection of Georgetown University School of Medicine, 1938, Medical School Files, Georgetown University Archives.

92. Untitled document announcing the cancer clinic held at the medical school, 12 April 1935, Medical School Files, Georgetown University Archives.

93. "New Clinic Opens at GU Hospital," *Washington Star*, 23 February 1938.

94. "Parran Addresses Medical Alumni," *Washington Star*, 18 September 1936. Also: Program of the Second Annual Alumni Extension Course, and O'Leary to Cahill, 5 October 1938, Medical School Files, Georgetown University Archives. Also: "Girl's Spleen Removed Successfully," *Washington Post*, 14 September 1938. Also: "A Miracle of Surgery," *Washington Herald*, 13 September 1938.

95. Samuel Zola, John A. Long, and Philip A. Caulfield, "Doctors at Providence Hospital," in *Providence Hospital Centennial Book, 1861–1961* (Washington, D.C., 1961), Also: Minutes, Executive Faculty, November 1934.

96. "D.C. Surgeon Details Operation to Restore Scalps Torn Away," *Washington Star*, 28 October 1937. Also: "New Scalps Grown: D.C. Surgeon Tells of Operations," *Washington Herald*, 28 October 1937.

97. Louis B. Wilson to ?, 14 July 1932, Medical School Files, Georgetown University Archives.

98. Personal communications from Robert J. Coffey.

99. Unsigned memorandum, 1935, Medical School Files, Georgetown University Archives.

100. Nevils to Phillips, 21 September 1934, Medical School Files, Georgetown University Archives.

101. "Outline Specification: Animal House for Georgetown University Medical School," 11 January 1932. Also: unsigned memorandum, 1935, Medical School Files, Georgetown University Archives.

102. Medical School Catalogue, 1938–39, Georgetown University Archives.

103. Personal communication from Robert J. Coffey.

104. Personal communications from Robert J. Coffey and Mary Catherine Coffey. Wedding report, *Washington Post*, 29 September 1939.

105. AAMC Report on Georgetown University School of Medicine, inspected 3–6 April 1938, Medical School Files, Georgetown University Archives.

106. Executive Medical Faculty to the President and Directors of Georgetown College, 17 November 1938, Medical School Files, Georgetown University Archives.

107. O'Leary to Executive Medical Faculty, 8 December 1938, Medical School Files, Georgetown University Archives.

108. Report on Georgetown University School of Medicine, inspected 13–15 November 1939, Medical School Files, Georgetown University Archives.

109. John C. Rose, "Dean's Page," *Georgetown Medical Bulletin* 18, no. 4 (May 1965): 198.

110. Fred C. Zapffe to O'Leary, 9 December 1939, Medical School Files, Georgetown University Archives. This favorable report seems odd, given that the AMA had inspected the school again in April 1939 and saw no reason to lift its confidential probation (see note 86); it did not restore Georgetown to full approval until 1949.

111. "Alumni to Honor Dr. John Moorhead," *Washington Times-Herald*, 23 March 1942. Also: "Surgery Divining Rod Used By Physician at Pearl Harbor," *Washington Star*, 24 March 1942.

112. O'Donnell to Bunn, 27 March 1953, Medical School Files, Georgetown University Archives.

113. Personal communication from Robert J. Coffey.

114. "D.C. Medical Schools Cooperate in Plans to Speed Graduations," *Washington Star*, 21 December 1941. Also: "Medical Colleges Plan 3-Year Study," *New York Times*, 22 December 1941. Also: "Petition" from six students, October 1942, Medical School Files, Georgetown University Archives.

115. "Medical School Faculties to Study Gas Warfare," *Washington Star*, 17 August 1942.

116. Luongo, 123.

117. "Dr. J. A. Cahill, Prominent Surgeon, Dies," *Washington Post*, 21 October 1942. Also: "Dr. J. A. Cahill Jr., Surgeon, Educator," *New York Times*, 21 October 1942.

118. *Ye Domesday Booke*, Georgetown University Yearbook (Washington, D.C., 1915), Georgetown University Archives.

119. *Who's Who in the Nation's Capital, 1938–39* (Washington, D.C., 1939), 734. F. R. Sanderson's curriculum vitae, Faculty Files, Georgetown University Archives.

120. "Dr. Fred Sanderson, 85, Dies; former Chief Surgeon at GU," *Washington Post*, 13 February 1979. Also: "Fred R. Sanderson dies at 85; Retired Surgeon," *Washington Star*, 13 February 1979.

121. "Dr. J. A. Cahill Critically Ill," *Washington Herald*, 3 February 1936. Also: "Dr. James Cahill Out of Danger," *Washington Post*, 5 February 1936.

122. "Dr. Sanderson Will Head D.C. Medical Group," *Washington Post*, 7 May 1942.

123. F. R. Sanderson Faculty File, Georgetown University Archives. Also: Personal communication from Mary Catherine Coffey.

124. Document headed: "Re: Georgetown Medical School rating in Journal of American Medical Association—May 8, 1943," later attached to 17 November 1938 letter from executive faculty to president and directors of Georgetown University, Medical School File, 1938, Georgetown University Archives.

125. Wall to McCauley, 12 June 1945; McCauley to Gorman, 15 June 1945; and Wall to Gorman, 19 June 1945, Medical School Files, Georgetown University Archives. Also: Luong, 125–6.

126. Wall to McCauley, 12 June 1945, asking McCauley to read it out in his absence at the executive faculty meeting on 14 June 1945, Medical School Files, Georgetown University Archives.

127. Yater to Gorman, 19 June 1945, Medical School Files, Georgetown University Archives.

128. McCauley to Gorman, 15 June 1945, Medical School Files, Georgetown University Archives. The annual bill for McCauley's services for the period 1 July 1944 to 30 June 1945 had been presented eighteen days earlier—Gorman to McCauley, 28 May 1945.

129. McCauley to Gorman, 14 June 1946, and Gorman to McCauley, 23 July 1946, Medical School Files, Georgetown University Archives.

130. Yater to Gorman, 24 September 1945, Medical School Files, Georgetown University Archives. Also: Luongo, 123–24.

131. Gorman to Yater, 28 September 1945, Medical School Files, Georgetown University Archives.

132. This handwritten draft, now attached to other correspondence relating to Yater's resignation in the Medical School Files, is unsigned and undated. The writing and text, however, reveal that it was written by Gorman soon after his meeting with Yater and Walsh in June 1945. In it, Gorman announced that "simultaneously with this letter" he was sending out a request to four people named by Yater "to suggest names for a full-time medical man qualified to act as Dean." Gorman also said he was appointing a five-man committee, headed by McCauley, "to push the question of a full-time Dean and gather the necessary information."

133. McCauley to Gorman, 7 July 1945, Medical School Files, Georgetown University Archives.

134. Wall to Gorman, 3 October 1945, Medical School Files, Georgetown University Archives.

135. Wall Faculty File, Georgetown University Archives. Also: Obituary, *Washington Times Herald*, 19 September 1952.

136. Robert C. Rush, secretary of the Georgetown Medical Alumni Club, to Gorman, 12 October 1945, Medical School Files, Georgetown University Archives.

137. John Rose to Mark Bauer, 23 September 1965, and Gerard Campbell to Yater, 22 November 1965, Yater Faculty File, Georgetown University Archives. Also: Yater to Campbell, 24 November 1965, Medical School Files, Georgetown University Archives.

138. Georgetown University School of Medicine commencement program, May 1976, Georgetown University Archives.

139. *The Old Georgetown University Hospital, 1898–1947*, unsigned, typescript, n.p., 42–43; Georgetown University Archives. Stephen W. Nealon Jr., "Georgetown University's New Hospital Opens," Georgetown University Medical Center *Bulletin* 1, no. 3 (October–November 1947).

CHAPTER 7

1. "Reverend McNally to Head GU Medical School," *Washington Post*, 15 September 1946. Curriculum vitae, Reverend Paul McNally's personal file, Georgetown University Archives.

2. Unsigned note, Reverend Paul McNally's personal file, Georgetown University Archives.

3. John F. Stapleton, *Upward Journey: The Story of Internal Medicine at Georgetown, 1851–1981* (Washington, D.C., 1996), 93–94.

4. Ibid., 95.

5. Personal communications from Robert J. Coffey and John C. Rose.

6. "Medical Men of Georgetown," *Georgetown Medical Bulletin* 21, no. 2 (November 1967): 87–88. Also: W. E. Baensch, "The Two Most Unforgettable Characters I've Ever Met," GUMC *Bulletin* 8, no. 1 (September 1954): 4–6. Also: Medical School Records, 1947 file, Georgetown University Archives. Also: Obituary, *Washington Post*, 3 November 1972.

7. Tuohy to Gorman, 10 March 1947, Medical School Files, Georgetown University Archives. Also: "Dr. Edward Tuohy, 51, Anesthesiologist, Dies," *Washington Evening Star*, 14 January 1959.

8. Murray Copeland, "Portraits of Georgetown: Charles Geschickter," GUMC *Bulletin* 12, no. 4 (March 1959): 163–65.

9. Faculty and Medical School Files, 1947, Georgetown University Archives. Also: "Dr. Copeland Decorated for Pacific War Service," *Washington Evening Star*, 15 March 1950. Also: Personal communication from Robert J. Coffey.

10. John W. Walsh, "Medical Men of Georgetown," *Georgetown Medical Bulletin* 20, no. 2 (November 1966): 113–15. Also: Personal communication from John C. Rose.

11. Personal communication from Robert J. Coffey. Edward Parker Luongo, *A Biography of Wallace Mason Yater, M.D.* (n.p., 1982), 134–43.

12. Personal communication from Robert J. Coffey. Also: Coffey to Hussey, 3 August 1961, R. J. Coffey Faculty File, Georgetown University Archives.

13. Personal communication from John C. Rose. Also: A memorandum to Dean McNally dated October 1946 (Medical School Files, Georgetown University Archives) noted that of 366 students enrolled, 158 were military veterans.

14. Six women enrolled in the 1947–48 freshman class. Report on student enrollment, 30 October 1947, Medical School Files, Georgetown University Archives. A seventh, Sarah Stewart, enrolled as a junior and in 1949 became the first woman to graduate in medicine from Georgetown. She was later acclaimed for outstanding contributions to cancer research and was twice nominated for the Nobel Prize. Obituaries: *Washington Star*,

4 December 1976, and *Washington Post*, 8 December 1976.

15. Caption to photograph in brochure celebrating the centennial of Georgetown medical school, 1950, Medical School Files, Georgetown University Archives.

16. Personal communication from John C. Rose.

17. Herbert Lansner, "Medical Society Plans to Televise Surgery Here," unidentified press report, 16 September 1947. Also: "Medical Center News," Georgetown University Medical Center *Bulletin* 1, no. 4 (December–January 1947–48): 176.

18. Personal communication from Robert J. Coffey.

19. Personal communication from Mary Catherine Coffey.

20. Medical School Catalogues, 1946–47 and 1950–51, Georgetown University Archives.

21. "Outline of Developments Since 1939 Survey," (report on department of surgery in the 1949 AMA/AAMC Report on Georgetown University School of Medicine), 32–33, Medical School Files, Georgetown University Archives. Also: personal communication from Robert J. Coffey.

22. "G.U. Medical School Graduate Gets Cahill Award in Surgery," *Washington Star*, 14 June 1949.

23. Medical School Catalogue, 1948–49, Georgetown University Archives.

24. Georgetown University Medical Center *Bulletin* 2, no. 2 (September, 1948). Also: Personal communication from Robert J. Coffey.

25. Allen O. Whipple, "Some Thoughts on the Training of the Surgeon," *Post Doctoral Education and Training of the Surgeon* (Princeton: Allen O. Whipple Surgical Society, 1957), 64–65.

26. Personal communication from Robert J. Coffey. Also: Stapleton, 119–32.

27. "Intern and Residency Training Program," Georgetown University Medical Center *Bulletin* 3, no. 1 (June–July 1949): 52–53.

28. "The Clinical Years" in *Journey's End*, Georgetown School of Medicine Yearbook, 1950, Georgetown University Archives.

29. Robert H. Moser, "Medical Grand Rounds," Georgetown University Medical Center *Bulletin* 6, no. 5 (May 1953): 134–36.

30. Personal communication from Robert J. Coffey.

31. AMA/AAMC's report of its survey carried out 14–18 March 1949: "Georgetown University School of Medicine: Outline of Developments Since 1939 Survey," report dated 27 May 1949, Medical School Files, Georgetown University Archives.

32. H. G. Weiskotten to McNally, 8 June 1949, Medical School Files, Georgetown University Archives.

33. Nevils to Guthrie, 9 July 1949, W. G. Morgan Faculty File, Georgetown University Archives.

34. Minutes, Executive Faculty, 9 September 1949, Medical School Files, Georgetown University Archives.

35. McNally to Guthrie, 17 March 1950, Medical School Files, Georgetown University Archives. Also: *Washington Post*, 10 June 1950.

36. Minutes, Executive Faculty, 9 September 1949, Medical School Files, Georgetown University Archives.

37. "Georgetown Medical Center Marks Centennial," *Hoya*, 20 December 1950.

38. Robert J. Coffey, from the foreword to *The Surgical Clinics of North America* 30, no. 6 (December 1950). The department of medicine's contributions were published in *The Medical Clinics of North America* the previous month.

39. Georgetown University Medical Center *Bulletin* 2, no. 2 (August–September 1948).

40. "Georgetown University Hospital Home Care Service for Cancer Patients," Georgetown University Medical Center *Bulletin* 4, no. 3 (October–November 1950): 76. Also: John F. Potter, "The Vincent T. Lombardi Cancer Research Center," *Georgetown Medical Bulletin* 31, no.1 (August 1977): 10. Also: personal communication from Robert J. Coffey.

41. Walter C. Hess, "The History of Georgetown University School of Medicine, 1930–1964," *Georgetown Medical Bulletin* 18, no. 1 (August 1964): 54.

42. Bernard J. Walsh, "The Surgical Treatment of Cardiovascular Disease," Georgetown University Medical Center *Bulletin* 1, no. 1 (June–July 1947).

43. Personal communication from Robert J. Coffey.

44. Charles Anthony Hufnagel, curriculum vitae, C. A. Hufnagel Faculty File, Georgetown University Archives.

45. Eleanor Roberts, "Dr. Hufnagel Got Inspiration in His Sleep," unidentified press report, n.d., circa 1948, Hufnagel scrapbook.

46. Steven M. Spencer, "Can We Rebuild Damaged Hearts?" *Saturday Evening Post* (November 1948) 6: 34–35, 120–24.

47. Charles A. Hufnagel, "Basic Concepts of Cardiac and Cascular Reconstruction," (presented as the George M. Kober Memorial Lecture, April 1959), published in *Georgetown Medical Bulletin* (November 1960): 90.

48. "Nation's Top Ten Young Men Named," newspaper clipping, 14 January 1949, Hufnagel scrapbook, Charles A. Hufnagel, curriculum vitae.

49. "An Interview with Dr. Charles Hufnagel," *Georgetown Medical Bulletin* 22, no. 2 (November 1968): 78. Also: "Doctors Reveal First Kidney Transplant Performed in 1947," *Staten Island, N.Y., Advance* (3 December 1971).

50. *Guiness Book of Records* (New York: Bantam, 1992), 189.

51. Frances D. Moore, *Transplant: The Give and Take of Tissue Transplantation* (New York, 1972), 39.

52. Personal communication from Robert J. Coffey.

53. Personal communication from Mrs. Kay Hufnagel.

54. Coffey to McNally, 16 October 1950, Medical School Files, Georgetown University Archives.

55. Personal communication from Linda Langan Kildea.

56. Wallace E. Clayton, "Surgical Aid—The Blood Vessel Bank," *Washington Star*, 2 February 1952.

57. "Medical Center News," *Georgetown University Medical Center Bulletin* 7, no. 2 (November 1953): 68. Also: Robert B. Brown and Charles A. Hufnagel, "Arterial Grafting in Military Surgery," *Journal of the American Medical Association* (29 January 1955): 419–42.

58. *Georgetown University Medical Center Bulletin* 4, no. 5 (February–March 1951). Also: N. S. Haseltine, "G.U. Surgeons 'Patch' Hearts with Plastic," *Washington Post*, 29 April 1951. Also: "Surgeons Button Up Hearts," *Science News Letter* (20 October 1951): 247.

59. Nate Haseltine, "Doctors Perfect Artificial Heart Valve," *Washington Post*, 4 March 1951.

60. Hufnagel had made two earlier attempts, but the patients had died—one of them on the operating table before the valve could be inserted. Herbert Yahraes, "New Parts for Ailing Hearts," *The Catholic Digest* (July 1956): 101. Also: "Woman's Death Disclosed in First 'Plastic Valve' Test," *Washington Post*, 11 October 1952. Also: See note 64.

61. Information on Martina Hall, unless otherwise indicated, from: Nate Haseltine, "Plastic Valve Installed in Woman's Heart by Georgetown Medical Center Surgeons," *Washington Post*, 9 October 1952. Also: John McKelway, "A New Heart Valve—and a New Life," *Washington Evening Star*, October 1952. Also: "Fixing a Leaky Valve," *Time*, 20 October 1952. Also: "Patient Fetes 4th Year of Rare Heart Surgery," *Washington Post and Times Herald*, 12 September 1956.

Also: "Surgeon's Artificial Heart Valve Saves Patients from Sure Death," *The Cincinnati Post*, 23 March 1956. Also: "Heart Valve Transplant Outwits Death," *Catholic Standard*, 4 April 1968.

62. Charles A. Hufnagel and W. Proctor Harvey, "The Surgical Correction of Aortic Regurgitation: Preliminary Report," *Georgetown University Medical Center Bulletin* 6, no. 3 (January 1953): 60–61. This was Hufnagel's first account of the Martina Hall operation, in which he was assisted by the cardiologist Proctor Harvey, then assistant professor of medicine at Georgetown. Also: Stephen L. Johnson, *The History of Cardiac Surgery, 1896–1955* (Baltimore, 1970), 106.

63. Ibid., 107.

64. Address by C. A. Hufnagel to the Society for Vascular Surgery, New York, reported in "Aortic Plumbing," *Pfizer Spectrum*, n.d., Hufnagel scrapbook.

65. Alton L. Blakeslee, "Surgeon Reveals Four Men Alive with Arteries Taken from Animals," *Associated Press*, 6 October 1953. Also: "Animal Arteries Transplanted 'Successfully' to Four Humans," *Washington Post*, 6 October 1953.

66. Nate Haseltine, "Georgetown U. Doctors Use Plastic Cylinder to Peer Into Heart Chamber, Scan Defects," *Washington Post*, circa June 1953.

67. "Orlon Artery Installed in Patient Here," unidentified press report, 1954, Hufnagel scrapbook. Also: Herbert Yahraes, "New Parts for Ailing Hearts," *Catholic Digest* (July 1956). Also: Personal communication from Mrs. Kay Hufnagel.

68. "Surgeon Designs a Plastic Heart," *Georgetown Record* 7, no. 6 (February 1958). Also: "Complete Plastic Heart Is Designed by D.C. Surgeon Who Devised Valve," newspaper clip, 30 January 1958, Medical School Files, Georgetown University Archives.

69. "Milestones in Cardiology," Franklin Institute Science Museum website, http://sln.fi.edu/biosci/history/firsts.html.

70. Minutes, Executive Faculty, 4 September 1953, Medical School Files, Georgetown University Archives. Also: "Carrel Collection Given to Medical Center," photo and caption, unidentified press report, circa August 1953. Also: "Medical Center News," *Georgetown University Medical Center Bulletin* (November 1953): 67. Also: Howard S. Madigan, "The Carrel Collection," *GUMC Bulletin* (January 1954): 74–75.

71. Personal communication from Linda Langan Kildea.

72. "$100,000 given Georgetown," *New York Times*, 10 June 1955. Also: "G.U. to Fulfill Dream of Carrel 'Organ Bank,'" *Sunday Star*, 12 June 1955. Also: personal communication from Robert J. Coffey.

73. "An Interview with Dr. Hufnagel," *Georgetown Medical Bulletin* (November 1968): 79.

74. Adele Chidakel, "He Mends Damaged Hearts," *Washington Sunday Star Magazine*, 24 February 1957.

75. Information throughout this section, unless otherwise indicated, relies on personal communications from Thomas C. Lee, Robert J. Coffey, Robert J. Coffey Jr., Anne Coffey Proctor, John F. Potter, and Linda Langan Kildea.

76. "Medical Center News and Announcements," Georgetown University Medical Center *Bulletin* (July 1956): 220.

77. Personal communication from Thomas C. Lee.

78. "Report on Special Meeting of AMA House of Delegates," *Medical Annals of the District of Columbia* (April 1965): 185. Also: "District Medical Society Elects Coffey President," *Washington Evening Star*, 21 November 1965. Also: Editorial, "Robert James Coffey, MD," *Medical Annals of the District of Columbia* (January 1966): 32. Also: Robert J. Coffey, "The Advent of Medicare," *Medical Annals of the District of Columbia* (April 1966).

79. "Medical Center News," *Georgetown Medical Bulletin* (August 1966): 69. Also: Robert J. Coffey, "The Tempo of Change," (presidential address presented at the Southern Surgical Association, Hot Springs, Va., 4 December 1967).

80. Personal communication from George Stephenson, archivist, American College of Surgeons; dates confirmed from Minutes, Conference Committee, n.p. Also: See note 169.

81. Robert J. Coffey's curriculum vitae.

82. "History of Surgeons' Travel Club," provided by Dr. John Butsch of New York, a current member of the STC.

83. Personal communication from Robert J. Coffey Jr.

84. "Dr. LeComte Dies—One of Founders of Medical Center Here," *Washington Evening Star*, 12 March 1954. Also: personal communication from Robert J. Coffey.

85. "Dr. Moran is Honored by Plastic Surgeons," *Washington Star*, 25 May 1959. Also: Moran to Bunn, 16 June 1958, R. E. Moran Faculty File, Georgetown University Archives. Also: Gipprich papers, Varia 1, box 4, folder 411, Georgetown University Archives. Also: personal communications from John C. Rose and Alfred Fleury.

86. Personal communications from La Salle D. Lefall Jr., John F. Potter, and Thomas C. Lee.

87. John C. Rose, "Dean's Report for the Academic Year 1968–69," *Georgetown Medical Bulletin* (November 1969): 56–58.

88. Roger Baker Faculty File, Georgetown University Archives.

89. Personal communication from William C. Maxted.

90. "Open-Kidney Surgery Made Safe, Simple," *Medical World News* (19 February 1965).

91. "D.C. Doctor Notes Gain on Cancer," *Washington Post*, 8 August 1965.

92. Baker to Rose, 27 December 1965, Medical School Files, Georgetown University Archives.

93. Peter Y. Evans, *The History of Ophthalmology at Georgetown University* (Washington D.C.: Georgetown University Medical Center for Sight, 1988). Also: personal communication from Dr. Evans.

94. George W. Hyatt Faculty File, Georgetown University Archives. Also: "News," *Georgetown Medical Bulletin* (February 1961): 248.

95. "Teddy's Ordeal," *Time Magazine*, 3 December 1973.

96. "News," *Georgetown Medical Bulletin* (May 1960): 251. Also: "An Interview with John F. Potter," *Georgetown Medical Bulletin* (November 1972): 4.

97. John F. Potter, "Program for the Development of a Cancer Research Institution in the Georgetown University Medical Center," 14 November 1961, Medical School Files, Georgetown University Archives, n.p. Also: Potter to Bunn, 14 November 1961, Medical School Files, Georgetown University Archives.

98. "An Interview with John F. Potter," *Georgetown Medical Bulletin* (November 1972): 11–12.

99. John F. Potter, documentation of events in establishment of Lombardi Cancer Center: "Report to John F. Griffiths, Executive Vice President for Health Sciences and Director of the Medical Center," 5 December 1986, Medical School Files, Georgetown University Archives, n.p.

100. Personal communication from Robert J. Coffey.

101. Personal communication from John F. Potter.

102. Alfred J. Luessenhop's curriculum vitae and Faculty File, Georgetown University Archives.

103. Alfred J. Luessenhop and William T. Spence, "Artificial Embolization of Cerebral Arteries: Report of Use in a Case of Arteriovenous Malformation," *Journal of the American Medical Association* 72, no. 11 (12 March 1960): 1153–55.

104. Personal communication from Alfred J. Luessenhop.

105. A. J. Luessenhop, F. Mora, and W. T. Sweet, "Intracranial Aneurysms and Arteriovenous Anomalies: Treatment by Cervical Carotid Occlusion—Pathogenesis and Treatment of Cerebrovascuar Disease," *Subarachnoid Hemorrhage* (1961): 516–56.

106. Personal communication from Alfred J. Luessenhop.

107. List of fiftieth anniversary honorees on Harvard's Department of Neurosurgery website. http://neurosurgery.mgh.harvard.edu/history.html.

108. The Luessenhop lecture and prize were established in 1997 jointly by the American Association of Neurological Surgeons' Section of Cerebral Vascular Surgery, the Congress of Neurological Surgeons, and the American Society of Therapeutic and Interventional Neuroradiology.

109. The first computerized axial tomography (CAT) scanner, invented by Godfrey N. Hounsfield and made by EMI Industries in England, was the greatest advance in radiology since the invention of the X ray. But this first scanner imaged only the brain and the purchase price was $450,000. At Georgetown, while surgeons pressed to buy one and the dean, John Rose, hesitated on grounds of cost. Robert Ledley said he could design not only a less costly version but one that would scan the whole body in color. According to Luessenhop, almost no one believed him. But Ledley made good his promise and invented the first whole-body scanner in 1973. Even Hounsfield, who received the Nobel Prize for his brain-scan in 1979, came to Georgetown to see it. Ledley received many honors for his invention, most recently the National Technology Award, presented by President Clinton in 1997.

110. Minutes, Executive Faculty, 19 June 1953. Georgetown University Hospital Files, Georgetown University Archives.

111. Personal communication from Robert J. Coffey.

112. "Father McNally, G.U., Dead of Heart Attack," *Washington Post*, 5 March 1955.

113. Georgetown University News Service, 18 June 1953. Also: Forster to Adler, 28 October 1953. Also Memorandum from Cohalan to Bunn, 22 July 1953. Medical School Files, Georgetown University Archives.

114. Personal communication from John Rose.

115. Reverend Thomas J. O'Donnell, "School of Medicine Report to the President of the University," 26 September 1953, Medical School Files, Georgetown

University Archives. Also: Georgetown University News Service, 2 May 1955.

116. "Medical Center News," G.U. Medical Center *Bulletin* (November 1953): 67. Also: Georgetown University News Service, 17 September 1956, Georgetown University Hospital Files, Georgetown University Archives.

117. Hussey to Collins, 24 August 1960, Medical School Files, Georgetown University Archives.

118. R. J. Glaser, J. Hirschboeck, W. S. Wiggins, and G. Caldwell, "Survey of the Georgetown University School of Medicine, Washington, D.C.," 3–6 March 1958, Medical School Files, Georgetown University Archives.

119. "Dean's Page," G.U. Medical Center *Bulletin* (May 1959): 178.

120. See note 118.

121. O'Donnell to Reverend Edward B. Rooney, S.J., 28 March 1955, Medical School Files, Georgetown University Archives.

122. "Dean's Annual Report for 1958–59," 30 June 1959, Medical School Files, Georgetown University Archives.

123. Personal communication from John Rose.

124. Probable grant proposal for Commonwealth Fund, 27 March 1957, Medical School Files, Georgetown University Archives.

125. "Report of Visit to Georgetown University School of Medicine, Washington, D.C." by the Liaison Committee on Medical Education, representing the AMA and AAMC, 25–26 April 1960, Medical School Files, Georgetown University Archives.

126. Bunn to Maloney, and Bunn to Hussey, both 3 November 1960, Medical School Files, Georgetown University Archives. Bunn appointed Reverend William F. Maloney, S.J. as Georgetown's first Vice President for Medical Center Affairs, giving him "line authority from the president and directors of the university in all units and areas of the medical center." Maloney became an ex-officio member of the executive faculties of the medical, dental, and nursing schools, a member of the executive staff of the hospital, and chairman of the hospital policy committee.

127. Bunn to Hussey, 21 September 1961, Medical School Files, Georgetown University Archives. Dr. Charles D. Shields was appointed the first executive director of the hospital.

128. Georgetown University News Service, 30 October 1962, Medical School Files, Georgetown University Archives. Also: "Medical Center News,"

Georgetown Medical Bulletin (November 1969): 74. Also: personal communication from John Rose.

129. "GU Appoints Dr. Rose Medical School Dean," *Washington Post*, 3 March 1963. Also: "Executive Faculty Committees," n.d., Medical School Files, January–March 1958, Georgetown University Archives. Also: "Dean's Report for Academic Year 1958–59," *Georgetown Medical Bulletin* (February 1960). Also: personal communication from John Rose.

130. "Dean's Report for Academic Year 1964–65," *Georgetown Medical Bulletin* (May 1966). Also: "From the Dean," *Georgetown Medical Bulletin* (May 1970). Also: "Dean's Report for Academic Year 1969–70," *Georgetown Medical Bulletin* (November 1970). Also: Clifton K. Himmelsbach, "Federal Support for Medical Education," *Georgetown Medical Bulletin* (August 1975).

131. Figures compiled from Dean's Reports, 1963–73.

132. "From the Dean," *Georgetown Medical Bulletin* (February 1972).

133. William C. McFadden, ed., *Georgetown at Two Hundred* (Washington, D.C., 1990), 307.

134. "Dean's Report for Academic Year 1969–70," *Georgetown Medical Bulletin* (November 1970).

135. "Dean's Report for Academic Year 1970–71," *Georgetown Medical Bulletin* (November 1971): 15–16.

136. Personal communication from John C. Rose, on this and other cited quotes from Dr. Rose throughout this section.

137. J. D. McCarthy, et. al., "Council on Medical Service: Conclusions and Recommendations," typescript, n.d., Medical School Files, July–December 1956, Georgetown University Archives. This was an AMA study, based on a survey of payment practices in medical schools across the nation, in which the CMS recommended that full-time clinical faculty be barred from private practice but instead be paid a salary. The recommendation was rejected by the AMA's House of Delegates in 1960 but endorsed by the AAMC. Also: Bergan to Rose, 11 January 1965, Medical School Files, Georgetown University Archives. The opinion of the AAMC at that time reflected Flexner's view, decades earlier, that salaried faculty would perform less clinical work, thus freeing them for more research and teaching. But this was not borne out in the later twentieth century because, as hospital costs rose, more clinical work was demanded in the university hospitals rather than less.

138. See notes 118 and 125.

139. Bauer to Bunn, 26 October 1964, Medical School Files, Georgetown University Archives.

140. Personal communication from John F. Potter, for this and other cited quotes from Dr. Potter throughout this section.

141. Memorandum, Rose to Coffey, "Annual Report of Time Spent in Private Practice and Income Derived from this Activity for Geographic Full-time Faculty," 4 January 1965, Medical School Files, Georgetown University Archives.

142. Personal communications from John Dillon, John F. Potter, and William Feller.

143. Baker to Forster, 1955, Roger Baker Faculty File, Georgetown University Archives.

144. Rose to Coffey, 4 January 1965, Medical School Files, Georgetown University Archives.

145. Personal communication from John Dillon, John F. Potter, and Thomas C. Lee.

146. Rose to Coffey, 4 January 1965, Medical School Files, Georgetown University Archives.

147. Personal communication from John Dillon.

148. Bergan to Rose, 11 January 1965, Medical School Files, Georgetown University Archives.

149. Minutes, Medical Center Council, 1 March 1965, Medical School Files, Georgetown University Archives.

150. Memorandum, Rose to Campbell and Bauer, "Our Problem," 5 March 1965, Medical School Files, Georgetown University Archives. This was a report of the meeting in Chicago the previous day and raised options on how a faculty practice plan could be introduced at Georgetown. In it, Rose wrote: "It is safe to say that the group in Chicago upheld the view of the Medical Center Council that, in the interests of the educational and research programs of the University, there should be some method of control or regulation over the private practice activities of the full-time faculty."

151. Campbell to Rose, 23 March 1965, Medical School Files, Georgetown University Archives.

152. Rose to Coffey, n.d., circa March 1965, Medical School Files, January–February 1965, Georgetown University Archives.

153. Ibid.

154. Personal communications from Thomas C. Lee and John Dillon.

155. Personal communications from John Dillon, Thomas C. Lee, and William Feller.

156. Personal communications from John F. Potter, John Dillon, and Thomas C. Lee.

157. Campbell to Rose, 23 March 1965, Medical School Files, Georgetown University Archives. This letter was read and discussed at the medical executive

faculty meetings in March and April of 1965. It provided the basis on which the Faculty Practice Plan committee was convened.

158. "Faculty Practice Plan, Preliminary Proposal," January 1967, Father Henle's office files, 1–2, Georgetown University Archives.

159. Rose to Coffey, 11 January 1967, Medical School Files, Georgetown University Archives. Also Rose to Campbell, 11 August 1967, Father Henle's office files, 1–2, Georgetown University Archives.

160. "Plan for Distribution of Fees from Medically Indigent Patients," Faculty Practice Plan Committee, May 1968, Father Henle's office files, 1–2, Georgetown University Archives.

161. Personal communications from John Rose and William Maxted.

162. Personal communications from John Rose, John Dillon, and Alfred Luessenhop.

163. Personal communication from Robert B. Wallace, chairman of the department of surgery 1980–97. The department's practice plan came into effect in October 1980. Two senior faculty members, Charles Hufnagel and John Potter, were grandfathered out of the plan and remained on a geographical full-time basis. Although he had opposed the plan in the 1960s, in 1978 Robert Coffey told John F. Stapleton, director of Georgetown University Hospital and professor of medicine, that he now agreed with the conversion to an absolute full-time system. Personal communication from Dr. Stapleton.

164. Personal communications from Thomas C. Lee, John F. Potter, Kathryn D. Anderson, Robert J. Coffey Jr., and Anne Coffey Proctor.

165. "Unmasking Dr. Coffey," *Georgetown Medical Bulletin* (November 1970): 4–11.

166. Personal communication from Thomas C. Lee.

167. Personal communications from Thomas C. Lee and Robert J. Coffey Jr.

168. Personal communication from Robert J. Coffey.

169. Personal communications from George Stephenson, archivist, American College of Surgeons, and from Robert J. Coffey. Also: "The ACS and History of Graduate Education in Surgery," *Bulletin of the American College of Surgeons* (February 1971): 15–37.

170. Personal communication from La Salle D. Lefall Jr.

171. "An Interview with Dr. Estelle Ramey," *Georgetown Medical Bulletin* (August 1970): 5–11.

172. Annie E. Rice (of Maine) and Jeannette J. Sumner (of Michigan) are listed in the 1881–82

Medical School Catalogue. At the end of that year, they transferred to the Women's Medical College of Pennsylvania where they graduated. See Gloria Moldow, "For Women, By Women: Women's Dispensaries and Clinics in Washington, 1882–1900," *Records of the Columbia Historical Society* (Washington, D.C., 1980), 50:297.

173. Dr. Elizabeth Blackwell, credited as the first woman to obtain a medical degree in the United States, entered Geneva Medical College, N.Y., in October 1847 and graduated in 1849. See Elizabeth Blackwell, *Pioneer Work in Opening the Medical Profession to Women: Autobiographical Sketches* (London and New York, 1895), 58–87.

174. "Five Women Get MDs from G.U.," *The Washington Post*, 10 June 1951. Also: Minutes, Executive Faculty, 9 November 1951. Also: Memorandum, McNally to Guthrie, 7 June 1951, Medical School Files, Georgetown University Archives. Also: *Catholic Standard*, 27 May 1955. The five were: Sister Frederic M. Niedfield, Ann Connolly, Mrs. G. Douglas Lockheart, Mrs. Vicky Cicviarella Halloran, and Frederika Donahue.

175. Personal communication from Sister Eileen Niedfield.

176. Personal communications from Robert J. Coffey and Thomas C. Lee.

177. Photo and caption accompanying "An Interview with Dr. Estelle Ramey," *Georgetown Medical Bulletin* (August 1970): 11.

178. *The Official ABMS Directory of Board Certified Medical Specialists* (New Providence, N.J., 1998). Also: *AMA Directory of Physicians in the United States* (Chicago, 1998).

179. Officers and Staff of the ACS, *Bulletin of the American College of Surgeons*, 1992–2000. Personal communication from Kathryn D. Anderson.

180. Personal communication from Mary Catherine Coffey.

181. Personal communication from Kathryn D. Anderson.

182. "From the Dean," *Georgetown Medical Bulletin* (August 1966): 3.

183. Compiled from annual Dean's Reports, 1960–70.

184. Research grants itemized in "Medical Center News," *Georgetown Medical Bulletin*, 1958–1970.

185. Hugh H. Hussey, "Report to Reverend T. Byron Collins, S.J. Regarding Activities, Georgetown University Hospital in Areas Undergoing Renovation," typescript, July 1960, Medical School

Files, Georgetown University Archives. This review of research at Georgetown noted that "removal of major parts of the liver in order to eradicate primary or secondary cancer of this organ has been under study for five years. Dr. Coffey's experience in this field has been the longest of any but one other group in the world."

186. R. J. Coffey, F. Niedfield, W. D. Byrne, J. J. Blumberg, and Michael F. Lapadula, "Vagectomy, Hemigastrectomy, and Gastroduodenostomy in Treatment of Duodenal Ulcer," *American Journal of Digestive Diseases* (April 1960): 324–38. Also: "Operation for Duodenal Ulcers Developed at Georgetown," Georgetown University News Service, 1 November 1967, Robert J. Coffey's Public Relations File, Georgetown University Archives. This noted that the procedure had been performed on four hundred patients since 1952, with only two patients suffering recurrence of duodenal ulcers.

187. Personal communications from Robert J. Coffey, Thomas C. Lee, and John C. Rose.

188. Robert J. Coffey, "The Management of Hyperparathyroidism," (presented at the forty-seventh annual Kober Lecture, Washington, D.C., 14 April 1971), published in the *Georgetown Medical Bulletin* (August 1971): 12–17.

189. Robert J. Coffey, Thomas C. Lee, and John J. Canary, "The Surgical Treatment of Primary Hyperparathyroidism: A twenty year experience," *Annals of Surgery* 185 (May, 1977): 518–23.

190. T. C. Lee, R. J. Coffey, J. Mackin, and J. J. Canary, "The Use of Propranolol in the Surgical Treatment of Thyrotoxic Patients," *Annals of Surgery* 177 (June 1973): 643–47.

191. T. C. Lee, R. J. Coffey, B. M. Currier, X. P. Ma, J. J. Canary, "Propranolol and Thyroidectomy in the Treatment of Thyrotoxicosis," (presented to the Southern Surgical Association, Hot Springs, Va., 7–9 December 1981), published in *Annals of Surgery* 195 (June 1982): 766–73.

192. Arlie Mansberger Jr. "One Hundred Years of Surgical Management of Hyperthyroidism," *The Southern Surgical Association: The First 100 Years,* 1887–1987 (Philadelphia, 1987), 356.

193. C. A. Hufnagel and P. Conrad, "Direct Approach for the Correction of Aortic Insufficiency," *Journal of the American Medical Association* 178 (2 October 1961): 320–21. Also: Charles G. Brooks, "G.U. Surgeons Replace Aortic Heart Valves," *Washington Evening Star,* 20 October 1961.

194. "Agent Curbs Clotting in Artificial Hearts," *Washington Post,* 8 February 1966.

195. Charles A. Hufnagel, "Basic Concepts of Cardiac and Vascular Reconstruction," (presented as the Kober Lecture, Washington, D.C., April 1959), published in *Georgetown Medical Bulletin* (November 1960): 88–96. Also: H. C. Urschel Jr., J. J. Greenberg, and C. A. Hufnagel, "Elective Cardioplegia by Local Cardiac Hypothermia," *New England Journal of Medicine* 261 (24 December 1959): 1330–32. Also: C. A. Hufnagel et al., "Profound Cardiac Hypothermia," *Annals of Surgery* 53, no. 5 (May 1961): 790–96. Also: "Rare Heart Surgery Lets Girl, 11, Walk Again," *Sunday Star,* 9 October 1960. Also: "Awards: Charles A. Hufnagel," *Modern Medicine,* 9 January 1961.

196. Personal communication from Linda Langan Kildea, as for all quotes from Mrs. Kildea in this section.

197. John Z. Bowers and Elizabeth F. Purcell, eds., *Advances in American Medicine: Essays at the Bicentennial* (New York, 1976), 2: 492–95, 655–56. Also: Roy Porter, *The Greatest Benefit to Mankind: A Medical History of Humanity* (New York and London, 1997), 617.

198. C. A. Hufnagel, J. McAlindon, and A. Vardar, "A Simplified Extra-Corporeal Pump Oxygenating System," *American Surgeon* 25 (May 1959): 314–20.

199. C. A. Hufnagel, J. F. Schanno, R. Pifarre, P. Conrad, and C. Hewson, "A Versatile Heat Exchanger for Use in Extracorporeal Bypass Systems," *Journal of Cardiovascular Surgery* 1 (March 1961): 158–64.

200. Nate Haseltine, "Drama of Operating Room: Surgeons Save Leg-to-Heart Bullet Victim," *Washington Post,* 6 May 1962.

201. William Grigg, "Kidney Transplant Patient Leaves GU," *Washington Evening Star,* May 1966. Also: "Successful Kidney Transplant," *Georgetown Medical Bulletin* (November 1966): 115.

202. "Dr. Charles A. Hufnagel to Receive Mendel Medal on 100th Anniversary of Mendelian Laws Discovery," *The Villanova University Alumnus* (May 1965): 2.

203. "Dean's Report for Academic Year 1968–69," *Georgetown Medical Bulletin* (November 1969): 68.

204. "Medical Center News," *Georgetown Medical Bulletin* (February 1967): 117–18.

205. Eleanor Nealon, "Dr. Charles Hufnagel Could Have Performed the First Heart Transplant: When He Does Do One, Expect the Patient to Live," *The Washingtonian,* November 1969, 64–67.

206. Press Release, Georgetown University News Service, 4 December 1967.

207. "Expert's Size-Up of Heart Transplants 'Evidence . . . Is Not Good Enough Yet,'" *U.S. News and World Report*, 22 January 1968.

208. Nealon, "Dr. Charles Hufnagel Could Have Performed the First Heart Transplant," 67,

209. Dirk van Zyll, age forty-four was operated on by Christiaan Barnard in Capetown in 1971 and survived twenty-three years and fifty-seven days until 7 July 1994. *Guinness Book of Records*, (New York Bantam Books, 1997).

210. Personal communications from Linda Langar Kildea, Robert J. Coffey, and Thomas C. Lee.

211. Personal communications from Robert J. Coffey and John F. Stapleton.

212. Personal communications from Robert J. Coffey and Kathryn D. Anderson. Also: "Blast Fatal to Patient in Surgery," *Washington Evening Star*, 1 March 1969.

213. Dean's Informational Bulletin, 43, 5 July 1960 Medical School Files, Georgetown University Archives.

214. Personal communication from Thomas C. Lee.

215. Personal communications from Robert J Coffey Jr., Thomas C. Lee, and John F. Potter.

216. Personal communication from Thomas C. Lee.

217. Campbell to the Board of Regents, 19 December 1967, Medical School Files, Georgetown University Archives.

218. Warren R. Young, "Hospital of the Future?" *Reader's Digest*, May 1967, 167. This article originally appeared in *Life*, 2 December 1966. Also: personal communications from Thomas C. Lee and Linda L. Kildea.

219. Ibid., 162.

220. Grant application HM 00390—01, "Research to Improve the Quality and Efficiency of Medical Care." Also: Assistant Surgeon General Harald M. Graning to Hufnagel, 22 April 1964, Medical School Files, Georgetown University Archives.

221. Nate Haseltine, "Georgetown U. Medical Unit Would Play Several Roles," *Washington Post*, 9 June 1963.

222. Young, 162.

223. "Resolution Concerning the Concentrated Care Center Loan and Grant," Georgetown University Board of Directors, 18 January 1974. Also: Breakdown of overall funding, Collins to Cotton, 26 September 1973, Concentrated Care Center Files, boxes 38 and 40, Healy Administration, Georgetown University Archives.

224. Personal communication from John F. Stapleton.

225. Personal communication from Linda L. Kildea.

226. The Executive Committee of the Georgetown University Board of Directors, meeting 15 December 1967, passed the following resolution: "The Board approves in principle separate incorporation and authorizes the President to prepare the necessary instruments for a separate incorporation of the Medical Center, leaving open at the time in question whether the School of Nursing with be part of the Medical Center or of the University." Campbell explained: "The need to proceed with the construction of the Concentrated Care Center, at a cost of $19 million, precipitated that discussion." Campbell to the Board of Regents, 19 December 1967, Medical School Files, Georgetown University Archives. Also: "GU to Explore Separate Incorporation of Its Medical Center," Georgetown University News Service, 11 January 1968.

227. "Dean's Informational Bulletin," 180, 1 April 1968, Medical School Files, Georgetown University Archives. John Rose headed the committee which explored the implications of separate incorporation.

228. Announcement by U.S. Department of Health, Education, and Welfare (HEW) Secretary Caspar Weinberger of further $15 million to complete Concentrated Care Center (CCC) construction: HEW News press release, 12 October 1973. Also: Henle to Collins, Kelly, McCormack, and McNulty, 1 January 1973, Concentrated Care Center Files, box 38, folder 1384, Healy Administration, Georgetown University Archives. Two key figures in the revival of the plans to build the CCC were Matthew McNulty, who in 1969 became the first non-Jesuit executive vice president for Medical Center Affairs, and Reverend T. Byron Collins, S.J., the university's vice president for Planning and Physical Plant. Also: Stapleton, 150—52.

229. The Concentrated Care Center was dedicated 26 June 1976. The main speaker was Donald S. Frederickson, director of HEW, U.S. Public Health Service, and National Institutes of Health.

230. Coffey to Campbell, 14 November 1967, R. J. Coffey Faculty File, Georgetown University Archives.

231. Campbell to Coffey, 22 November 1967, R. J. Coffey Faculty File, Georgetown University Archives.

232. Dean's Informational Bulletin, 117, 26 January 1968, Medical School Files, Georgetown University Archives.

233. "From the Dean," *Georgetown Medical Bulletin* (August 1968): 3.

234. Hufnagel took over as chairman of the surgery department 1 January 1969. He was chairman for ten

years, during which time he headed the medical panel selected to judge former President Richard M. Nixon's fitness to testify at the Watergate cover-up trial (November 1974). Hufnagel resigned as chairman in 1979, after his surgical dexterity had waned and his cardiac program came under criticism. He died 31 May 1989, ironically of failure of the heart and kidneys, his two main fields of research. Today, his place in the pantheon of medical pioneers is recognized, among many other places, at Philadelphia's Franklyn Institute Science Museum where, in its major exhibit on the heart, Hufnagel is among the fourteen scientists listed as having achieved "milestones in cardiology."

235. Personal communication from Thomas C. Lee.

236. *Georgetown Medical Bulletin* (August 1970): 36.

237. *Georgetown Medical Bulletin* (November 1970). Thomas Lee, aside of his surgical duties, edited the *Bulletin* from 1968 to 1980. An accomplished artist, he also painted the portraits of many of his Georgetown colleagues; some of these paintings hang in the Georgetown University Medical Center.

238. See note 188.

239. Coffey Distinguished Chair of Surgery Correspondence, 1972–76, Hugh Grant Files, box 59, folder 2005, Georgetown University Archives.

240. Grant to Collins, 28 November 1972, Hugh Grant Files, box 59, folder 2005, Georgetown University Archives.

241. Coffey to Collins, 26 September 1972. Also: Georgetown University press release, 25 May 1973. Also: McCormack to Edwards, 5 December 1972, Hugh Grant Files, box 59, folder 2005, Georgetown University Archives. Also: McNulty to Henle, 18 June 1973, and Henle to Hufnagel, 13 August 1973, Robert J. Coffey Chair Folder, Henle Administration, box 27, folder 833, Georgetown University Archives.

242. Henle to LaBarre, 14 March 1974, Endowed Chairs File, Henle Administration, folder 24.10, Georgetown University Archives. Georgetown University Medical Center's first endowed chair, the Schering Chair of Pharmacology, was established in 1966.

243. McNulty to Grant, 12 December 1972, Hugh Grant Files, box 59, folder 2005, Georgetown University Archives.

244. Personal communication from Mary Catherine Coffey.

245. Valerie Strauss, "Georgetown's Medical Center Gets $60 Million," *Washington Post*, 12 June 1997.

Index